Gender and Dermatology

Ethel Tur • Howard I. Maibach
Editors

Gender and Dermatology

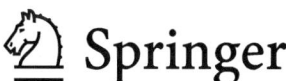 Springer

Editors
Ethel Tur
Tel Aviv University
Tel Aviv
Israel

Howard I. Maibach
Department of Dermatology
UCSF Medical Center
San Francisco
CA
USA

ISBN 978-3-319-72155-2   ISBN 978-3-319-72156-9   (eBook)
https://doi.org/10.1007/978-3-319-72156-9

Library of Congress Control Number: 2018936629

Printed on acid-free paper

This Springer imprint is published by the registered company Springer International Publishing AG part of Springer Nature
The registered company address is: Gewerbestrasse 11, 6330 Cham, Switzerland

Preface

The nature of certain diseases is different between women and men. Genetic and hormonal differences affect skin structure and function, thus affecting disease processes. In addition, exogenous factors differ according to differences in lifestyle between the sexes. In the last two decades it has been recognized that women are more different medically than previously appreciated, and studies started being conducted accordingly. Methodologies used in dermatological research have improved substantially, providing means of objective evaluation of skin function and characteristics, leading to improvement in treatment and disease outcome.

Diseases differ between men and women in terms of prevention, clinical signs, therapeutic approach, prognosis, and psychological and social impacts.

This book outlines several aspects of differences between the skin of women and men in health and disease, based on available data. It is not designed to be exhaustive in its coverage of the subject, but rather to highlight certain aspects of it. We wish and hope that this book will ignite more interest in the topic of gender dermatology.

The editors are grateful to all our contributing authors for their efforts and cooperation in applying their knowledge and skill.

Special thanks to our team at Springer: Mr. Grant Weston, Responsible Editor, Mr. Andre Tournois, Project Coordinator, Mr. Karthik Periyasamy, Production editor, and Mr. Dinesh Vinayagam, Project Manager, for their meticulous work.

Tel Aviv, Israel   Ethel Tur
San Francisco, CA, USA   Howard I. Maibach

Contents

Effects of Gender on Skin Physiology and Biophysical Properties

Richard Randall Wickett and Greg G. Hillebrand

Abbreviations

N.S. No significant difference
SC Stratum corneum
TEWL Transepidermal water loss

1.1 Introduction

This chapter will review the literature on gender differences in skin physiology focusing on non-invasive biophysical measures of skin function. While there are countless studies on the biophysical properties of human skin, there are fewer that examine gender differences. Many studies are sponsored by the cosmetic industry and not surprisingly focus on women and often compare effects of aging or photoaging. Unfortunately, the literature that explores gender differences does not always present a clear picture as will be seen. This contribution will review sebum production, skin pH, barrier function as assessed by transepidermal water loss (TEWL), stratum

corneum (SC) hydration measured by electrical properties, skin viscoelasticity and facial skin wrinkling.

1.2 Sebum Production

On average sebum production is approximately the same between men and women up to about age 50. However, there is extreme variability between individuals. Pochi et al. measured sebum production rates in men and women between the ages of 40 and 79 over a three-hour period using absorbent paper on the forehead [1]. Results are presented in Table 1.1.

Sebum production clearly drops off in women after age 50 probably because of menopause. In all age groups, even 70–79, there was considerable overlap between the ranges measured with higher sebum producing women producing more sebum in 3 h than lower producing men.

A more comprehensive study of gender differences in skin sebum production is that by Luebberding et al. [2]. The authors investigated 300 women and men between the ages of 20 and 74. Sebum production was measured on the cheeks and foreheads using the Sebumeter [3]. Mean values and standard deviations and statistical significance levels (p values) for each age range and over the entire age range are given in Table 1.2. There were 30 subjects of each sex in each age range.

R. R. Wickett (✉)
James L. Winkle College of Pharmacy,
University of Cincinnati, Cincinnati, OH, USA
e-mail: wicketrr@ucmail.uc.edu

G. G. Hillebrand
Global Discovery, Research and Development,
Amway Corporation, Ada, MI, USA
e-mail: greg.hillebrand@Amway.com

© Springer International Publishing AG, part of Springer Nature 2018
E. Tur, H. I. Maibach (eds.), *Gender and Dermatology*,
https://doi.org/10.1007/978-3-319-72156-9_1

Table 1.1 Sebum production rates and ranges in female and male subjects

Age range	Number F/M	Female[a]	Range[a]	Male[a]	Range[a]
40–49	31/50	1.86	0.12–4.80	2.39	0.54–5.14
50–59	21/14	1.08	0.07–2.38	2.43	1.05–4.36
60–69	18/14	0.88	0.22–1.62	2.42	0.83–4.95
70–79	12/13	0.85	0.33–2.19	1.69	0.63–3.23

[a]Sebum production in mg/10 cm^2 of skin in 3 h data from Pochi et al. [1]

Table 1.2 Sebum levels on the forehead for females and males

Age range	Female[a]	SD	Male[a]	SD	p
20–29	115.50	57.13	120.77	50.24	NS
30–39	114.82	63.60	127.53	53.87	NS
40–49	130.77	63.74	125.93	50.27	NS
50–59	96.73	61.25	125.93	59.66	<0.05
60–74	66.89	43.68	139.10	66.84	<0.001
20–74	105.45	61.66	105.45	61.66	<0.001

[a]Sebum measurement in μg/cm^2 data from Luebberding et al. [2]

While the overall mean was smaller for women than men, significant differences were not seen before the 50–59 age group in agreement with the results of Pochi et al. above. Note the large standard deviations indicating the large variation in sebum production across the sample populations. Sebum production on the cheek was lower than on the forehead but age and sex differences showed very similar trends. Firooz et al. [4] also reported lower sebum production in females compared to males in pooled data from several age groups and body sites. Among all the skin parameters reviewed in this work, lower sebum production in females compared to males above the age of 50 was observed most consistently.

1.3   Skin Surface pH

pH is defined as 'the negative logarithm of the hydrogen ion concentration'. The most common method for measuring the skin's surface pH is to apply a flat surface membrane electrode hydrated with distilled water to the skin surface and measure the apparent pH. This leads to the definition of skin surface pH in bioengineering terms as: 'apparent pH as measured by a flat glass elec-trode at the skin surface with a hydrated skin-electrode interface [5]. In healthy skin, surface pH is lower than physiological pH ranging from about 4.5–5.5 on most body sites under most conditions. There has been increasing interest in the role of skin surface pH in maintaining a healthy stratum corneum barrier [5].

Measurements of gender differences in skin pH have not produced completely consistent results though there is a trend for females to have slightly higher pH than males. Table 1.3 shows a summary of results from several labs comparing the skin surface pH in men vs. women at various body sites and age groups. Table 1.3 doesn't present specific pH values because in some cases the authors only provide graphical data so exact numerical values are not available. Luebberding et al. present numerical pH data and found that males have significantly lower pH on every body site for every age group [2]. The overall averages were 5.12 for females and 4.58 for males. This was among the largest differences seen in any of the papers reviewed. Zlotogorski [6] found 5.1 on the cheek for males and 5.2 on the cheek for females and the difference was not statistically significant. In contrast Ehlers and Ivens [7] reported higher skin pH in males (5.8) compared to females (5.5) on the forearm.

In a large cross-sectional study of skin condition, Hillebrand and colleagues measured cheek and forearm skin surface pH in 450 subjects (191 males, 259 females) ranging in age for 9–78. The subjects were art festival goers (ArtPrize 2015, Grand Rapids Michigan) who happened to walk by the study venue and volunteered to be participants. Thus, subjects were literally recruited *off the street* and represent a *real world* sampling of the local population. Furthermore, the skin was not washed or prepared in any manner prior to making the measurement in order to measure an

Table 1.3 Skin pH results from various authors

Age range	Number F/M	Body site	Result	Reference
20–60	292/282	Forehead	M = F	Zlotogorski [6]
20–60	292/282	Cheek	M = F	Zlotogorski [6]
21–37	37/46	Face	M < F	Kim [8]
13–70	354/304	Forehead	M < F	Man [9]
0–12	142/128	Forearm	M < F	Man [9]
36–50	82/60	Forearm	M < F	Man [9]
51–70	28/31	Forearm	M < F	Man [9]
70+	31/24	Forearm	M = F	Man [9]
70+	31/24	Forehead	M = F	Man [9]
20–74	150/150	Forehead	M < F	Luebberding [2]
20–74	150/150	Cheek	M < F	Luebberding [2]
20–74	150/150	Neck	M < F	Luebberding [2]
20–74	150/150	Forearm	M < F	Luebberding [2]
20–74	150/150	Hand	M < F	Luebberding [2]
Not reported	6/6	Forearm	M > F	Ehlers [7]
9–78	259/191	Forearm	M < F	Hillebrand[a]
9–78	259/191	Cheek	M = F	Hillebrand[a]

[a]G. G. Hillebrand unpublished data

unadulterated apparent pH. Skin pH ranged as low as pH 3.1 to as high as pH 6.8 or nearly 4 orders of magnitude in hydronium ion concentration! While there was no significant gender-dependent difference in cheek skin pH (mean ± SD: 5.28 ± 0.43 for males and 5.23 ± 0.47 for females), males showed significantly ($p < 0.001$) lower forearm skin pH compared to females (mean ± SD: 4.59 ± 0.61 for males vs. 4.78 ± 0.65 for females). Figure 1.1 shows the percentage of males and females in specific pH ranges from pH 3 to pH 7. Females tend to skew to higher pH in accord with the difference in the population means. What is noteworthy is the large overlap in the wide bell curves for skin pH frequencies between males and females. Thus, the difference in mean pH between genders is small compared to the variance for the entire population (Hillebrand, unpublished data).

1.4 Transepidermal Water Loss

Measurement of TEWL [10] has been shown to be a valid method to evaluate skin barrier function in-vivo [11]. Several researchers have investigated possible gender differences in TEWL with varying results. Some of the results are presented in Table 1.4. Luebberding et al. [2] reported higher TEWL in males than in females with significant differences on the forehead, cheek, neck and forearm. Chilcott and Farrar [12] reported higher TEWL in males compared to females on the forearm and Firooz et al. [4] also reported higher TEWL in males in pooled data from eight body sites. Wilhelm et al. [13] and Hadi et al. [14] did not observe any significant effect of gender on TEWL.

Chilcott and Farrar [12] used the ServoMed EP-2 Evaporimeter (ServoMed, Kinna, Sweden) to measure TEWL while Luebberding et al. [2] used the TEWAmeter® TM300 (Courage & Khazaka, Cologne, Germany). This may in part explain the higher forearm results seen by Luebberding. While results from the two instruments correlate very well, TEWAmeter data tend to be up to two times higher than ServoMed data [11, 15]. Li et al. [16] also reported lower TEWL in female subjects compared to males in Chinese subjects from two age groups, 18–25 and 40–50 on various body sites.

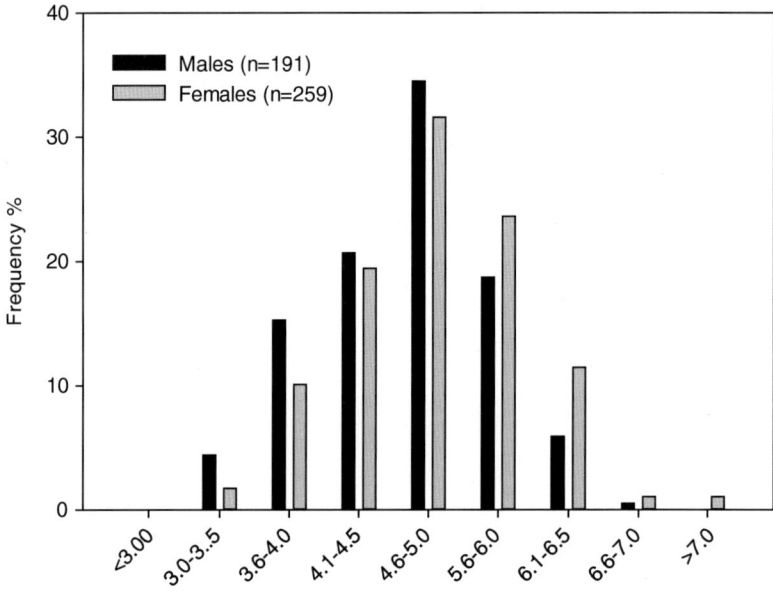

Fig. 1.1 Percent of subjects (frequency %) having forearm pH values in a specific pH range

Table 1.4 TEWL females and males

Ages	No. (F/M)	Body site	Female	Male	P	Reference
20–74	150/150	Forehead	10.51	9.29	P < 0.01	Luebberding [2]
20–74	150/150	Cheek	11.15	10.34	P < 0.05	Luebberding [2]
20–74	150/150	Neck	9.25	6.96	P < 0.001	Luebberding [2]
20–74	150/150	Forearm	9.10	5.50	P < 0.001	Luebberding [2]
20–74	150/150	Hand	11.52	10.92	N.S.	Luebberding [2]
18–28	10/8	Forearm	4.68	4.98	P < 0.05	Chilcott [12]
10–60	25/25	8 sites	9.52	15.49	P < 0.05	Firoz [4]

N.S. no significant difference

1.5 Stratum Corneum Hydration

The stratum corneum needs to maintain proper hydration in order to function properly and lack of adequate moisture in the SC can lead to dry skin. Instrumental methods to measure SC hydration in-vivo rely on measuring either surface conductance or capacitance [17–20]. Luebberding et al. [2] measured skin hydration with the CM 825® (Courage & Khazaka, Cologne Germany) on five body sites on 150 subjects of each gender broken into five age groups. Results from each body site, pooled by age are presented in Table 1.5.

Females showed higher hydration on the cheek and hand while males had higher values on the neck. Differences on the forehead and forearm

Table 1.5 Capacitance by body site and gender[a]

Body site	Female	Male	P value
Forehead	52.94	50.94	N.S.
Cheek	60.81	57.62	P < 0.05
Neck	54.34	59.62	P < 0.001
Forearm	44.07	43.10	N.S.
Hand	38.62	32.49	P < 0.001

[a]Data from Luebberding et al. [2]. 150 subjects of each sex in each age group. Age range = 20–74. *N.S.* no significant difference

were not statistically significant. Li et al. [16] found females to haves significantly higher hydration on the décolletage are but no other body sites. Neither Firooz et al. [4] nor Wilhelm et al. [13] reported significant gender differences in hydration.

1.6   Elasticity

Skin is a viscoelastic material. It has the unique ability to rebound after being stretched allowing itself to return to its initial size and maintain a tight covering over the body surface. Unfortunately, skin elasticity declines after the third decade in both men and women, especially on chronically sun-exposed skin sites [21–23]. This loss in elasticity is likely the major driver for visible facial skin wrinkling and sagging [24]. Skin elasticity is commonly measured using the non-invasive suction method [25–27]. The Cutometer® is one of the more widely used suction-based skin elasticity instruments because of its portability, speed and simplicity (Courage + Khazaka Electronic, Koln, Germany). The stress/strain curve can be divided into different regions such as maximum deformation (Uf) and immediate retraction (Ur). Ratios of these absolute parameters yield relative parameters of skin elasticity (e.g. Ur/Uf or R7) that are independent of skin thickness. Nedelec et al. [28] used the Cutometer MPA 580 with a 6-mm probe to measure skin elasticity at 16 body sites on 121 males and 120 females who were mostly Asian or Caucasian and aged between 20 and 85 years old. They found no consistent trend for gender differences in skin elasticity (R7) across age groups. Cua et al. [29] also did not observe a significant difference in skin elasticity between males and females though their sample size was very small. Ishikawa et al. [30] compared skin elasticity on men vs. women in a large subject sample on multiple skin sites. Specifically, they used the Cutometer SEM 474 to measure skin elasticity on the forearm, hand, finger and chest of 96 males and 95 females ages 9–87. Again, there was no significant difference in skin elasticity between males and females. Luebberding et al. [31] used the Cutometer MPA 580 to measure skin elasticity on the cheek, neck and dorsum of the hand in 150 males and 150 females ages 20–74. Skin elasticity (Ur/Uf) declined with age in both genders, but was only slightly higher in women than in men. The authors noted that there was a more rapid decline in elasticity in women after 40 years of age. Firooz et al. [4] also used the Cutometer

MPA 580 to measure skin elasticity in 25 females and 25 males ages 10–60. While women had slightly higher elasticity than men, the difference was not statistically significant. More recently, Hadi et al. [14] used the DermaLab® Combo to measure the skin elasticity on the forearm of 50 males and 50 females, ages 18–27. Females showed slightly higher skin elasticity than males but the difference was not statistically significant. Finally, Ma et al. [32] used the Cutometer MPA 580 to measure skin elasticity on the forehead and cheek of 240 healthy male and female volunteers living in Shanghai, aged 20–70 years. There was no significant difference in forehead skin elasticity between the genders. However, the researchers did observe lower cheek skin elasticity (both R5 and R7) in older (age 50–70) males than females. In summary, while skin elasticity declines with age in both males and females, gender-associated differences in skin elasticity at any given age are small and likely not clinically meaningful.

1.7   Facial Wrinkling

When it comes to facial wrinkling, which sex ages faster, men or women? Chung et al. [33] assessed facial wrinkling on 236 men and 171 women using standardized visual grading scales. The results suggest that while the pattern of facial wrinkling is similar between the sexes, women showed more severe wrinkles after adjusting for age, sun exposure and smoking. Gender-dependent differences in facial wrinkling should also consider facial location. In the perioral region (upper lip), women exhibit more and deeper wrinkles than men [34]. However, on the forehead, men show an earlier onset and more severe wrinkling at every age than women [32]. Hamer et al. [35] measured facial wrinkling using digital imaging in 3831 Europeans (58% female) aged 51–98. Men had higher wrinkle area than women in the younger age groups (<75) but women showed more wrinkles in the older age group (>75). Chien et al. [36] developed photographic scales for perioral and crow's feet wrinkles that were gender specific meaning that there was a scale for men and a scale for women. They used the grading scales to assess facial wrinkling on 71 men and 72 women, aged 21–91 years. All subjects were graded using both scales. Interestingly, a participant's score on the female-specific scale differed significantly from the male-specific scale score showing that it is important to use gender-specific scales for the visual grading of facial wrinkling. The researchers found that perioral wrinkling was more severe in women than men. For participants older than 45 years, there was even greater gender disparity. Tsukahara et al. measured facial wrinkling in 173 Japanese men and women [37]. Men showed increased forehead wrinkles compared with women at all ages. However, the difference in facial wrinkle severity tended to disappear in the older age groups and there were no gender-related differences at any age for upper eyelid wrinkles. In related work, 3D analysis of skin replicas found that the depth of eye wrinkles in men showed an annual variation with more wrinkles at the corner of the eye in the fall compared to the spring; no such annual variation was observed in women [38]. The varying density of sebaceous glands on the face may partly explain the variation in facial wrinkling at different facial sites. Tamatsu et al. [39] looked at cadaver skin specimens from females and males ranging in age from the 20s to 90s at age of death. The found a negative correlation between wrinkle depth and

sebaceous gland density. Sebaceous gland density was found to be significantly lower in the lateral canthus than in the forehead on both males and females. However, while the sebaceous gland density was significantly lower in females than in males in both facial regions, there was no significant gender-dependent difference in wrinkle depth.

In a cross-sectional study of skin condition, Hillebrand and colleagues measured facial wrinkling in the periorbital area (under eye and crow's feet wrinkles) on 147 Caucasian males and 183 Caucasian females, aged 10–78. Regression analysis showed that both *gender* and *age* to be significant ($p < 0.05$) factors in describing the variance in wrinkle severity (Fig. 1.2a). However, when other factors are considered in the regression analysis, like the subject's body mass index, smoking history in pack years and years working outside, gender drops out as a significant factor suggesting that some of the variance initially explained by gender can be explained by other gender-associated confounding factors. We will discuss confounding factors more later in the chapter. Figure 1.2b shows the data in Fig. 1.2a replotted as age group means for males and females. While females had higher wrinkles than men in all age groups, none of the pairwise comparisons between males and females in any given age group were significantly different (one-way ANOVA, Tukey Test).

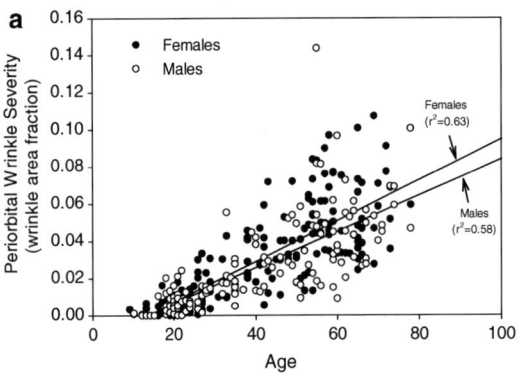
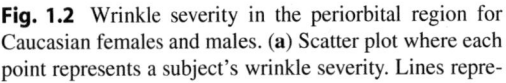
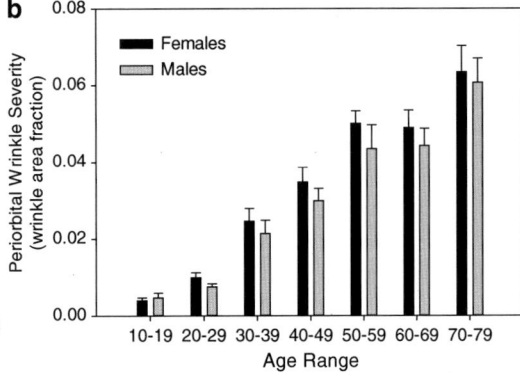

Fig. 1.2 Wrinkle severity in the periorbital region for Caucasian females and males. (**a**) Scatter plot where each point represents a subject's wrinkle severity. Lines represent best fit linear regression curves. (**b**) Age group means ± standard error

1.8 Confounding Factors

The differences observed between male and female skin may be ascribed to intrinsic factors like hormones [40] and other genetically determined variables or extrinsic factors like differences in smoking, diet, sun protection and skin care routines. Even differences in facial expression patterns may differ between the sexes and influence skin condition, especially facial wrinkling [41]. Below we discuss confounding factors that should be considered when designing and interpreting clinical data for men and women.

1.8.1 Smoking History

Smoking has been shown to increase facial wrinkling [34]. A report by Okada et al. involving identical twins underscores the risk of smoking on appearance and health. They compared facial wrinkling in identical twins and showed that a 5-year difference in smoking history can have a noticeable effect on skin aging [42]. Similar observations were reported by Doshi et al. [43]. The exact mechanism for how smoking affects skin wrinkling is not understood but may involve changes in skin barrier function and associated changes in chronic skin dryness caused both by smoking and exposure to *second-hand* smoke [44] which is associated with having more wrinkles [41, 43, 44]. Since men are more likely to smoke than women (Centers for Disease Control and Prevention [45], smoking needs to be considered as a confounding variable when comparing the skin condition of males to females.

1.8.2 Diet and Nutrition

Consuming an adequate amount of fruit and vegetables has been shown to reduce the risk of excess weight gain, type 2 diabetes, cardiovascular disease, and specific cancers [46, 47]. Pezdirc et al. [47] has recently reviewed the summation of evidence linking diet and skin health. The majority of studies conducted in this space focus on the effect of dietary supplements on skin condition and most enroll only females. In a cross-sectional study of 4025 women ages 40–74, Cosgrove et al. found that higher intakes of vitamin C and linoleic acid and lower intakes of fats and carbohydrates are associated with better skin-aging appearance [48]. Higher intakes of vegetables, fruit, olive oil, and legumes may cause less skin wrinkling and are protective against actinic damage [49]. Iizaka et al. measured nutritional status and habitual dietary intact, stratum corneum hydration and xerosis in 118 older (>65) Japanese subjects, mostly females [50]. They concluded that a dietary pattern characterized by higher vegetable and fruit intake was associated with a better skin condition. Since men's daily intake of fruits and vegetables is less than that of women [51], dietary differences in the sample population should be considered in interpretation and analysis of clinical results as well as in clinical design.

1.8.3 Skin Care Habits and Practices

A person's daily skin care routine will undoubtedly affect their skin condition. Regular use of moisturizers will improve skin barrier function, skin hydration, and lessen the advancement of wrinkling [14, 41]. Those who regularly protect their skin from acute and chronic sun exposure will slow the advancement of skin aging. Male facial skin is largely influenced by beard grooming routines [52, 53]. In this regard, many of the differences observed between male and female skin may be attributable to differences in skin care habits and practices, especially differences on the face [54].

1.8.4 Sun Exposure

Sun exposure is well known to be a major cause of wrinkling, especially in facial skin [23, 55–57]. When discussing gender differences in facial wrinkles the relative tendency for sun exposure and the frequency of sunscreen application should be considered as regular sunscreen use may provide some protection against the signs of photoaging [58, 59]. Haluza et al. reported that Australian men are more likely to suffer sun exposure and less likely to use sunscreen compared to their female counterparts [60]. This may explain the earlier onset [35] and more severe wrinkling seen in men on the forehead [37] but is not consistent with the higher levels of perioral wrinkles seen in women [36].

1.9   Summary

One of most important and difficult questions whenever comparing measured properties between two groups is whether statistically significant differences are clinically relevant. We have reviewed and summarized many of the studies aimed at improving our understanding of the similarities and differences between male and female skin with particular attention to differences in biophysical skin properties. We noted that results depended on the method used, the body site being measured, the age of the subjects, and their prior history of smoking, sun exposure, and use of skin care products. The most consistent difference between the genders reported in this review is lower sebum production in women, especially over the age of 50. However, because of the high individual variability in sebum output there is overlap between the high sebum producing females and low sebum producing males (Table 1.1). Thus care must be taken when drawing conclusions from the differences reported in the studies summarized here.

Acknowledgements The authors wish to thank Aimee Herbel (Amway Corporation) for her help in collecting the pH data in Fig. 1.1.

References

1. Pochi PE, Strauss JS, Downing DT. Age-related changes in sebaceous gland activity. J Invest Dermatol. 1979;73(1):108–11.
2. Luebberding S, Krueger N, Kerscher M. Skin physiology in men and women: in vivo evaluation of 300 people including TEWL, SC hydration, sebum content and skin surface pH. Int J Cosmet Sci. 2013;35(5):477–83.
3. Ogoshi K. Optical measurement of sebum excretion using opalescent film imprint. The Sebumeter. In: Handbook of non-invasive methods and the skin. Boca Raton: Taylor and Francis; 2006. p. 841–6.
4. Firooz A, Sadr B, Babakoohi S, Sarraf-Yazdy M, Fanian F, Kazerouni-Timsar A, et al. Variation of biophysical parameters of the skin with age, gender, and body region. Sci World J. 2012;2012:386936.
5. Fluhr JW, Bankova L, Dikstein S. Skin surface pH: mechanism, measurement, importance. In: Serup J, GBE J, Grove GL, editors. Handbook of non-invasive methods and the skin. 2nd ed. Boco Raton: Taylor and Francis; 2006. p. 411–20.
6. Zlotogorski A. Distribution of skin surface pH on the forehead and cheek of adults. Arch Dermatol Res. 1987;279(6):398–401.
7. Ehlers C, Ivens UI, Møller ML, Senderovitz T, Serup J. Females have lower skin surface pH than men. Skin Res Technol. 2001;7(2):90–4.
8. Kim MK, Patel RA, Shinn AH, Choi SY, Byun HJ, Huh CH, et al. Evaluation of gender difference in skin type and pH. J Dermatol Sci. 2006;41(2):153–6.
9. Man MQ, Xin SJ, Song SP, Cho SY, Zhang XJ, Tu CX, et al. Variation of skin surface pH, sebum content and stratum corneum hydration with age and gender in a large Chinese population. Skin Pharmacol Physiol. 2009;22(4):190–9.
10. Nilsson GE. Measurement of water exchange through the skin. Med Biol Eng Comput. 1977;15:209–18.
11. Fluhr JW, Feingold KR, Elias PM. Transepidermal water loss reflects permeability barrier status: validation in human and rodent in vivo and ex vivo models. Exp Dermatol. 2006;15(7):483–92.
12. Chilcott RP, Farrar R. Biophysical measurements of human forearm skin in vivo: effects of site, gender, chirality and time. Skin Res Technol. 2000;6(2):64–9.
13. Wilhelm KP, Cua AB, Maibach HI. Skin aging. Effect on transepidermal water loss, stratum corneum hydration, skin surface pH, and casual sebum content. Arch Dermatol. 1991;127(12):1806–9.
14. Hadi H, Awadh AI, Hanif NM, Md Sidik NF, Mohd Rani MR, Suhaimi MS. The investigation of the skin biophysical measurements focusing on daily activities, skin care habits, and gender differences. Skin Res Technol. 2016;22(2):247–54.
15. Barel AO, Clarys P. Study of the stratum corneum barrier function by transepidermal water loss measurements: comparison between two commercial instruments: Evaporimeter and Tewameter. Skin Pharmacol. 1995;8(4):186–95.
16. Li X, Galzote C, Yan X, Li L, Wang X. Characterization of Chinese body skin through in vivo instrument assessments, visual evaluations, and questionnaire: influences of body area, inter-generation, season, sex, and skin care habits. Skin Res Technol. 2014;20(1):14–22.
17. Barel AO, Clarys P. In vitro calibration of the capacitance method (Corneometer CM 825) and conductance method (Skicon-200) for the evaluation of the hydration state of the skin. Skin Res Technol. 1997;3:107–13.

18. Berardesca E. EEMCO guidance for the assessment of stratum corneum hydration: electrical methods. Skin Res Technol. 1997;3:126–32.
19. Fluhr JW, Gloor M, Lazzerini S, Kleesz P, Grieshaber R, Berardesca E. Comparative study of five instruments measuring stratum corneum hydration (Corneometer CM 820 and CM 825, Skicon 200, Nova DPM 9003, DermLab). Part II. In vivo. Skin Res Technol. 1999;5:171–8.
20. Tagami H, Ohi M, Iwatsuki K, Kanamaru Y, Yamada M, Ichijo B. Evaluation of the skin surface hydration in vivo by electrical measurement. J Invest Dermatol. 1980;75(6):500–7.
21. Agache PG, Monneur C, Leveque JL, de RJ. Mechanical properties and Young's modulus of human skin in vivo. Arch Dermatol Res. 1980;269(3):221–32.
22. Diridollou S, Vabre V, Berson M, Vaillant L, Black D, Lagarde JM, et al. Skin ageing: changes of physical properties of human skin in vivo. Int J Cosmet Sci. 2001;23(6):353–62.
23. Kligman AM. Early destructive effect of sunlight on human skin. JAMA. 1969;210(13):2377–80.
24. Imokawa G, Nakajima H, Ishida K. Biological mechanisms underlying the ultraviolet radiation-induced formation of skin wrinkling and sagging II: overexpression of neprilysin plays an essential role. Int J Mol Sci. 2015;16(4):7776–95.
25. Barel AO, Courage W, Clarys P. Suction method for measurement of skin mechanical properties: the Cutometer. In: Serup J, Jemec GBE, editors. Handbook of non-invasive methods and the skin. Ann Arbor: CRC Press; 1995. p. 335–40.
26. Murray BC, Wickett RR. Sensitivity of cutometer data to stratum corneum hydration level. Skin Res Technol. 1996;2:167–72.
27. O'Goshi KI. Suction chamber methods for measurement of skin mechanics: the Cutometer. In: Serup J, Jemec GBE, Grove GL, editors. Handbook of non-invasive methods and the skin. 2nd ed. Boco Raton: Taylor and Francis; 2006. p. 579–91.
28. Nedelec B, Forget NJ, Hurtubise T, Cimino S, de Muszka F, Legault A, et al. Skin characteristics: normative data for elasticity, erythema, melanin, and thickness at 16 different anatomical locations. Skin Res Technol. 2016;22(3):263–75.
29. Cua AB, Wilhelm KP, Maibach HI. Elastic properties of human skin: relation to age, sex, and anatomical region. Arch Dermatol Res. 1990;282(5):283–8.
30. Ishikawa T, Ishikawa O, Miyachi Y. Measurement of skin elastic properties with a new suction device (I): relationship to age, sex and the degree of obesity in normal individuals. J Dermatol. 1995;22(10):713–7.
31. Luebberding S, Krueger N, Kerscher M. Mechanical properties of human skin in vivo: a comparative evaluation in 300 men and women. Skin Res Technol. 2014;20(2):127–35.
32. Ma L, Tan Y, Zheng S, Li J, Jiang C, Chen Z, et al. Correlation study between image features and mechanical properties of Han Chinese facial skin. Int J Cosmet Sci. 2017;39(1):93–100.
33. Chung JH, Lee SH, Youn CS, Park BJ, Kim KH, Park KC, et al. Cutaneous photodamage in Koreans: influence of sex, sun exposure, smoking, and skin color. Arch Dermatol. 2001;137(8):1043–51.
34. Paes EC, Teepen HJ, Koop WA, Kon M. Perioral wrinkles: histologic differences between men and women. Aesthet Surg J. 2009;29(6):467–72.
35. Hamer MA, Pardo LM, Jacobs LC, Ikram MA, Laven JS, Kayser M, et al. Lifestyle and physiological factors associated with facial wrinkling in men and women. J Invest Dermatol. 2017;137(8):1692–9.
36. Chien AL, Qi J, Cheng N, Do TT, Mesfin M, Egbers R, et al. Perioral wrinkles are associated with female gender, aging, and smoking: development of a gender-specific photonumeric scale. J Am Acad Dermatol. 2016;74(5):924–30.
37. Tsukahara K, Hotta M, Osanai O, Kawada H, Kitahara T, Takema Y. Gender-dependent differences in degree of facial wrinkles. Skin Res Technol. 2013;19(1):e65–71.
38. Tsukahara K, Osanai O, Kitahara T, Takema Y. Seasonal and annual variation in the intensity of facial wrinkles. Skin Res Technol. 2013;19(3):279–87.
39. Tamatsu Y, Tsukahara K, Sugawara Y, Shimada K. New finding that might explain why the skin wrinkles more on various parts of the face. Clin Anat. 2015;28(6):745–52.
40. Makrantonaki E, Zouboulis CC. Androgens and ageing of the skin. Curr Opin Endocrinol Diabetes Obes. 2009;16(3):240–5.
41. Hillebrand GG, Liang Z, Yan X, Yoshii T. New wrinkles on wrinkling: an 8-year longitudinal study on the progression of expression lines into persistent wrinkles. Br J Dermatol. 2010;162(6):1233–41.
42. Okada HC, Alleyne B, Varghai K, Kinder K, Guyuron B. Facial changes caused by smoking: a comparison between smoking and nonsmoking identical twins. Plast Reconstr Surg. 2013;132(5):1085–92.
43. Doshi DN, Hanneman KK, Cooper KD. Smoking and skin aging in identical twins. Arch Dermatol. 2007;143(12):1543–6.
44. Muizzuddin N, Marenus K, Vallon P, Maes D. Effect of cigarette smoke on skin. J Soc Cosmet Chem. 1997;48:235–42.
45. Jamal A, King BA, Whitmill JBSD, Graffimder C. Current cigarette smoking among adults - United States, 2005-2015. Morb Mortal Wkly Rep. 2016;65:1205–11.
46. Boeing H, Bechthold A, Bub A, Ellinger S, Haller D, Kroke A, et al. Critical review: vegetables and fruit in the prevention of chronic diseases. Eur J Nutr. 2012;51(6):637–63.
47. Pezdirc K, Hutchesson M, Whitehead R, Ozakinci G, Perrett D, Collins CE. Can dietary intake influence perception of and measured appearance? A systematic review. Nutr Res. 2015;35(3):175–97.
48. Cosgrove MC, Franco OH, Granger SP, Murray PG, Mayes AE. Dietary nutrient intakes and skin-aging appearance among middle-aged American women. Am J Clin Nutr. 2007;86(4):1225–31.

49. Purba MB, Kouris-Blazos A, Wattanapenpaiboon N, Lukito W, Rothenberg EM, Steen BC, et al. Skin wrinkling: can food make a difference? J Am Coll Nutr. 2001;20(1):71–80.

50. Iizaka S, Nagata S, Sanada H. Nutritional status and habitual dietary intake are associated with frail skin conditions in community-dwelling older people. J Nutr Health Aging. 2017;21(2):137–46.

51. Blanck HM, Gillespie C, Kimmons JE, Seymour JD, Serdula MK. Trends in fruit and vegetable consumption among U.S. men and women, 1994-2005. Prev Chronic Dis. 2008;5(2):A35.

52. Draelos ZD. Male skin and ingredients relevant to male skin care. Br J Dermatol. 2012;166(Suppl 1):13–6.

53. Oblong JE. Male skin care: shaving and moisturization needs. Dermatol Ther. 2012;25(3):238–43.

54. Mizukoshi K, Akamatsu H. The investigation of the skin characteristics of males focusing on gender differences, skin perception, and skin care habits. Skin Res Technol. 2013;19(2):91–9.

55. Battie C, Jitsukawa S, Bernerd F, Del BS, Marionnet C, Verschoore M. New insights in photoaging, UVA induced damage and skin types. Exp Dermatol. 2014;23(Suppl 1):7–12.

56. Gilchrest BA. Skin aging and photoaging: an overview. J Am Acad Dermatol. 1989;21(3 Pt 2):610–3.

57. Kligman LH, Kligman AM. The nature of photoaging: its prevention and repair. Photo-Dermatology. 1986;3(4):215–27.

58. Green AC, Hughes MC, McBride P, Fourtanier A. Factors associated with premature skin aging (photoaging) before the age of 55: a population-based study. Dermatology. 2011;222(1):74–80.

59. Iannacone MR, Hughes MC, Green AC. Effects of sunscreen on skin cancer and photoaging. Photodermatol Photoimmunol Photomed. 2014;30:55.

60. Haluza D, Simic S, Holtge J, Cervinka R, Moshammer H. Gender aspects of recreational sun-protective behavior: results of a representative, population-based survey among Austrian residents. Photodermatol Photoimmunol Photomed. 2016;32(1):11–21.

Racial and Gender Influences on Skin Disease

2

Daniel Callaghan and Neelam A. Vashi

2.1 Introduction

Skin of color typically refers to individuals of African, Afro-Caribbean, Asian, Hispanic, Native American, Middle Eastern and Pacific Island backgrounds. In the United States, individuals from these groups made up 38% of the population in 2014, which is expected to increase to 56% by 2060 [1].

Due to differences in skin physiology as well as to different cultural practices, there are several dermatologic conditions that affect these populations at a higher rate compared to Caucasians. Furthermore, there are a number of diseases that disproportionately affect males and females within these populations. In this chapter, we will discuss categories of diseases that are more commonly seen in these ethnic groups, including follicular, scarring, and pigmentary disorders with a special focus on their epidemiology and pathogenesis.

2.1.1 Physiologic Differences

2.1.1.1 Skin Physiology

Skin is routinely characterized by the Fitzpatrick scale, a classification scheme based on how one reacts to sun exposure. Type I skin is fair, burns easily and does not tan. Type VI skin is dark brown or black, tans and never burns. Although large variation exists within the SOC population (SOC), generally speaking, SOC is generally represented by Fitzpatrick types III–VI skin.

The hallmark feature of skin of color is the amount and distribution of melanin. Darker skin phenotypes have larger, non-aggregating melanosomes distributed throughout the epidermis. Conversely, fairer skinned individuals have smaller, aggregated melanosomes which are not present in the upper layers of the epidermis [2]. Due to this increased melanin, Black skin transmits only 7.4% of ultraviolet (UV) radiation, compared to 29.4% in Caucasian skin [3]. While this pigmentation offers protection against some diseases seen more commonly in Caucasians, such as non-melanoma skin cancer, it makes those with darkly pigmented skin more susceptible to other diseases, particularly pigmentary disorders.

The stratum corneum in skin of color is more compact due to greater intercellular cohesion. Although there is no difference in dermal thickness, Black skin has more numerous and larger fibroblasts, which is thought to partially explain why they are at an increased risk of keloid

D. Callaghan
Boston University Medical Center, Boston, MA, USA
e-mail: daniel.callaghan@bmc.org

N. A. Vashi (✉)
Dermatology, Boston University Center for Ethnic Skin, Boston University School of Medicine, Boston, MA, USA
e-mail: nvashi@bu.edu

© Springer International Publishing AG, part of Springer Nature 2018
E. Tur, H. I. Maibach (eds.), *Gender and Dermatology*,
https://doi.org/10.1007/978-3-319-72156-9_2

formation. Additionally, Black skin has collagen fibers that are smaller but more closely stacked together. Of note, studies regarding physiologic differences in eccrine, apocrine and sebaceous glands in different races have demonstrated conflicting results [2, 4].

2.1.1.2 Hair Physiology
Individuals of African descent have hair that is characterized by flat, elliptical strands with curved follicles, which leads to tightly spiraled hair. Blacks also have fewer elastic fibers anchoring hair follicles to the dermis. Conversely, Asian hair is rounder, with the largest cross-sectional area relative to other ethnicities, resulting in hair that is generally straighter [5, 6]. These variations account in part for the different clinical characteristics seen in the hair of these ethnic groups. African Americans tend to have hair that is drier, slower growing and more fragile compared to Caucasians. Conversely, Asian hair tends to be thicker in diameter with faster growth [7, 8].

2.1.2   Cultural Differences

Due to these physiologic differences, cultural differences exist in terms of how the SOC population cares for their skin and hair. For example, African Americans may braid their hair in cornrows as a symbol of cultural identity and because it offers a lower maintenance hairstyle. Hair extensions and weaves are used to give the hair a longer, straighter or more voluminous appearance. Given the curly nature of Black hair, it is also common for them to straighten their hair with chemicals or heat such as hot combs, flat irons and blow dryers. Alternatively, Sikh men and women do not cut their hair but rather allow it to grow as a symbol of devotion to God. They also wear turbans to care for their hair and as a sign of identity and equality. Over time, many of these hair styling practices can lead to irritation and follicular damage which propagates the inflammatory cascade. Ultimately, these different physiologic and cultural differences have been implicated in the pathogenesis of several diseases seen more commonly in skin of color.

2.2   Follicular and Scarring Disorders

2.2.1   Central Centrifugal Cicatricial Alopecia

2.2.1.1 Introduction
Central centrifugal cicatricial alopecia (CCCA), formerly known as hot comb alopecia or follicular degeneration syndrome, is a disease seen almost exclusively in African American women, characterized by scarring hair loss first seen on the vertex of the scalp.

2.2.1.2 Epidemiology
CCCA is the most common scarring alopecia among African American women and is rarely reported in other ethnic groups. Large population based studies are lacking, but one study of African American women in the Southeastern United States found the incidence of CCCA to be 5.6% [9]. Although it is predominantly seen in women, it has been reported in African American men [10].

2.2.1.3 Pathogenesis
CCCA is an inflammatory disorder which ultimately results in scarring; however, the specific reasons why this inflammation occurs remain elusive and are likely multifactorial.

Skin of Color
Despite the fact that the specific pathogenesis of CCCA is unclear, one prevailing theory is that it is due in part to traumatic hair styling practices, which are much more common in Blacks. These include tight braids, weaves, or cornrows and the use of chemical relaxers, texturizers, and/or heat. Although this theory has been reinforced by studies in which a significant association between CCCA and hairstyling practices was observed, other studies were unable to find a similar association [9, 11].

It has also been suggested that there is a genetic component to the development of CCCA, as it has been described to run in families. Dlova et al. observed 14 South African families in which an autosomal dominant pattern of CCCA was demonstrated. Furthermore, 20% of these individuals reported no history of traumatic hair-styling, which suggests that there is more to the pathogenesis of CCCA than these practices, and a genetic component may also be at play [12].

Gender

Males rarely use the hair styling practices which have been implicated in the pathogenesis of CCCA, which may explain why it is far less common for them to be affected. However, the fact that it has been seen in males, particular African American males, supports the claim that there may be an underlying genetic component to the disease [10].

2.2.1.4 Clinical Features

As the name suggests, CCCA generally begins on the crown or vertex of the scalp, and slowly expands centrifugally. In early stages, mild hair thinning may make the disease difficult to distinguish from androgenetic alopecia. Although it typically expands slowly, it can eventually progress centrifugally to affect the entire crown of the scalp. Left untreated, scarring occurs and the scalp becomes smooth and shiny, with follicular dropout and preservation of a few short, brittle hairs [13].

Patients may complain of mild pruritus or tenderness in the area that is affected, which can be a sign of disease activity. In certain cases, patients may present with superimposed folliculitis decalvans, with pustules and crusting.

2.2.1.5 Histology

Depending on the stage of the disease, CCCA demonstrates a follicular lichenoid lymphocytic infiltrate when caught early, which leads to follicular fibrosis as it progresses. Features that help make the diagnosis include follicular miniaturization, premature desquamation of the inner root sheath, focal preservation of sebaceous glands, naked hair shafts, compound follicular structures, perifollicular fibrosis and/or inflammation, and lamellar hyperkeratosis and parakeratosis in the hair canal [14].

2.2.1.6 Treatment

There are limited treatment options available for CCCA, and results are often unsatisfactory. As it can ultimately lead to scarring, treatment should

be started as soon as possible. It is important to discuss and set expectations with the patient, including the fact that it is challenging to predict the course of the disease. Furthermore, if scarring has already occurred, it is important to make the patient aware that regrowth will be quite limited. Unless these expectations are outlined early and clearly, at future visits, patients may be frustrated with their management.

Given the implication of certain hair styling techniques in the pathogenesis of CCCA, it should be stressed to patients to avoid such practices, even if they have denied using them in the past. Being a disease of inflammation, topical or intralesional steroids are typically used. Oral tetracyclines have also been used in the treatment of CCCA. Other therapies that have been reported anecdotally include antimalarials, topical calcineurin inhibitors, minoxidil, thalidomide, cyclosporine and mycophenolate mofetil [13].

Patients may present to clinic specifically inquiring about the effectiveness of hair transplantation, and in some cases may have already consulted with a hair transplant surgeon. Although hair transplantation has been reported to be successful in patient who have had stable disease for at least 9–12 months, patients should be educated on the potential need for multiple hair transplant sessions, the need for continued medical therapy, and the possibility of disease recurrence [15].

2.2.2 Traction Alopecia

2.2.2.1 Introduction

Traction alopecia (TA) is another form of scarring alopecia that is most prominently seen in women of color. It develops in the setting of hair styling techniques that create prolonged tension or repetitive pulling on hair.

2.2.2.2 Epidemiology

TA is almost exclusively reported in women and is most frequently seen in African Americans. That said, it has also been described in other ethnic groups, and the prevalence rate has also been reported to be relatively high in Hispanics [16].

Although it is far less commonly described in males, they can also be affected; for example, TA has been reported among Sikh males who wear their hair twisted tightly under turbans [17]. One study looking at 874 South African adults found that 31.7% of women had TA compared with just 2.2% of men [18].

2.2.2.3 Pathogenesis

Traction alopecia develops when hairstyling practices cause tension on the hair follicle, which over time leads to inflammation, fibrosis and permanent alopecia.

Skin of Color

The increased prevalence of TA in Blacks is explained both by cultural and physiologic differences. As described before, Black hair grows in a tight spiral pattern, making it more susceptible to breakage when manipulated. Furthermore, Blacks more commonly use hair styling techniques such as braids, weaves, chemical relaxers and heat, which puts more tension on their hair and increases their risk of developing TA. For instance, it has been shown that chemically processed hair has a greater risk of developing TA [19]. TA can also be seen in Hispanics who wear their hair in tight ponytails. Japanese women have also been reported to get TA on the occipital or temporal scalp from wearing their hair in a tight bun [16].

Gender

The increased prevalence in women is explained by the fact that they are far more likely to style their hair using the aforementioned practices.

2.2.2.4 Clinical Features

TA is most commonly seen in the frontal and temporal region of the scalp but can present anywhere depending on the hair styling practice. When caught early, there may be perifollicular erythema, papules or pustules. In a study involving 41 patients with TA, including 12 Hispanic patients, Samrao et al. reported clinically evident inflammation in 54% of African American women compared with 17% of Hispanic women [16].

Although clinical history is crucial in making this diagnosis, it is not uncommon for patients to deny styling their hair in a manner that predisposes them to TA. When the history does not support the diagnosis, the clinician may look for the fringe sign to help identify the disease. The 'fringe sign' describes the presence of short retained hairs along the hairline and can help distinguish TA from other forms of hair loss such as ophiasis alopecia areata. It has been reported in up to 100% of women with TA affecting the frontal or temporal hairlines [16].

2.2.2.5 Histology

Histologically, early TA demonstrates decreased follicular number but preservation of the sebaceous glands. Features of trichomalacia, including twisting or deformation of anagen bulbs can also be seen when caught early. Depending on the stage, follicular scarring may or may not be present. As the disease progresses, the number of sebaceous glands may be reduced and hair follicles become surrounded by a lymphocytic infiltrate and fibrosis [20]. However, these findings are not pathognomonic and clinicopathologic correlation is necessary to make an accurate diagnosis.

2.2.2.6 Treatment

The first step in the treatment of TA is cessation of any hairstyling technique which may be contributing to the disease process. It may be difficult to convince patients to change their hairstyling practices, which they have often been using for years. As the hair styling practices that lead to TA are often started in childhood, it is important to also educate parents about this risk to help prevent the disease.

In the setting of active inflammation, topical or intralesional steroids can be used. Intralesional administration of steroids should be performed at the periphery of the hair line to prevent retained hair from being lost. Oral antibiotics are also utilized in cases of TA when there is clinically apparent inflammation.. With patients who have lost hair as a result of TA but have not yet developed scarring, topical minoxidil may be beneficial [21].

As with other scarring alopecias that are difficult to manage medically, camouflage techniques can be effective and can help improve patients' quality of life. Surgical options, including follicular unit transplantation and mini- or micrografting have also been reported to be effective in the appropriately selected patient [22].

2.2.3 Acne Keloidalis Nuchae

2.2.3.1 Introduction

Acne keloidalis nuchae (AKN) is a form of chronic folliculitis most frequently seen in Black males. It is characterized by papules and pustules on the occipital scalp and posterior neck, which over time can develop into keloid-like plaques and scarring alopecia.

2.2.3.2 Epidemiology

AKN has been described in all races but is most frequently seen in Black men after adolescence and under the age of 55. In decreasing incidence it also affects Hispanic, Asian and Caucasian males [23]. Knable et al. studied 453 male football players between the ages of 14 and 27, and found that while AKN was seen in 24% of black players, no white players were affected [24]. Although 20 times more common in men, women can also be affected by it [25].

2.2.3.3 Pathogenesis

Despite its name, AKN is not a variant of acne vulgaris, and the name folliculitis keloidalis nuchae has been suggested. The exact etiology is unknown, but it is a result of chronic inflammation which ultimately leads to scarring and keloid-like plaques.

The development of AKN is typically attributed to chronic trauma to the follicular scalp. Most investigators believe that AKN is a result of mechanical injury from friction and hair styling practices, such as the use of electric razors and shaving, which leads to irritation, occlusion, trauma and inflammation [26].

Some propose that AKN is a primary cicatricial alopecia resulting from an immune response against antigens on the follicular epithelium, intrafollicular canal or sebaceous glands. Antigens that have been implicated include normal skin flora, demodex, desquamated keratinocytes, sebum and cosmetics [27, 28]. This inflammation results in damage to the hair shaft, with the resulting clinical changes described in AKN. Other reported etiologic factors have included seborrheic dermatitis, *Staphylococcus aureus* infection, and elevated serum testosterone levels [29].

Skin of Color

Previously, AKN was thought to be the result of inward growth of hair leading to a foreign body reaction and subsequent inflammation. The spiraled nature of hair in Blacks would make them more susceptible and explains why they are more commonly affected by the disease. That being said, there is no clinical or histologic evidence to substantiate this claim. For instance, one South African study did not find an association between the prevalence of AKN and the use of clippers as opposed to razors [18]. Furthermore, one author observed that ingrown hairs are not commonly seen in AKN as they are in PFB [27, 30].

If this theory is to be disregarded, it is unclear why there is an increased prevalence of AKN in Blacks. If one subscribes to the thought that AKN is a primary cicatricial alopecia resulting from immune dysregulation, it may be that there is a genetic component which predisposes these individuals to the disease.

Gender

Similarly, our lack of understanding of the pathogenesis of AKN makes it difficult to explain why it is almost exclusively seen in males. However, that observation alone, coupled with the fact that it is rare before puberty or after the age of 55, has led some to propose that there is a hormonal component involved. An increase in androgen levels, androgen receptor sensitivity or increased activity of sebaceous glands may play a role [30].

2.2.3.4 Clinical Features

AKN initially presents as inflammatory papules on the nape of the neck and posterior scalp, which over time result in fibrosis and keloid-like plaques. These patients can also develop secondary infection with pustules, subcutaneous abscesses and sinus drainage. Repeated inflammation leads to the destruction of hair follicles, fibrosis and ultimately scarring alopecia. Furthermore, the keloid-like plaques that develop are usually devoid of hair.

These changes can be a significant cosmetic concern to patients and negatively affects their quality of life [23, 31]. Similar to other inflammatory disorders, these patients also complain of pruritus, and the lesions can be painful and tender to palpation.

2.2.3.5 Histology

Histologic characteristics of AKN include perifollicular, lymphocytic and plasmacytic inflammation most intense at the level of the isthmus and lower infundibulum, lamellar fibrosis, loss of sebaceous glands, thinning of the follicular epithelium and total epithelial destruction with residual "naked" hair fragments [28]. These histologic findings closely resemble other forms of cicatricial alopecia, which is what has led some to propose it to be a form of primary cicatricial alopecia.

2.2.3.6 Treatment

Early treatment correlates with a good prognosis; however, as the disease progresses, it can be more difficult to treat and more invasive measures must be utilized.

Management is typically first directed at avoiding any inciting factors that may be causing irritation. Mild disease can be managed medically with topical or intralesional steroids, topical or oral antibiotics, particularly tetracyclines, and retinoids [26].

Light and laser therapies, including the 1064-nm neodymium-doped yttrium aluminum garnet (Nd:Yag) laser and targeted UVB light, have offered promising results with mild side effects including transient erythema and mild burning. These treatment options work to destroy the hair follicle and decrease the inflammation implicated in the pathogenesis of the disease.

Surgical or cryosurgical treatment with secondary intention healing may be an effective treatment option; however, the risk of scarring is an obvious concern. Unfortunately, the risk of at least mild recurrence is nearly 50%, typically within weeks to months of medication discontinuation [26].

2.2.4 Pseudofolliculitis Barbae

2.2.4.1 Introduction

Pseudofolliculitis barbae (PFB) is a chronic, non-infectious, inflammatory follicular disorder which results in erythematous papules most frequently found in the beard area. Given the similarities in appearance of AKN and PFB, the two diseases were previously thought to be on the same spectrum, with the difference being the location they affected. However, the two diseases are now thought to be separate entities, each with a different pathogenesis.

2.2.4.2 Epidemiology

PFB is most often found in Black males, with the reported incidence varying from 45% to 83%. It is also seen in other populations who may have more tightly curled hair, including Hispanics and Middle Easterners. It is less commonly observed in women [32].

2.2.4.3 Pathogenesis

PFB occurs because of ingrown hairs, which induce a foreign body inflammatory reaction upon re-entering the skin through extrafollicular or transfollicular penetration. Certain hair styling techniques, such as pulling the skin taut while shaving and/or cutting the tip to a sharp point, can make re-entry more likely.

Skin of Color

Blacks have tightly spiraled hairs, which curve in such a manner to emerge almost parallel to the skin. Rather than continue to grow outward, this orientation puts them at risk to curl and re-enter the skin. Beyond this, some individuals may have a genetic predisposition to developing PFB, which was demonstrated by Winter et al. who found that a defect in a hair follicle keratin increased the risk of developing PFB by a factor of 6.12 [33].

Gender

PFB is thought to affect males more so than females because of its close association with shaving. That being said, women can also develop PFB. One study found that hormonal disorders leading to hyperandrogenism and hirsutism is a risk factor for women to develop PFB [34].

2.2.4.4 Clinical Features

PFB presents as firm, follicular or perifollicular papules most often found on the neck and cheeks in men. Some papules may contain visible hairs. When it does affect women, the chin is the most commonly area affected, especially in hirsute women who shave or pluck unwanted hairs. Although it is associated with shaving in men, it should be noted that the mustache and nuchal areas are rarely affected [32, 35].

Although secondary infection can occur, pustules are rare in PFB, which can help distinguish it from acne vulgaris. No comedonal lesions are seen in PFB, which also helps distinguish it from acne.

PFB must also be distinguished from traumatic folliculitis, more commonly known as razor burn. Traumatic folliculitis occurs when shaving is performed too closely. It presents as painful follicular papules which may be confused for PFB but disappear within 24–48 h. PFB, conversely, persists for weeks after cessation of shaving.

PFB may be associated with pruritus and pain and may be complicated by postinflammatory hyperpigmentation (PIH), scarring, and formation of keloids [32].

2.2.4.5 Histology

Histopathologically, PFB is characterized by a foreign body inflammatory response to hair re-entering the skin. Epidermal penetration shows invagination with an inflammatory infiltrate, which becomes more intense as the hair reaches the dermis [21].

2.2.4.6 Treatment

Given its pathogenesis, the first recommendation in the management of PFB is often cessation of shaving, the only curative treatment, or use of electric shavers. However, that can be an inconvenience for individuals who prefer to be closely shaved, and is impractical for others who may be required to be closely shaved. For those who are able to stop shaving, remission is often seen within 30 days [36].

For men who are unable or unwilling to avoid shaving, shaving techniques that have been proposed to help reduce the burden of PFB include shaving regularly to prevent hair from growing long enough to re-enter the skin, preparing the skin beforehand with warm water and a gentle cleanser to soften the hair, applying shaving foam or gel to provide a protective anti-friction layer, keeping the skin relaxed rather than pulling taut, and using a technologically advanced multiblade razor or foil-guarded manual single-blade razor. The use of after-shave products containing moisturizing ingredients also help rehydrate and comfort the skin [35].

For PFB that cannot be controlled by nonmedical interventions, retinoids have been reported to improve the disease, with the thought that they relieve hyperkeratosis and remove the thin covering of epidermis that the hair becomes embedded in when re-entering the skin. Mild topical corticosteroids can also be used temporarily to reduce inflammation [32]. In addition, topical eflornithine hydrochloride cream can be used to slow hair growth.

For severe disease, especially in the setting of frequent superinfection with the development of pustules and abscess formation, topical or oral antibiotics may be indicated, with tetracyclines commonly employed [35]. Laser therapy has been used successfully, with the Nd:YAG 1064 nm lasers having the best safety and efficacy profile for use in SOC patients.

2.2.5 Dissecting Cellulitis

2.2.5.1 Introduction

Dissecting cellulitis of the scalp (DCS) is a form of primary neutrophilic cicatricial alopecia. It is a chronic inflammatory disorder resulting in scarring alopecia more frequently seen in Black males. It makes up a component of the follicular occlusion tetrad, which also includes hidradenitis suppurativa (HS), acne conglobata, and pilonidal cysts.

2.2.5.2 Epidemiology

DCS is most commonly seen in Black males between their third to fifth decades of life, with only 10% of cases involving Caucasians [37]. Although it can affect women, it is rare. A retrospective study of 51 patients with DCS in France found that 65% were skin type IV or above, and only 1 was female [38]. One third of patients with DCS have coexisting acne conglobata or hidradenitis suppurativa, and are thought to be at an increased risk for developing HLA-B27 negative spondyloarthropathy [21].

2.2.5.3 Pathogenesis

The overlying pathogenesis of DCS is thought to be the result of a defect in follicular keratinization, which leads to occlusion of the pilosebaceous unit and accumulation of sebaceous and keratinous material. This leads to subsequent follicular expansion and inflammation. Dilated follicles can rupture, further propagating the inflammation with a neutrophilic and granulomatous response. Secondary infection can occur with the development of folliculitis. Ultimately, chronic inflammation results in nodules and abscesses which can form interconnecting sinus tracts and can also result in scarring and alopecia. These sinus tracts can serve as niduses for bacterial overgrowth and inflammation, resulting in a cyclical inflammatory and scarring process that can be difficult to control [21, 39].

The inciting factor for this process has yet to be fully elucidated. One theory that has been proposed is it is the result of loss of immune tolerance to alloantigens in the hair follicle, which leads to the inflammatory response seen [38].

Skin of Color

It is unclear why DCS is seen more frequently in Blacks. The role of hair type and hair styling practices has also been suggested to be implicated in the pathogenesis of DCS; however, strong evidence supporting this is sparse. As there have been cases of familial DCS in the literature, it suggests that there is a genetic risk factor, which may be predisposing Black patients to the disease disproportionately [40].

Gender

It is also unclear why males are affected more predominantly than females. Hormones have been suggested to play a role in its pathogenesis, and one retrospective review found that 3/21 (14%) of patients associated the onset of their disease with use of anabolic-androgenic steroids [41].

2.2.5.4 Clinical Features

Dissecting cellulitis typically begins as a follicular pustule on the occipital or vertex of the scalp. Patients may develop multiple pustules which can evolve into nodules and abscesses that form interconnecting sinus tracts. Over time, if untreated, the scalp takes on a cerebriform, boggy appearance with resulting overlying scarring alopecia. This can be further complicated by hypertrophic scarring and keloids. Patients' quality of life can be severely affected as the lesions can be both painful and disfiguring [4, 37, 39].

2.2.5.5 Histology

Similar to other inflammatory, scarring diseases, the histopathologic features of DCS demonstrate great variability based on the stage of the disease examined. In early lesions, dilatation of the infundibula is observed, with a surrounding perifollicular, mixed, neutrophilic and lymphoplasmacytic infiltrate, particularly affecting the lower portion of the infundibula. As the disease progresses, deep-seated abscesses in the adventitial dermis and subcutis form and follicular destruction results, with eventual fibrosis. Sinus tracts can be seen which are lined with squamous epithelium [42].

2.2.5.6 Treatment

Management of DSC remains challenging. Therapy is initially managed medically, with topical or intralesional steroids, antibacterial cleansers, topical or oral antibiotics, prednisone and isotretinoin as monotherapy or in combination with rifampin. Although relapse is common after discontinuation, there are some reports of isotretinoin causing a sustained remission for up to 2.5 years [43]. TNF-α inhibitors, which have been used to treat HS and acne conglobata, have been reported to show improvement in some patients with refractory DSC; however, not all patients show a response [44, 45].

Resistant DCS has been successfully treated with laser therapy, including an 800 nm pulsed diode laser and the 1064 nm long-pulse Nd:YAG laser [21].

Though medical options can be valuable in stabilizing the disease process, some feel they can never offer a sustainable response as they are unable to address the existing sinus tracts, which serve as a nidus for infection, drainage, and continued inflammation. For this reason, severe disease has been treated with complete scalp excision followed by split-thickness skin grafting, although side effects and recurrence have been reported to occur. More recently, Powers et al. reported benefit from a staged excision, which provides the benefits of more targeted focus of disease control and preservation of hair-bearing portions of the scalp, leading to better outcomes [37, 39].

2.3 Disorders of Pigmentation

2.3.1 Nevus of Ota

2.3.1.1 Introduction
Dermal melanocytoses comprise a group of melanocytic lesions which can be congenital or acquired. Nevus of Ota, acquired bilateral nevus of Ota-like macules (ABNOM, also known as Hori's nevus) and acquired unilateral nevus of Ota-like macules (also known as Sun's nevi) are three facial dermal melanocytoses which are far more commonly found in Asian females. Controversy exists as to whether or not these lesions belong on a spectrum or are clinically separate entities [46]. Histology and treatment of all lesions are similar.

2.3.1.2 Epidemiology
Nevus of Ota primarily affects Asian populations but can also be seen in Africans and Indians. It is rarely seen in Caucasian patients. Approximately 0.034% of the Asian population is affected by nevus of Ota, and it is five times more likely to be seen in women than men [47, 48]. They have been reported to be unilateral in 90% of cases and bilateral in 5–10% of cases [48]. Dermal melanocytoses can be congenital or acquired. Nevus of Ota is typically congenital; however, may appear during puberty. When small lesions are acquired, they are called Sun's nevus if unilateral, and Hori's nevus if bilateral. A population-based study in Taiwan described the overall incidence of ABNOM to be 0.8% [46].

2.3.1.3 Pathogenesis
Nevus of Ota is thought to be the result of migration arrest of melanocytes on their way from the neural crest to the epidermis [49]. It has been hypothesized that the acquired variant of these lesions may be related to reactivation of existing dermal melanocytes which were previously misplaced during embryological development [50]. One recent review of 102 patients found sun exposure (47.1%), pregnancy (32.0%), cosmetics (29.4%), sensitive skin (22.6%) and positive family histories (21.6%) to be highly related to the development of ABNOM [51]. Given the higher prevalence among Asians, a genetic component likely exists. It has also been suggested that hormones play a role in the pathogenesis as pregnancy has been associated with the development of ABNOM.

2.3.1.4 Clinical Features
Nevus of Ota presents as a bluish or gray-brown discoloration in areas innervated by the first two branches of the trigeminal nerve. Roughly two-thirds of patients will have characteristic involvement of the ipsilateral sclera.

ABNOM present as blue-brown and/or slate-gray macules occurring in a speckled pattern bilaterally on the malar regions, and can also involve the forehead, upper eyelids, cheeks and nose [46]. Although some consider these lesions to be on the same spectrum of Nevus of Ota, others distinguish them by their adult onset, speckled and bilateral pattern, and lack of mucosal involvement [52].

Patients with nevus of Ota are at increased risk for glaucoma, and therefore should be followed with routine eye exams [53]. Malignant transformation of dermal melanocytoses is rare. A recent review found a total of 14 cases of cutaneous melanoma arising in dermal melanocytoses, with 10 of those arising within nevi of Ota, and 4 arising within nevi of Ito. Interestingly, of the 10 reported cases of cutaneous melanoma arising in association with nevus of Ota, 8 of the patients were Caucasian, with the race/ethnicity of the two additional patients not being reported [54]. Although asymptomatic, as nevus of Ota can be cosmetically disfiguring, patients can suffer from severe emotional or psychological distress [47].

2.3.1.5 Histology
Lesions demonstrate irregularly shaped melanocytes dispersed throughout the dermis.

2.3.1.6 Treatment
As with other pigmentary disorders, photoprotection is a cornerstone of therapy. Cosmetic camouflage may also be utilized to help reduce the burden of disease. Laser therapy is the treatment of choice for nevus of Ota. Traditionally Q-switched (QS) lasers, including the 694 nm QS ruby, 755 nm QS alexandrite, and both the 532 and 1064 nm QS Nd:YAG lasers showed the most favorable clearance rates with the fewest side effects [47].

More recently, picosecond lasers have been shown to be safe and effective in the treatment of these lesions [55]. Although not all lesions respond to treatment, but for those that do respond, recurrence rate after treatment is rare (0.8–2.1%) [56]. When the appropriate patient and laser are selected, side effects are infrequent; however, risk of post-inflammatory hyperpigmentation should always be considered in the SOC population.

2.3.2 Melasma

2.3.2.1 Introduction
Melasma is a common disorder of hyperpigmentation with higher prevalence in females along with Fitzpatrick skin types III–IV and/or those of Hispanic descent. It is thought to be the result of a complex interplay of genetics, hormones, and exposure to ultraviolet and visible light.

2.3.2.2 Epidemiology
The prevalence of melasma varies widely based on the ethnic and geographic composition of the population. When populations of skin of color have been studied, the prevalence of melasma has ranged from 8.8% to 41% [57]. Most studies report the incidence of melasma being highest in skin types III–V. It predominantly affects women, with one population based study out of Brazil reporting it in 6% of men [58].

2.3.2.3 Pathogenesis
Pathophysiology remains unclear. Ultraviolet and visible light exposure, pregnancy, sex hormones, use of oral contraceptives, steroids, inflammation and photosensitizing drugs are known triggers that have been implicated in its pathogenesis. In addition, melanocytes associated with melasma lesions are more biologically active when compared to normal skin; this is evidenced by increased mitochondria, Golgi complex, and rough endoplasmic reticulum [59]. The growing knowledge on melasma pathogenesis suggests a complex cellular interplay involving melanocytes, keratinocytes, dermal fibroblasts, increased vascularity and increased mast cells.

Skin of Color
Although melasma is found in all ethnic groups, studies have shown a higher prevalence in more pigmented populations including Hispanic, Japanese, Korean, Chinese, Indian, Pakistani, Middle Eastern, and Mediterranean-African individuals [60, 61]. It may also be seen more in these populations because of a genetic influence, which has been theorized based on its tendency to run in families, with over 40% of patients reporting having relatives affected with the disease [57].

Gender
There is a clear association between hormones and the development of melasma as it is most commonly seen among women and with the use

of oral contraceptives and during pregnancy. Despite this strong association, the specific role hormones play in its pathogenesis is poorly understood. However, it is known that human melanocytes have estrogen and progesterone receptors, and the expression of estrogen receptors appears to be increased in skin affected by melasma [62, 63].

2.3.2.4 Clinical Features

Melasma presents as hyperpigmented macules coalescing into irregularly shaped patches most commonly found on the cheeks, upper lip, forehead, nose, cheek and chin. Extra-facial disease on sun-exposed areas can also occur. Under dermoscopy, when limited to the stratum corneum melasma presents as a well-defined brown to dark brown network. When it involves the lower epidermis, it appears as lighter shades of brown with a more irregular network. When there is also involvement of the dermis, it demonstrates a blue or bluish-gray color [57].

Melasma can cause a significant amount of psychological stress in patients and negatively affects their quality of life [64].

2.3.2.5 Histology

Melasma is characterized by hypertrophic melanocytes and an increased amount of melanin seen in all layers of the epidermis along with a possible increased number of melanophages. An increased number of melanocytes are not observed [59].

2.3.2.6 Treatment

There are a wide variety of treatment options for melasma, and while many patients respond favorably, it can be resistant to treatment in others. Treatment is aimed at reducing the amount of epidermal melanin and blocking solar radiation. Melasma that is seen more intensely under Wood's lamp examination typically responds better to topical treatments [57].

The mainstay of treatment for melasma is preventative therapy, including strict photoprotection with sunscreen and sun avoidance. This is especially valuable to reinforce in this patient population, that may not be accustomed to wear-

ing sunscreen [65]. In women who note the onset of melasma after beginning oral contraceptives, they should be stopped if possible [52]. Topical agents including hydroquinone, retinoids and azelaic acid have been reported with good success in the treatment of melasma. Combination creams have been shown to be more successful than monotherapy [66].

Chemical peels may be useful for patients with moderate to severe melasma that is resistant to topical therapy. Superficial peels, including glycolic acid and salicylic acid peels, have been shown to be effective with few adverse effects [67].

Laser and light based therapies, including intense pulsed light, QS Nd:YAG and pulse dye lasers, have been shown to be effective in severe or refractory disease. These therapies are limited by the fact that they demonstrate a high relapse rate and carry the risk of side effects including PIH, particularly in darker skin types [66]. Newer lasers, such as those using picosecond technology, show promising results and limited side effects.

Oral agents have been used for the treatment of melasma, with oral tranexamic acid showing the most promising results [68, 69]. Other agents with a good safety profile that may have efficacy include Polypodium leucotomos extract, carotenoid, melatonin and procyanidin. However, these agents are most commonly used as supplements to other treatments options and are rarely considered to be effective as monotherapy.

Conclusion

Differences in cultural practices, particularly hair styling practices, as well as physiologic differences, such as an increased amount of melanin, are implicated in many of the dermatologic conditions that are more commonly seen in skin of color. Similarly, differences in hair styling practices between men and women, as well as differences in hormone levels, may explain why there is a discrepancy in the incidence of some diseases in different genders. More research must be performed to further illustrate the pathogenesis behind these conditions, which will allow for more targeted and effective treatment options. Skin of color represents an incredibly heterogeneous group of individuals, and care must be taken to avoid making generalizations about patients, but rather each patient must be treated individually for optimal results.

References

1. Colby SL, Ortman JM. Projections of the size and composition of the US population: 2014 to 2060; 2015. P25-1143.
2. Taylor SC. Skin of color: Biology, structure, function, and implications for dermatologic disease. J Am Acad Dermatol. 2002;46(2). https://doi.org/10.1067/mjd.2002.120790.
3. Kaidbey KH, Agin PP, Sayre RM, Kligman a M. Photoprotection by melanin—a comparison of black and Caucasian skin. J Am Acad Dermatol. 1979;1(3):249–60. https://doi.org/10.1016/S0190-9622(79)70018-1.
4. Zaidi Z. Skin of colour: characteristics and disease. J Pak Med Assoc. 2017;67(2):292–9.
5. Montagna W, Carlisle K. The architecture of black and white facial skin. J Am Acad Dermatol. 1991;24(6):929–37. https://doi.org/10.1016/0190-9622(91)70148-U.
6. Lindelöf B, Forslind B, Hedblad MA, Kaveus U. Human hair form. Morphology revealed by light and scanning electron microscopy and computer aided three-dimensional reconstruction. Arch Dermatol. 1988;124(9):1359–63. https://doi.org/10.1001/archderm.1988.01670090015003.
7. Lewallen R, Francis S, Fisher B, et al. Hair care practices and structural evaluation of scalp and hair shaft parameters in African American and Caucasian women. J Cosmet Dermatol. 2015;14(3):216–23. https://doi.org/10.1111/jocd.12157.
8. Loussouarn G, Lozano I, Panhard S, Collaudin C, El Rawadi C, Genain G. Diversity in human hair growth, diameter, colour and shape. An in vivo study on young adults from 24 different ethnic groups observed in the five continents. Eur J Dermatol. 2016;26(2):144–54.
9. Olsen EA, Callender V, McMichael A, et al. Central hair loss in African American women: incidence and potential risk factors. J Am Acad Dermatol. 2011;64(2):245–52. https://doi.org/10.1016/j.jaad.2009.11.693.
10. Davis EC, Reid SD, Callender VD, Sperling LC. Differentiating central centrifugal cicatricial alopecia and androgenetic alopecia in African American men report of three cases. J Clin Aesthet Dermatol. 2012;5(6):37–40.
11. Kyei A. Medical and environmental risk factors for the development of central centrifugal cicatricial alopecia. Arch Dermatol. 2011;147(8):909. https://doi.org/10.1001/archdermatol.2011.66.
12. Dlova NC, Jordaan FH, Sarig O, Sprecher E. Autosomal dominant inheritance of central centrifugal cicatricial alopecia in black South Africans. J Am Acad Dermatol. 2014;70(4):679–82. https://doi.org/10.1016/j.jaad.2013.11.035.
13. Herskovitz I, Miteva M. Central centrifugal cicatricial alopecia: challenges and solutions. Clin Cosmet Investig Dermatol. 2016;9:175–81.
14. Miteva M, Tosti A. Dermatoscopic features of central centrifugal cicatricial alopecia. J Am Acad Dermatol. 2014;71(3):443–9. https://doi.org/10.1016/j.jaad.2014.04.069.
15. Callender VD, Lawson CN, Onwudiwe OC. Hair transplantation in the surgical treatment of central centrifugal cicatricial alopecia. Dermatol Surg. 2014;40(10):1125–31. https://doi.org/10.1097/dss.0000000000000127.
16. Samrao A, Price VH, Zedek D, Mirmirani P. The "fringe sign" - a useful clinical finding in traction alopecia of the marginal hair line. Dermatol Online J. 2011;17(11):1.
17. James J, Saladi RN, Fox JL. Traction alopecia in Sikh male patients. J Am Board Fam Med. 2007;20(5):497–8. https://doi.org/10.3122/jabfm.2007.05.070076.
18. Khumalo NP, Jessop S, Gumedze F, Ehrlich R. Hairdressing and the prevalence of scalp disease in African adults. Br J Dermatol. 2007;157(5):981–8. https://doi.org/10.1111/j.1365-2133.2007.08146.x.
19. Khumalo NP, Jessop S, Gumedze F, Ehrlich R. Determinants of marginal traction alopecia in African girls and women. J Am Acad Dermatol. 2008;59(3):432–8. https://doi.org/10.1016/j.jaad.2008.05.036.
20. Donovan JC, Mirmirani P. Transversely sectioned biopsies in the diagnosis of end-stage traction alopecia. Dermatol Online J. 2013;19(4):11.
21. Madu P, Kundu RV. Follicular and scarring disorders in skin of color: presentation and management. Am J Clin Dermatol. 2014;15(4):307–21. https://doi.org/10.1007/s40257-014-0072-x.
22. Callender VD, McMichael AJ, Cohen GF. Medical and surgical therapies for alopecias in black women. Dermatol Ther. 2004;17(2):164–76. https://doi.org/10.1111/j.1396-0296.2004.04017.x.
23. Kundu RV, Patterson S. Dermatologic conditions in skin of color: part II. Disorders occurring predominately in skin of color. Am Fam Physician. 2013;87(12):859–65. http://www.ncbi.nlm.nih.gov/pubmed/23939568
24. Knable ALJ, Hanke CW, Gonin R. Prevalence of acne keloidalis nuchae in football players. J Am Acad Dermatol. 1997;37(4):570–4. https://doi.org/10.1016/S0190-9622(97)70173-7.
25. Kelly AP. Pseudofolliculitis barbae and acne keloidalis nuchae. Dermatol Clin. 2003;21(4):645–53. https://doi.org/10.1016/S0733-8635(03)00079-2.
26. Maranda EL, Simmons BJ, Nguyen AH, Lim VM, Keri JE. Treatment of acne keloidalis nuchae: a systematic review of the literature. Dermatol Ther (Heidelb). 2016;6(3):363–78. https://doi.org/10.1007/s13555-016-0134-5.

27. Herzberg AJ, Dinehart SM, Kerns BJ, Pollack SV. Acne keloidalis. Transverse microscopy, immunohistochemistry, and electron microscopy. Am J Dermatopathol. 1990;12(2):109–21. http://www.ncbi.nlm.nih.gov/pubmed/2331046

28. Sperling LC, Homoky C, Pratt L, et al. Acne keloidalis is a form of primary scarring alopecia. Arch Dermatol. 2016;136(4):479–84. https://doi.org/10.1001/archderm.136.4.479.

29. Lee A, Cho S, Yam T, Harris K, Ardern-Jones M. Staphylococcus aureus and chronic folliculocentric pustuloses of the scalp - cause or association? Br J Dermatol. 2016;175(2):410–3.

30. Ogunbiyi A. Acne keloidalis nuchae: prevalence, impact, and management challenges. Clin Cosmet Investig Dermatol. 2016;14(9):483–9.

31. Salami T, Omeife H, Samuel S. Prevalence of acne keloidalis nuchae in Nigerians. Int J Dermatol. 2007;46(5):482–4. https://doi.org/10.1111/j.1365-4632.2007.03069.x.

32. Alexis A, Heath CR, Halder RM. Folliculitis keloidalis nuchae and pseudofolliculitis barbae: are prevention and effective treatment within reach? Dermatol Clin. 2014;32(2):183–91. https://doi.org/10.1016/j.det.2013.12.001.

33. Winter H, Schissel D, Parry DAD, et al. An unusual Ala12Thr polymorphism in the 1A alpha-helical segment of the companion layer-specific keratin K6hf: evidence for a risk factor in the etiology of the common hair disorder pseudofolliculitis barbae. J Invest Dermatol. 2004;122(3):652–7. https://doi.org/10.1111/j.0022-202X.2004.22309.x.

34. Nguyen TA, Patel PS, Viola KV, Friedman AJ. Pseudofolliculitis barbae in women: a clinical perspective. Br J Dermatol. 2015;173(1):279–80. https://doi.org/10.1111/bjd.13644.

35. Gray J, McMichael AJ. Pseudofolliculitis barbae: understanding the condition and the role of facial grooming. Int J Cosmet Sci. 2016;38:24–7. https://doi.org/10.1111/ics.12331.

36. Conte M, Lawrence J. Pseudofolliculitis barbae. No "pseudoproblem". JAMA. 1979;241(1):53–4.

37. Mundi J, Marmon S, Fischer M, Kamino H, Patel R, Shapiro J. Dissecting cellulitis of the scalp. Dermatol Online J. 2012;18(12):8.

38. Badaoui A, Reygagne P, Cavelier-Balloy B, et al. Dissecting cellulitis of the scalp: a retrospective study of 51 patients and review of literature. Br J Dermatol. 2016;174(2):421–3. https://doi.org/10.1111/bjd.13999.

39. Powers M, Mehta D, Ozog D. Cutting out the tracts: staged excisions for dissecting cellulitis of the scalp. Dermatol Surg. 2017;43:738.

40. Bjellerup M, Wallengren J. Familial perifolliculitis capitis abscedens et suffodiens in two brothers successfully treated with isotretinoin. J Am Acad Dermatol. 1990;23(4 Pt 1):742–3.

41. Segurado-Miravalles G, Camacho-Martínez FM, Arias-Santiago S, et al. Epidemiology, clinical presentation and therapeutic approach in a multicentre series of dissecting cellulitis of the scalp. J Eur Acad Dermatol Venereol. 2016;31:e199–200. https://doi.org/10.1111/jdv.13948.

42. Bernárdez C, Molina-Ruiz AM, Requena L. Histologic features of alopecias: part II: scarring alopecias. Actas Dermosifiliogr. 2015;106(4):260–70. https://doi.org/10.1016/j.ad.2014.07.006.

43. Scerri L, Williams H, Allen B. Dissecting cellulitis of the scalp: response to isotretinoin. Br J Dermatol. 1996;134(6):1105–8.

44. Mansouri Y, Martin-Clavijo A, Newsome P, Kaur MR. Dissecting cellulitis of the scalp treated with tumour necrosis factor-α inhibitors: experience with two agents. Br J Dermatol. 2016;174(4):916–8. https://doi.org/10.1111/bjd.14269.

45. Sand FL, Thomsen SF. Off-label use of TNF-alpha inhibitors in a dermatological university department: retrospective evaluation of 118 patients. Dermatol Ther. 2015;28(3):158–65. https://doi.org/10.1111/dth.12222.

46. Park JM, Tsao H, Tsao S. Acquired bilateral nevus of Ota-like macules (Hori nevus): etiologic and therapeutic considerations. J Am Acad Dermatol. 2009;61(1):88–93. https://doi.org/10.1016/j.jaad.2008.10.054.

47. Shah VV, Bray FN, Aldahan AS, Mlacker S, Nouri K. Lasers and nevus of Ota: a comprehensive review. Lasers Med Sci. 2016;31(1):179–85. https://doi.org/10.1007/s10103-015-1834-2.

48. Magarasevic L, Abazi Z. Unilateral open-angle glaucoma associated with the ipsilateral nevus of ota. Case Rep Ophthalmol Med. 2013;2013:924937. https://doi.org/10.1155/2013/924937.

49. Saha A, Bandyopadhyay D. Nevus of Ota. Indian Pediatr. 2014;51(6):510.

50. Hori Y, Kawashima M, Oohara K, Kukita A. Acquired, bilateral nevus of Ota-like macules. J Am Acad Dermatol. 1984;10(6):961–4.

51. Zhang Q, Tan C, Jiang P, Yang G. Clinical profile and triggering factors for acquired, bilateral nevus of Ota-like macules. Cutan Ocul Toxicol. 2017;36:327–30.

52. Vashi N, Kundu R. Facial hyperpigmentation: causes and treatment. Br J Dermatol. 2013;169(Suppl 3):41–56.

53. Teekhasaenee C, Ritch R, Rutnin U, Leelawongs N. Glaucoma in oculodermal melanocytosis. Ophthalmology. 1990;97(5):562–70.

54. Tse JY, Walls BE, Pomerantz H, et al. Melanoma arising in a nevus of Ito: novel genetic mutations and a review of the literature on cutaneous malignant transformation of dermal melanocytosis. J Cutan Pathol. 2016;43(1):57–63. https://doi.org/10.1111/cup.12568.

55. Levin MK, Ng E, Bae Y-SC, Brauer JA, Geronemus RG. Treatment of pigmentary disorders in patients with skin of color with a novel 755 nm picosecond, Q-switched ruby, and Q-switched Nd:YAG nanosecond lasers: a retrospective photographic review. Lasers Surg Med. 2016;48(2):181–7. https://doi.org/10.1002/lsm.22454.

56. Lee HS, Kim M, Kang HY. Recurrence of nevus of Ota after successful laser treatment: possible role of dermal stem cells. Ann Dermatol. 2016;28(5):647–9.

57. Handel AC, Miot LDB, Miot HA. Melasma: a clinical and epidemiological review. An Bras Dermatol. 2014;89(5):771–82.   https://doi.org/10.1590/abd1806-4841.20143063.

58. Ishiy P, Silva L, Penha M, Handel A, Miot H. Skin diseases reported by workers from the campus of UNESP Rubião Jr, Botucatu-SP (Brazil). An Bras Dermatol. 2014;89:529–31.

59. Kang W, Yoon K, Lee E, Kim J, Lee K, Yim H. Melasma: histopathological characteristics in 56 Korean patients. Br J Dermatol. 2002;146: 228–37.

60. Taylor SC. Epidemiology of skin diseases in ethnic populations. Dermatol Clin. 2003;21(4):601–7. https://doi.org/10.1016/S0733-8635(03)00075-5.

61. Sheth VM, Pandya AG. Melasma: a comprehensive update: part I. J Am Acad Dermatol. 2011;65(4):689–97. https://doi.org/10.1016/j.jaad.2010.12.046.

62. Lieberman R, Moy L. Estrogen receptor expression in melasma: results from facial skin of affected patients. J Drugs Dermatol. 2008;7:463.

63. Jang YH, Lee JY, Kang HY. Oestrogen and progesterone receptor expression in melasma: an immunohistochemical analysis. J Eur Acad Dermatol Venereol. 2010;24:1312.

64. Yalamanchili R, Shastry V, Betkerur J. Clinico-epidemiological study and quality of life assessment in melasma. Indian J Dermatol. 2015;60(5):519.

65. Maymone M, Neamah H, Wirya S, Patzelt N, Zancanaro P, Vashi N. Sun-protective behaviors in patients with cutaneous hyperpigmentation: a cross-sectional study. J Am Acad Dermatol. 2017;76:841.

66. Rivas S, Pandya AG. Treatment of melasma with topical agents, peels and lasers: an evidence-based review. Am J Clin Dermatol. 2013;14(5):359–76. https://doi.org/10.1007/s40257-013-0038-4.

67. Grimes P. The safety and efficacy of salicylic acid chemical peels in darker racial-ethnic groups. Dermatol Surg. 1999;25:18.

68. Zhou LL, Baibergenova A. Melasma: systematic review of the systemic treatments. Int J Dermatol. 2017;56(9):902–8. https://doi.org/10.1111/ijd.13578.

69. Lee HC, Thng TGS, Goh CL. Oral tranexamic acid (TA) in the treatment of melasma: a retrospective analysis. J Am Acad Dermatol. 2016;75(2):385–92. https://doi.org/10.1016/j.jaad.2016.03.001.

Aging of the Skin

Enzo Berardesca, Norma Cameli, and Maria Mariano

Skin aging is generally classified as intrinsic aging and photoaging based on the mechanism of action and the skin site [1]. Intrinsic aging is characterized by thinning of the epidermis and fine wrinkles caused by cellular aging [1, 2], while photoaging is characterized by deep wrinkles, skin laxity, telangiectasias, and appearance of lentigines, and is mainly caused by exposure to UV and other environmental factors [1, 3]. At the cellular level skin aging has been attributed to the loss of mature collagen and increased matrix metalloproteinase (MMP) expression [1–3]. MMP-1 is known as an initiator collagenase responsible for collagen fragmentation in skin aging process, and MMP-2 and -9 are known to be responsible for further degradation of collagen [1, 3]. Impaired TGF-β signaling caused reduction of collagen synthesis is another reason for collagen loss in aged skin [2, 4, 5].

More recently, other environmental factors have been recognized being involved in the aging process known as the 'exposome' concept; it is generally agreed that both external and internal factors as well as the response of the human body to these factors all add up to define the exposome. Specifically, these can be conducted to: (1) sun radiations: ultraviolet radiation, visible light and infrared radiation, (2) air pollution, (3) tobacco

smoke, (4) nutrition, (5) a number of less well studied, miscellaneous factors, as well as (6) cosmetic products [6]. Basically all these damage epidermal living cells and metabolism by increasing reactive oxygen species formation (ROS) inducing changes in cell metabolism and function.

From a clinical point of view an important change is the thinning of the epidermis. Starting at about age 30, the epidermis decreases in thickness at about 6.4% per decade [7]. Changes in epidermal thickness are most pronounced in exposed areas, such as the face, neck, upper part of the chest and the extensor surface of the hands and forearms [8] due to the accumulation of intrinsic aging and extrinsic aging. Flattening of the dermal–epidermal junction due to a retraction of the rete pegs is also a feature of aged skin [7]. The skin becomes less resistant to shearing forces and more vulnerable to insult [9]. Changes in microcirculation and blood supply can be responsible decreased basal cell proliferation and alterations in transcutaneous penetration [7, 10] With aging, epidermal turnover diminishes resulting in a smaller number of cell layers [11].

3.1 Changes in Stratum Corneum with Age

The water content of the SC decreases progressively with age and eventually falls below the level necessary for effective desquamation. This

E. Berardesca (✉) · N. Cameli · M. Mariano
San Gallicano Dermatological Institute, Rome, Italy
e-mail: berardesca@berardesca.it

© Springer International Publishing AG, part of Springer Nature 2018
E. Tur, H. I. Maibach (eds.), *Gender and Dermatology*,
https://doi.org/10.1007/978-3-319-72156-9_3

causes corneocytes to pile up and adhere to the skin surface, which accounts for the roughness, scaliness and flaking that accompanies xerosis in aged skin. The integrity of the SC barrier is dependent on an orderly arrangement of critical lipids [7]. The total lipid content of the aged skin decreases dramatically, and this alteration in the lipid barrier results in dryer skin [12]. Age-related changes in the amino acid composition reduce the amount of cutaneous NMF, thereby decreasing the skin's water-binding capacity [13].

There have been few attempts to measure the rate of corneocyte loss and desquamation in relation with the ageing process. This is odd because desquamation is a very important process. Corneocyte size and renewal (or turnover) depends not only by the rate of input into the system (epidermopoiesis) but also on the rate at which cells are lost (desquamation). The epidermis shows a linear decrease in thickness with age, both in absolute terms and in cell number. The reduction in epidermal population size suggests that there may be also a decrease in the rate on production of epidermal cells, and the apparent lengthening of the stratum corneum renewal time seems to confirm it. In addition, there is some evidence that the rate of reepithelization of wounds decreases with age. Using tritiated thymidine and an autoradiographic labelling method Kligman [14] reported a reduced value for an elderly cohort compared to a younger group; in a study comparing the effects of ageing between sun exposed and non exposed sites this has not been detected [15]. In a more sensitive but complicated assay using the FACS fluorescent assay it was demonstrated an age related decrease in the DNA synthesis and so in a longer cell cycle through the stratum corneum [16]. Stratum corneum cell turnover and replacement time have been evaluated using also the dansyl chloride staining technique. Dansyl chloride is a fluorescent dye which penetrates the full thickness of the stratum corneum and, when applied topically to the skin in vivo, becomes florescent under Wood's light [17]. The time the fluorescente takes to disappear corresponds to the turnover cycle of the stratum corneum; these studies have shown a progressive increase in the turnover

time of the stratum corneum associated with increasing age [18]. The lengthening of the turnover implies a reduction in the desquamation rate but this is not as large as thought. The reason for this is the increase of corneocyte size during ageing. Thus there are fewer corneocytes in an old individual's stratum corneum compared to a young one per volume unit. Studies measuring the release of corneocytes from the skin showed also that there is a decrease of corneocyte loss at least measured under these experimental conditions [19].

The evolution of corneocyte size during the ageing process has been studied by several authors; there is a consensus that the size progressively increases with age, even though there are body site variations and seasonal variations (changes due to hormonal status will be discussed later in this document). The more investigated sites are the arm and the forearm and data shows a progressive increase of corneocyte size from birth to age [20–23].

Some differences have been reported between sunexposed and non sunexposed areas [24] where in general UV irradiation increases epidermal turnover leading to smaller corneocytes compared to a similar photoprotected site. Indeed, seasonal variations in corneocyte size have been reported with smaller corneocytes in summer as a consequence of prolonged solar irradiation [25]. In a study on professional cyclists it was found that the size of corneocytes from the area of the arm protected by the shirt was "normal", while in the adjacent exposed area the area of the cells was significantly smaller [26].

In conclusion there is a correlation and an inverse relationship between stratum corneum turnover and dimensions of corneocytes.

3.2 Changes in the Dermis with Age

At the dermal level, all three major extracellular components of the dermis (collagen, elastin, and hyaluronic acid) are depleted in older skin. Collagen content decreases at about 2% per year [27], due to both a decrease in collagen synthesis

[28] and an increase in the degradation of collagen [29]. The relative proportions of collagen types are also disrupted in aged skin. The proportion of Type I collagen to Type III collagen in young skin is approximately 6:1, a ratio which drops significantly over the lifespan as Type I collagen is selectively lost [30], and Type III synthesis increases [31]. Collagen fibers become thicker and collagen bundles more disorganized than in younger skin [27]. Collagen cross-links stabilize resulting in a loss of elasticity.

Functional elastin declines in the dermis with age. Elastin becomes calcified, elastin fibers degrade and turnover declines [28]. The loss of structural integrity of the dermis leads to increased rigidity and diminished elasticity [32]. This damage is more pronounced in women than in men [33].

Other changes occur at the level of the dermal extracellular matrix (ECM). In the ECM of the dermis, extracellular HA is bound to itself or Proteoglycans (PG), playing space-filling and shock-absorbing roles [34]. Dermal hyaluronic acid (HA) is mainly synthesized by dermal fibroblasts, which show a tenfold higher production rate than epidermal keratinocytes, and shows the strongest staining in the papillary dermis [34, 35]. Crosslinking of HA with matrix proteins such as the collagen network results in the formation of linked structures and increases tissue stiffness [34]. Intensity of HA staining decreased in both the epidermis and dermis in older adults [36].

3.3 Influence of Sex Hormones

Menopause, and the effects of postmenopausal estrogen deficiency, can have profound effects on skin. Estrogens affect several skin functions including hair growth, pigmentation, vascularity, elasticity, and water-holding capacity (as reviewed by [37]). There is a strong correlation between skin collagen loss and estrogen deficiency due to menopause [33]. It has been demonstrated the postmenopausal women have decreased amounts of types I and III collagen, and a decreased type III/I ratio in comparison

with premenopausal women [37]. Women with a premature menopause have accelerated degenerative changes in dermal elastic fibers [33]. In addition, decreased estrogens after menopause also affect the water-holding capacity of the skin. Estrogens clearly have a key role in skin aging, and menopause may accelerate the decline in skin appearance and function.

The influences of sex hormones on morphologic and functional parameters of the epidermis ar of increasing interest. The effects of hormones and ageing on stratum corneum structure, function and composition are not yet known in detail. Although age-dependent factors have been studied, few data are available concerning changes in perimenopausal women [38] with a significantly decreased sebum content of the forehead in menopausal women and higher stratum corneum hydration of the forehead in late menopausal women. Influences of female hormones on the composition of stratum corneum sphingolipids have been described, as well as the negative impact of age on the biosynthesis of sphingolipids [39]. With age a decline occurs in hormone levels, especially in sex hormones like estrogen, testosterone, dehydroepiandrosterone and growth hormones [40, 41]. Hormone replacement therapy leads to an increase in collagen content [42]. Under basal conditions the physiologic functions of stratum corneum seems to remain unchanged with age. Under stressed conditions, however, aged skin is more susceptible to barrier disruption than younger skin, i.e. an aged epidermal permeability barrier shows decreased cohesion as well as delayed barrier repair with age under stress conditions [43, 44].

In a recent study [45] corneocyte size in pre and post-menopausal women of the same age group (40–50 years age range) was investigated and compared to men of the same decade using a videomicroscopic technique: despite the close age range, the significantly smaller corneocytes in premenopausal women vs. postmenopausal women or men are likely to be attributed to the different levels of female sex hormones. The detected differences support the hypothesis that sexual hormones have an impact on corneocyte surface area. Female sex hormone levels of premenopausal women are supposed to be higher than those of non-hormonal substituted post-menopausal women or men, and thus the smaller corneocyte surface area could be explained by the influence of female sex hormones. The barrier function and the stratum corneum hydration parameters are not involved in this mechanism as no correlation between these parameters and corneocyte surface area was detectable. In this study, no other major differences in barrier function or stratum corneum water holding properties have been detected (maybe for the close chronological age range of the groups investigated), even though there some reports in the literature on the positive impact of hormone replacement therapy on cutaneous mechanical properties and waterholding capacity [46, 47]. Further investigation is necessary to study the physiology of perimenopausal skin especially under stress conditions. The role of hormonal replacement has been documented in a study [48] where menopausal women who had been treated for at least 5 or 10 years, the biophysical measurements were significantly higher for the parameters evaluating hydration and sebum secretion, which generally decrease after the menopause, associated with higher values for the yellow intensity parameter and the skin relief parameters on the forehead. The skin relief parameters on the forehead were significantly higher in menopausal women since at least 5 years and taking HRT. This study is one of the few studies who have demonstrated an effect of exposure to HRT on skin colour assessed by colorimetry, and on skin relief with an increase of the roughness parameters on the forehead. An investigation assessed the effect of HRT on the skin, using high frequency diagnostic ultrasound combined with computerised image analysis. The study was a cross-sectional observational study carried out on 84 women (comprising 34 HRT users, 25 post-menopausal controls and 25 premenopausal controls). The time that volunteers had been taking HRT varied from 6 months to 6 years. The skin was shown to be thicker in the HRT group than in the post-menopausal control group [49]. An additional study evaluating the severity of facial wrinkling by an eight-point photographic scale in a sample of Korean women,

estimated the HRT exposition impact among 85 post-menopausal, comprising 15 taking HRT. HRT was found to be associated with a lower risk for facial wrinkling in the post-menopausal women group [50]. These results support the subjective impression and the clinical evaluation concerning the impact of HRT on the development and the severity of some properties associated with skin ageing after menopause [51].

References

1. Zeng JP, Bi B, Chen L, Yang P, Guo Y, Zhou YQ, et al. Repeated exposure of mouse dermal fibroblasts at a sub-cytotoxic dose of UVB leads to premature senescence: a robust model of cellular photoaging. J Dermatol Sci. 2014;73:49–56.
2. Purohit T, He T, Qin Z, Li T, Fisher GJ, Yan Y, et al. Smad3-dependent regulation of type I collagen in human dermal fibroblasts: impact on human skin connective tissue aging. J Dermatol Sci. 2016;83(1):80–3.
3. Xia W, Quan T, Hammerberg C, Voorhees JJ, Fisher GJ. A mouse model of skin aging: fragmentation of dermal collagen fibrils and reduced fibroblast spreading due to expression of human matrix metalloproteinase-1. J Dermatol Sci. 2015;78:79–82.
4. Walraven M, Beelen RH, Ulrich MM. Transforming growth factor-beta (TGF-beta) signaling in healthy human fetal skin: a descriptive study. J Dermatol Sci. 2015;78:117–24.
5. Lee DH, Oh J-H, Chung JH. Glycosaminoglycan and proteoglycan in skin aging. J Dermatol Sci. 2016;83(3):174–81.
6. Krutmann J, Bouloc A, Sore G, Bernard BA, Passeron T. The skin aging exposome. J Dermatol Sci. 2017;85(3):152–61.
7. Waller JM, Maibach HI. Age and skin structure and function, a quantitative approach (I): blood flow, pH, thickness, and ultrasound echogenicity. Skin Res Technol. 2005;11:221–35.
8. Boss GR, Seegmiller JE. Age-related physiological changes and their clinical significance. West J Med. 1981;135:434–40.
9. Grove GL. Physiologic changes in older skin. Clin Geriatr Med. 1989;5:115–25.
10. Sudel KM, Venzke K, Mielke H, Breitenbach U, Mundt C, Jaspers S, Koop U, Sauermann K, Knussman-Hartig E, Moll I, Gercken G, Young AR, Stab F, Wenck H, Gallinat S. Novel aspects of intrinsic and extrinsic aging of human skin: beneficial effects of soy extract. Photochem Photobiol. 2005;81:581–7.
11. Holt DR, Kirk SJ, Regan MC, Hurson M, Lindblad WJ, Barbul A. Effect of age on wound healing in healthy human beings. Surgery. 1992;112:293–7; discussion 297-8.

12. Seyfarth F, Schliemann S, Antonov D, Elsner P. Dry skin, barrier function, and irritant contact dermatitis in the elderly. Clin Dermatol. 2011;29:31–6.
13. Jackson SM, Williams ML, Feingold KR, Elias PM. Pathobiology of the stratum corneum. West J Med. 1993;158:279–85.
14. Kligman AM. Perspectives and problems in cutaneous gerontology. J Invest Dermatol. 1979;73:39–56.
15. Marks R, et al. The effects of phoageing and intrinsic ageing on epidermal structure and function. G Ital Chir Dermatol Oncol. 1987;2:252–63.
16. Marks R. The epidermal engine. A commentary on epidermopoiesis, desquamation and their interrelationships. Int J Cosmet Sci. 1986;8:135–44.
17. Jansen LH, Hojyo-Tomoko MT, Kligman AM. Improved fluorescence staining technique for estimating turnover of the human stratum corneum. Br J Dermatol. 1974;90:9–14.
18. Roberts D, Marks R. Determination of age variations in the rate of desquamation. A comparison of four techniques. J Invest Dermatol. 1979;74:13–6.
19. Marks R. Measurement of biological ageing in human epidermis. Br J Dermatol. 1981;104:627–33.
20. Plewig G. Regional differences in cell sizes in the human stratum corneum II. Effect of sex and age. J Invest Dermatol. 1970;54:19–23.
21. Marks R, Nicholls S, King CS. Studies on isolated cornocytes. Int J Cosmet Sci. 1981;3:251–8.
22. Grove GL, Lavker RM, Hoelzle E, Kligman AM. Use of noon intrusive tests to monitor age associated changes in human skin. J Soc Cosmet Chem. 1981;32:15–26.
23. Leveque JL, Corcuff P, DeRigal J, Agache P. In vivo studies on the evolution of physical properties of the human skin with age. Int J Dermatol. 1984;23:322–9.
24. Corcuff P, Leveque JL. Corneocyte changes after acute UV irradiation and chronic solar exposure. Photo-Dermatology. 1988;5:110–5.
25. Hermann S, Scheuber E, Plewig G. Exfoliative cytology: effects of seasons. In: Marks R, Plewing G, editors. Stratum corneum. Beriln: Springer; 1983. p. 181–5.
26. Leveque JL, Porte G, DeRgal J, Corcuff P, Francois AM, Saint-Leger D. Influence of chronic sun exposure on some biophysical parameters of the human skin; an in vivo study. J Cutan Aging Cosmet Dermatol. 1988;1:123–7.
27. Fenske NA, Lober CW. Structural and functional changes of normal aging skin. J Am Acad Dermatol. 1986;15:571–85.
28. Duncan KO, Leffell DJ. Preoperative assessment of the elderly patient. Dermatol Clin. 1997;15:583–93.
29. Ashcroft GS, Horan MA, Herrick SE, Tarnuzzer RW, Schultz GS, Ferguson MW. Age-related differences in the temporal and spatial regulation of matrix metalloproteinases (MMPs) in normal skin and acute cutaneous wounds of healthy humans. Cell Tissue Res. 1997;290:581–91.
30. Oikarinen A. The aging of skin: chronoaging versus photoaging. Photodermatol Photoimmunol Photomed. 1990;7:3–4.
31. Savvas M, Bishop J, Laurent G, Watson N, Studd J. Type III collagen content in the skin of postmenopausal women receiving oestradiol and testosterone implants. Br J Obstet Gynaecol. 1993;100:154–6.
32. Brincat MP, Baron YM, Galea R. Estrogens and the skin. Climacteric. 2005;8:110–23.
33. Calleja-Agius J, Muscat-Baron Y, Brincat MP. Skin ageing. Menopause Int. 2007;13:60–4.
34. Anderegg U, Simon JC, Averbeck M. More than just a filler - the role of hyaluronan for skin homeostasis. Exp Dermatol. 2014;23:295–303.
35. Oh JH, Kim YK, Jung JY, Shin JE, Chung JH. Changes in glycosaminoglycans and related proteoglycans in intrinsically aged human skin in vivo. Exp Dermatol. 2011;20:454–6.
36. Meyer LJ, Stern R. Age-dependent changes of hyaluronan in human skin. J Invest Dermatol. 1994;102:385–9.
37. Verdier-Sevrain S, Bonte F, Gilchrest B. Biology of estrogens in skin: implications for skin aging. Exp Dermatol. 2006;15:83–94.
38. Ohta H, Makita K, Kawashima T, Kinoshita S, Takenouchi M, Nozawa S. Relationship between dermato-physiological changes and hormonal status in pre-, peri-, and postmenopausal women. Maturitas. 1998;30:55–62.
39. Denda M, Koyama J, Hori J, Horii I, Takahashi M, Hara M, Tagami H. Age- and sex-dependent change in stratum corneum sphingolipids. Arch Dermatol Res. 1993;285:415–7.
40. Tazuke S, Khaw KT, Barrett-Connor E. Exogenous estrogen and endogenous sex hormones. Medicine (Baltimore). 1992;71:44–51.
41. Roshan S, Nader S, Orlander P. Review: ageing and hormones. Eur J Clin Investig. 1999;29:210–3.
42. Sauerbronn AVD, Fonseca AM, Bagnoli VR, Saldiva PH, Pinotti JA. The effects of systemic hormonal replacement therapy on the skin of postmenopausal women. Int J Gynaecol Obstet. 2000;68:35–41.
43. Ghadially R, Brown BE, Sequeira-Martin SM, Feingold KR, Elias PM. The aged epidermal permeability barrier. Structural, functional, and lipid biochemical abnormalities in humans and a senescent murine model. J Clin Invest. 1995;95:2281–90.
44. Reed JT, Ghadially R, Elias PM. Skin type, but neither race nor gender influence epidermal permeability barrier function. Arch Dermatol. 1995;131:1134–8.
45. Fluhr JW, Pelosi A, Lazzerini S, Dikstein S, Berardesca E. Differences in corneocyte surface area in pre- and post-menopausal women: assessment with the noninvasive videomicroscopic imaging of corneocytes method (VIC) under basal conditions. Skin Pharmacol Appl Ski Physiol. 2001;14(Suppl 1):10–6.
46. Pierard-Franchimont C, Letawe C, Goffin V, Pierard GE. Skin waterholding capacity and transdermal estrogen therapy for menopause: a pilot study. Maturitas. 1995;22:151–4.
47. Pierard GE, Letawe C, Dowlati A, Pierard-Franchimont C. Effect of hormone replacement therapy for menopause on the mechanical properties of skin. J Am Geriatr Soc. 1995;43:662–5.

48. Guinot C, et al. Effect of hormonal replacement therapy on skin biophysical properties of menopausal women. Skin Res Technol. 2005;11:201–4.

49. Chen L, Dyson M, Rymer J, et al. The use of high frequency diagnostic ultrasound to investigate the effect of hormone replacement therapy on skin thickness. Skin Res Technol. 2001;7:95–7.

50. Youn CS, Kwon OS, Won CH, et al. Effect of pregnancy and menopause on facial wrinkling in women. Acta Derm Venereol. 2003;83:419–24.

51. Farage MA, Miller KW, Elsner P, Maibach HI. Intrinsic and extrinsic factors in skin ageing: a review. Int J Cosmet Sci. 2008;30:87–95.

Hair and Scalp Variation Related to Gender

4

Ferial Fanian and Alexandre Guichard

4.1 Introduction

By evoking hair variations related to gender, the first elements which come to mind are hair length, hair beauty, hair style or androgenic alopecia. However, sex steroids have a much more tremendous impact on skin and hair by modulating epidermal and dermal thickness as well as immune system function, skin surface pH, quality of wound healing, sebaceous gland excretions, hair growth and response to treatment, among so many others [1].

In dermatology there has been increasing interest in studying gender differences in skin and hair to learn more about the physiology, the environment, diseases pathogenesis and to discover more effective and adapted treatments.

4.2 Normal/Physiologic Conditions: Is There Any Difference Between Both Sexes?

The hair follicle represents an attractive experimental system because of its accessibility, dispensability, and self-renewal capacity [2]. Hair

performs no vital function but its psychological functions are inestimable. Hair follicles populate the entire cutaneous surface, with the exception of palms, soles, glans penis and mucocutaneous junctions. They are formed before birth and no new follicles develop after birth. Hair is morphologically and biologically different in different parts of the body, and varies in structure, rate of growth and response to stimuli. Eyebrows and eyelashes do not respond to sex hormones, whereas pubic, axillary and facial hair, do [3].

4.2.1 Hair Structure and Compositions

There is no important structural differences between female and male hair, however we can find some little gender differences:

4.2.1.1 Estrogen Receptors (ERs)

Very little gender difference has been found in the expression of the 2 ERs (ie, ERα, and Erβ in non-balding scalp skin [4], but it is not known whether there is a gender difference in ERs in balding skin [1]. In the hair follicle, no specific nuclear staining has been observed for ERα [4, 5] while ERb is widely expressed in the hair follicle. Strong nuclear staining was detected in dermal papilla cells, inner sheath cells, matrix cells, and outer sheath cells including the buldge region Erβ has widespread localization in the hair follicle, espe-

F. Fanian (✉)
Laboratoires FILORGA/FILL-MED, Paris, France
e-mail: ferial.fanian@chu-besancon.fr

A. Guichard
Expert in Trichology, Independent Consultant, Lyon, France

© Springer International Publishing AG, part of Springer Nature 2018
E. Tur, H. I. Maibach (eds.), *Gender and Dermatology*,
https://doi.org/10.1007/978-3-319-72156-9_4

cially in the dermal papilla cells, inner sheath cells, matrix cells and the specialized bulge region of the outer root sheath, and appears to be the main receptor for estrogen's effect on hair growth [1, 5].

In the study of Wehner and Schweikert published in 2013 [6], substantial rates of estrogen formation [sum of Estron (E1) and estradiol (E2)] from estron sulfate (E1S) were found in anagen hair samples of men and women from all investigated sites (anagen and telogen hair roots were obtained from various sites of the scalp (frontal, occipital, and temporal) and the body (axilla and pubes), and in men, anagen hair roots were also obtained from the beard). In general, E1 and E2 accounted for around 97% and 3% of the formed estrogens, respectively. Estrogen formation in anagen hair roots from the scalp was significantly lower in men than in women <50 years of age. In contrast, comparable levels of estrogen formation were observed in male and female body hair and male beard hair. The estrogen production in hair roots from all these sites was higher than in those from the scalp of men aged <50 years. Scalp hair of women aged >50 years showed a significantly lower estrogen production than hair from women aged <50 years. Contrary to this, estrogen formation in scalp hair roots was significantly higher in men than in women aged >50 years. The results concerning the age dependency of E2 formation reflects a gender difference of STS activity. The conversion rates of E1–E2 in hair from men aged <50 years were 2.7% ± 0.21% and in hair from those aged >50 years 2.9% ± 0.23% (mean ± SEM, P < 0.2, nonsignificant). The conversion rates in the corresponding group of women aged <50 years were 2.2% ± 0.3% and in those aged >50 years, 3.2% ± 0.3% (P < 0.01; significant) [6].

4.2.1.2 Androgen Receptors (ARs)

In the hair follicle, no AR immunoreactivity could be detected in the epithelial cells of the outer root sheath including the bulge region and the inner root sheath. On the other hand, the majority of dermal papillar cells expressed AR so the AR expression is restricted to dermal papillar cells [5].

4.2.1.3 Progestron Receptors (PRs)

Graham and Clarke reported the expression of PR in a large variety of tissues and cells, but there was no mention that skin could express PR [7]. While Schmidt et al. detected PR in pubic hair in pre- and postmenopausal women by radio-receptor assay [8]. They observed nuclear and cytoplasmic staining for PR within the dermal papilla of hair follicles in 30% of cases of androgenic alopecia [5].

4.2.1.4 Trace Metal Composition

Many researchers have demonstrated the usefulness of human scalp hair as an indicator of the distribution and exposure of trace metal metabolism in human body [9]. It is recognized that metal distribution in human hair has marked dependence on age and gender [10].

In the study of Khalique et al., 88 human scalp hair samples, both from male and female donors, with ages from 3 to 100 years, were collected in rural area of district Chakwal, Pakistan [12]. Levels of 10 metals (Ca, Mg, Fe, Zn, Cu, Mn, Cd, Co, Cr and Ni) were determined by ICP-AES (Inductively Coupled Plasma Atomic Emission Spectrophotometry) in the scalp hair of male and female donors. In total, 58 male and 30 female hair samples were analyzed in triplicate. The results revealed that calcium showed the highest concentration of 462 µg/g in the hair of males and 870 µg/g in those of females followed by Zn, at 208 and 251 µg/g for the two sexes. For male donors, Cd showed the lowest concentration (1.15 µg/g) while for female donors Co remained at minimum level (0.92 µg/g). The order of decreasing metal concentration in the hair of male donors was: Ca > Zn > Mg > Fe > Cu > Mn > Ni > Cr > Co > Cd while that for female donors it was: Ca > Zn > Mg > Fe > Cu > Mn > Cr > Ni > Cd > Co. The female group exhibited enhanced levels of all selected metals except Fe and Co in their hair as compared with the male counterparts. A strong bivariate positive correlation was found between Fe and Zn (r = 0.841) for the hair samples from male category while for the female category, strong positive correlations were observed between Ca–Mg (r = 0.617), Ca–Zn (r = 0.569), Ca–Mn (r = 0.565), Mg–Mn (r = 0.655), Cr–Cu (r = 0.655) and Cr–Ni (r = 0.685). The distribution of metals in the hair of donors with respect to different age groups was also investigated for both genders. The study showed that in case of males, the concentration of all selected metals decreased with increasing age except for Cu, Co and Cr. However, for females the hair metal levels increased with age, except for Co for which the concentration decreased with age. No appreciable change in the metal concentration was observed as a function of age for the combined sexes. The observed variations of metal concentrations in two sexes with different age groups reflect the impact of multivariable role of metals regulating and controlling the metabolism in human body. Data from the present study are in agreement with those reported earlier from other parts of the world [11]. Any differences observed in the levels of selected metals in the present study were indicative of the individual variability, sex specificity, age dependence, individual metabolic activity, occupational exposure, geological location and food habits of the donors [12].

Tamburo et al., examined a total of 943 hair samples from adolescents of 11 to 14 years old, which were analyzed for their content of Al, As, Ba, Cd, Co, Cr, Cu, Li, Mn, Mo, Ni, Pb, Rb, Sb, Se, Sr, U, V and Zn [13]. Donors were 537 females and 406 males, all of them responding to the following exclusion criteria: non-Caucasian ethnicity; living in the selected area for b5 years; presence of diseases; habitual use of cigarettes; recent surgery or orthodontic treatment; colored hair or recent use of hairstyling products. The results shows that, in spite of the wide overlapping of the distributions, differences exist for most chemical elements. It is worth noting that the coverage intervals of Cd, Co, Cu, Mn, Ni, Sr, V and Zn are much wider for females than males, as well as those of Li and U computed formales extend far beyond those for females (p < 0.01) [13]:

- Sr: Hair of female donors contained, on the base of median value, 3.8 times more Sr (6.6 µg/g) than males (1.7 µg/g) [13–16] (2.5 times more [17]).
- Zn: Females hair contained higher level of hair Zn than in males [13, 14].

- Ni: Hair of female donors contained, on the base of the median value, 2.5 times more Ni (0.32 µg/g) than males (0.13 µg/g) [13, 16].
- Hair of females contained 3 times more Ba than men [17]
- Hair of females contained 2 times more Cu and Si than men [17]
- Hair of females contained 88% more La tahn men [17]
- Hair of females contained 86% more Ca and Mg than males [17]

Gender difference acts as confounding factor and therefore it should be better explored in hair biomonitoring methods [13].

Zaichick and Zaichick revealed that higher Au, Ca, Mg, and Sr mass fractions as well as lower Cl, Fe, I, Sc, Se, and Sm content were typical of female scalp hair as compared to those in male hair [18].

4.2.2 Hair Growth

4.2.2.1 Children
During the 1960s, Barman et al. reported that the average monthly growth rate in children is 10 mm (range 8–10.4 mm), with a 5–10% slower growth rate in females, compared to males [19].

4.2.2.2 Adults
In 2016, Van Nestand Rushton evaluated total of 59,765 anagen hairs in Caucasian controls (24,609) and patients with pattern hair loss (35,156) employing the validated, non-invasive, contrast-enhanced-phototrichogram with exogen collection and computer assisted image analysis (CE-PTG-EC) [20]. The results revealed that the mean growth rate of the thinner fibres was lower than thicker fibres (P < 0.0001). However, for the thicker hair (≥60 µm), there was a slightly faster mean growth rate in females as compared to males [20].

4.2.2.3 Vellus Hair
For the vellus hairs, Blume et al. demonstarted in 1991 that vellus hair growth is not affected by age or sex. The growth of vellus hair and the

secretion of sebum from vellus hair follicles were measured on the forehead, cheek, chest, shoulder and back of healthy men and women aged 15–30 years. Hair growth was assessed by computerized image-analysis of photographs and sebum excretion by the use of Sebutape followed by image analysis [21].

4.2.2.4 African Hairs

Loussouarn et al. evaluated 38 young adults (19 women, 19 men, mean ± SD age 27 ± 10 years). Phototrichograms were performed in order to record three parameters of hair growth: hair density, telogen percentage and rate of growth. For each volunteer, three regions of the scalp, namely vertex, temporal and occipital areas, were assessed. Hair density varied from 90 to 290 hairs per cm^2, with higher counts on the vertex and without any significant difference between men and women. Telogen percentage showed wide variations, from 2 to 46%, with higher levels on the temporal area and in men. The rate of growth fluctuated from 150 to 363 μm per day with no difference related either to gender or to scalp region.

4.2.2.5 Conclusion

The published studies supports that there is not any difference in hair growth rate between genders. However there are some evidences to reveal a slight slower hair growth rate in female children.

4.2.3 Hair Graying

4.2.3.1 Gender Difference According the Zone

Gray hair is a conspicuous sign of ageing. It is known to usually occur in the fourth decade regardless of gender, but the age at onset varies from one person to the next [22]. Jo et al. studied 1002 korean subjects in 2011 (522 men and 480 women) between 12 and 91 years old. Evaluation was based on a subjective questionnaire and a photographic scale showing increasing reference degrees of graying (grade 1 to 5) for the extent of grayness. An analysis of questionnaire responses

revealed that the temporal area was significantly more involved in men than in women whereas the frontal and parietal areas were affected more in women. Interestingly, according to the investigator's examination results, the temporal and occipital involvements were significantly more common in men than in women [23].

4.2.3.2 Graying Rate

In the same study, multivariate logistic linear regression analysis showed that age and smoking behavior were significantly correlated with hair graying. In contrast, gender, drinking history, hair loss, a history of a skin disease of the scalp, and a concurrent medical disease were not significantly correlated with graying [23].

4.2.4 Hair and Endogenous Hormones

4.2.4.1 Prolactin

The role of prolactin in hair growth regulation has been intensely studied in mammals with seasonally dependent cycles of pelage replacements. Prolactin has been shown to stimulate hair growth, moulting, and shedding in sheep and mink, and contradictory data report of induction of both anagen (hair growth) and catagen (hair follicle regression) in seasonal dependent hair follicles by prolactin [24]. Interestingly, administration of bromocriptine, a dopaminergic inhibitor of pituitary prolactin secretion, induces telogen effluvium in women, but not in men [25]. This is likely to be due to premature catagen induction. This raises the possibility that, in women, PRL may actually be a hair-growth-promoting/anagen-maintaining factor [26].

Lu et al. in 2007 demonstrated that the predominantly hair-growth-inhibitory effect seen in (female) mice is recapitulated in the serum-free organ culture of human air follicles [27], which has been previously confirmed by Philpott et al. in 1990 [28]: high-dose prolactin (400 ng mL^{-1}, a level that can be found in patients with macroprolactinoma) stimulated premature catagen development and inhibited hair shaft production and hair matrix keratinocyte proliferation in microdissected hair follicless from male occipital scalp skin [24].

Surprisingly, Langan et al. in 2010 found that, in a repeat hair follicle organ culture experiment, using a small number of hair follicles derived from female frontotemporal scalp skin, the same dose of prolactien (400 ng mL^{-1}) resulted in significant hair follicle shaft elongation. They repeated these experiments with a larger number of female hair follicles, derived from frontotemporal scalp skin specimens from additional donors, used a well-characterized specific prolactin receptor antagonist [29], by assissing prolactin receptor expression immunohistologically, and using microarray technology to examine the modulation of intrafollicularly expressed genes. In these repeat analyses, they found again that prolactin treatment (400 ng mL^{-1}) of female frontotemporal scalp hair follicles significantly promoted hair shaft elongation in serum-free hai follicle organ culture. This effect was reduced in the presence of a pure prolactin receptor antagonist (del1-9-G129R-hPRL, 4 μg mL^{-1}) introduced by Bernichtein et al. in 2003 [30]. In contrast to the prominent catagen-inducing effects seen in male occipital scalp hair follicles [24], prolactin did not have such an effect in female frontotemporal hair follicles. Moreover, treatment with prolactin receptor antagonist alone significantly inhibited both hair follicle and hair shaft production and spontaneous catagen development. According to this catagen-promoting effect of the used prolactin receptor antagonist, Langan et al. suggested that endogenous, intrafollicular prolactin production actually maintains human female frontotemporal scalp hair follicles in anagen VI. These data were independently confirmed by calculation of the hair cycle score and by the microarray-based demonstration that prolactin downregulated the steady-state transcript levels for a number of catagen-associated genes [26].

On this basis, we could consider that intracutaneous prolactin effects are highly gender and/or site dependent. Conversely, this may be related to gender- and/or location-dependent differences in the distribution of prolactin receptors. This differential response may depend on the post-receptor signal transduction pathways that are predominantly used by the same cell populations in different genders/skin locations, and/or on gender- and/or site-specific differences in the key target genes, whose expression is up- or down-regulated after prolactin receptor stimulation. This can account for diametrically opposed functional effects of prolactin and prolactin receptor antagonists on identical peripheral target organs, such as the skin and its appendages [26]. Thus, Langan et al. proposed that the distinct hair-growth-modulatory effects of prolactin in female frontotemporal versus male occipital scalp hair follicles [24] are the manifestation of gender- and/or location-dependent differential responses to prolactin.

4.2.4.2 Cortisone

In a prospective cohort carried out in Rotterdam, hair samples were collected from 2484 children of 6 years old in order to measure the hair cortisol and cortisone concentration to identify the potential association of child and family characteristics with cortisol and cortisone concentration. The results revealed that boys have a higher hair cortisol concentration ($p < 0.05$) [31].

In another study on 283 elderly participants (65–85 years), Manenschijn et al. confirmed that the hair cortisol levels are significantly higher in men than in women (median, 26.3 pg/mg hair [interquartile range (IQR), 20.6–35.5 pg/mg hair] vs 21.0 pg/mg hair [IQR, 16.0–27.0 pg/mg hair]; p value <0.001). High hair cortisol levels were associated with an increased cardiovascular risk (odds ratio, 2.7; $p = 0.01$) and an increased risk of type 2 diabetes mellitus (odds ratio, 3.2; $p = 0.04$). There were no associations between hair cortisol levels and noncardiovascular diseases [32].

4.2.5   Hair Modification Occurring in Transgender People

Given the complexities of the transitioning process, transgender individuals may face unique dermatologic needs. In addition to hormonal supplementation, many individuals undergo one or more gender-affirming surgical procedure.

As essential phase to initiate the transition process is hormone supplementation, which has notable effects on skin and hair. Women most commonly take estrogens and specifically estradiol, often associated with an antiandrogen such as spironolactone or a 5-alpha reductase inhibitor [33]. Estrogens rapidly and persistently reduce hair and skin sebum production [34]. Estrogens also lead to a reduction in quantity and density of body hair, which is often a desired effect. Moreover, it has been reported that in transgender woman with androgenetic alopecia, a regrow of scalp hair after ~6 months on oral estradiol and spironolactone therapy achieving testosterone levels within normal female range [35]. On the contrary, men, who take testosterone, experience opposite effects such as significant increase in sebum production, an increase in body hair but also are more likely to present male-pattern androgenic alopecia [34, 36].

In addition to hormonal supplementation, the transitioning process is associated with surgeries. After the forehead, the hairline pattern represent the second most important feature of gender identification within the upper third of the face. Therefore, autologous hair transplant to redefine hairline is an important esthetic surgery to consider in the field of facial feminization surgery which can be performed simultaneously with forehead reconstruction in a single operation [37]. With respect to persistent facial hair, especially in women, laser hair removal remains the gold standard.

4.2.6   Hair Based Gender Identification

Hair can yield DNA evidence, which can be of interest in forensic medicine. Hair, pulled out by the root, as in some violent struggles, contain root pulp which is a good source of nuclear DNA. Fluorescence In Situ Hybridization (FISH) technique using nonradioactive fluorescently labeled chromosome specific DNA probes, can rapidly identify the presence of a chromosome(s), chromosome region(s), or gene(s) in cells. The technique is accurate, rapid, sensitive, easily per-

formed, and readily available. By using FISH, Prahlow et al. easily identified the presence of the number of copies of the X and Y chromosome signals in hair bulb and determined exactly genders of several samples [38]. Interestingly, it has been demonstrated that sex identification is possible up to 8 months when samples are stored in a dried condition [39].

4.2.7   Ethnicity and Hair Specificity

Certain scalp disorders are preferentially associated with ethnicity especially in Africans, which can be explained by hair phenotypes, traditional hairstyles and current trend.

Compare to male, female with afro-textured hair are more likely to develop central centrifugal cicatricial alopecia, traction alopecia, hot-comb alopecia in which the fragility of the hair shaft is increased, likewise with chemical relaxers which can also induce local contact irritation and local chemical burns [40, 41]. Heat sources commonly used such as blow-dryers and hood dryers can become extremely hot and cause fragility of hair and damage to the tensile strength of the hair shaft.

On the other hand, due to frequent haircuts, male are more likely to develop acne (folliculitis) keloidalis nuchae in male [41, 42].

With respect to body hair, female living in Mediterranean basin are more likely to present hypertrichosis and hirsutism [43].

4.3   Hair, Gender and Environment

4.3.1   Heavy Metals and Pollution

Hair is a stable substance that, depending on its length, is capable of retaining years of information. Therefore, plethora of articles reported hair as a biomarker to determine occupational or industrial exposures to trace elements, pollutant or drugs intake.

Human hair is stable, easily accessible for sampling (non-invasive) and analysis [44].

Thanks to its rapid (approximately 0.35 mm per day), and continual growth [45], hair analysis enables the monitoring of long-term exposure and its dating. Metal cations bind to sulphur molecules within keratin present in the hair matrix [46], and this characteristic makes hair a useful sample for environmental health surveys.

A study performed in Brazil showed that women had significantly lower total mercury in hair than men [10]. Based on previous studies, authors suggested that the decrease in hair mercury concentrations in female hair might be due to pregnancy and lactation [47, 48]. Gender differences in hair mercury varies greatly among reports.

A study performed in Russia aimed to determine the contents or an upper limit of contents of 37 chemical elements in human scalp hair samples of healthy adults [18]. It was shown that higher Au, Ca, Mg, and Sr mass fractions as well as lower Cl, Fe, I, Sc, Se, and Sm content were typical of female scalp hair as compared to those in male hair. Results were consistent with the literature specifically regarding Au, Ca, Cl, I, Mg, and Sr. The higher content of Au might be explained by its extensive use in jewelry. Elevated levels of Ca and Mg and low Fe in the scalp hair of women compared with men can be attributed to the physiological characteristics of the female body related to reproduction. A high content of Sr in the hair of women is likely due to differences in the ratio of nutrition foods of animal and plant origin. Usually, women consume more plant foods, which is the main supplier of Sr in the human body.

In Pakistan, 8 on 10 metals are higher in female. Authors reported twofold more Ca, Cu and Mg in female than in male hair. Authors assumed that this could be explained on the basis of differences in metabolism and physiological role of the metals for two genders [12].

Trace elements such as Ag, Sr, Mg, M, Mo, Sn, K and Pb become available for endogenous binding in hair mainly through sweat glands in hair follicles [49, 50]. Time profile of element contents in hair of a given person showed that the level changed significantly (even several fold) with changes of living habits or environmental

exposure [50]. Moreover, Chojnacka et al. demonstrated that the effect of living habits on the level of a given element was found to be stronger than the influence of either gender or family relationship. This inter- and intra-individual variation of the elements contents in hair, which is unique, is a part of a more global concept called exposome which encompasses the totality of human environmental (i.e. non-genetic) exposures from conception onwards, complementing the genome. Based on these findings, Huang et al. tried another approach by analyzing the relative concentrations of the elements in the hair rather a quantification. By coupling specific analytical method (ETV-ICP-OES) with statistical method (linear discriminant analysis), authors were able to infer gender in 15 samples by analyzing the relative proportions of magnesium, sulfur, strontium and zinc in hair [51].

Lead (Pb) was studied in different articles as it is a ubiquitous persistent environmental contaminant (e.g. metal products, pigments, chemical, batteries), a measureable and a neurotoxin that can affect brain development. Interestingly, Pb amount contented on hair varies according to gender. In Spanish adolescents, Peña-Fernández et al. reported a significant difference in Pb levels in male and female hair (0.53 vs. 0.77 μg/g) (p < 0.001) [52]. This result is consistent with findings reported by Sanna et al. [53] and Evrenoglou et al. [54]. Although the exact cause of this gender dependence level of Pb in hair is not known several assumptions were proposed such as an effect of the hormonal system in the mineral excretion through hair [55] or dietary habits especially fish and seafood [56]. Although, it seems that females tend to accumulate Pb in the hair more than males; a review of the literature revealed contradictory studies [53].

Despite sensitive methods and well-designed studies, this review of the literature reveals that hair elements contents varies greatly among reports. However, despite this difference of proportion or quantification, all studies reported a significant difference between male and female. Therefore it seems not relevant to consider the absolute quantification of elements content in hair but simply be aware that the gender impacts significantly the proportion of elements in hair. Any differences observed in the levels of selected metals between studies could be explained by the difference of environmental exposure, food and hair care habits, socio-economical, geographical (even within the same country) and health status.

Thus, when analyzing indicators of pollution or intoxication, gender, age and the latter factors may have a significant impact on the result. Moreover, another the limitation in the analysis of elements content in hair is to determine whether the element comes from consumption or from exposure from the environment.

4.3.2 Alcohol

Alcohol abuse is an underlying cause for a number of public health issues such as liver disease, heart disease, cerebro-vascular disease, cancer, unintentional injury, and Fetal Alcohol Spectrum Disorders [57]. Traditionally, alcohol abuse screening has been performed using a number of self-administered questionnaires and alcohol biomarkers (indirect which detect the effects of excessive alcohol consumption or direct such as alcohol metabolites). Among them, the quantification of ethyl glucuronide (ETG) in hair represents a relevant indicator of excessive, as well as chronic, alcohol abuse extensively reported in the literature over the past 10 years. ETG is a minor alcohol metabolite that accumulates in hair and is proposed as a stable marker for the detection of chronic and excessive alcohol consumption above a cut-off level of 30 pg/mg hair [58]. However, Jones et al. in a study which aimed to compare fingernails and hair ETG content, interestingly reported that concentrations of ETG in female hair were notably less than the ETG found in male hair [59]. The mean ETG concentration in the hair of the male participants was 17.4 ± 32.6 pg/mg and 4.85 ± 10.4 pg/mg in the hair of female participants. Moreover, the correlation of matched fingernail and hair ETG concentration for males was much higher (r = 0.782, P < 0.01) than the correlation for female matched pairs (r = 0.249, P < 0.01), suggesting a gender

bias. According to the authors this discrepancy might be explained by an exposure to hydrogen peroxide and ammonium hydroxide, which are common constituents of cosmetic hair treatments [60]. A higher frequency of hair care treatment among the female participants may be one explanation for the diminished ETG concentrations in female hair and the weak correlation between female ETG hair and fingernail. The higher concentrations of ETG in fingernail and the observed gender bias of hair ETG suggested that fingernail may be the preferred specimen type for long-term ETG detection.

However, Crunelle et al. in a study on 36 alcohol dependent patients (25 males and 11 females) demonstrated that there is no significant effect of gender and age on ETG concentration in this group [58].

4.4 Hair and Scalp Disorders with Gender Approach

4.4.1 Pattern Hair Loss

Pattern hair loss describes the miniaturization of large, pigmented terminal scalp hairs into small, nonpigmented vellus hairs [61]. In a review published by Olsen et al. in 2005, the authors provided some information on the potential pathophysiology, clinical presentation, and histology of pattern hair loss in men and women [62]. These differences are summarized in Table 4.1.

4.4.2 Hair Pain (Trichodynia)

The term "trichodynia" has recently been proposed for discomfort, pain or paresthesia of the scalp related to the complaint of hair loss [63]. Rebora et al. [63] found that 34.2% of female patients, who had their hair consultation because of hair loss, complained of this phenomenon. In a subsequent survey, Grimalt et al. [64] claimed that 14% of their patients reported trichodynia. Willimann and Trüeb [65] evaluated 403 patients seeking advice for hair loss in the hair consultation clinic between 1997 and 1999. Patients either

Table 4.1 Summarized caracterisations of pattern hair loss in men and women [62]

	Male pattern hair loss (MPHL)	Female pattern hair loss (FPHL)
Age trait	Increasing	Increasing
Androgen	Clearly dependent	Less certain
Pattern of hairloss	Bitemporal, frontal, mid scalp, and vertex regions (Hamilton-Norwood patterns)	Diffuse central thinning or frontal accentuation, there is not usually any recession of the frontal hairline (Christmas tree" pattern)
Family history	Commonly positive on either side of the family (paternal influence higher than maternal), no family history in 20% of patients	Less likely than men
Distribution	Central scalp	Central scalp ± sides of scalp
Onset	Anytime post-puberty, usually by age 40 (14% of healthy boys aged 15–17 years old show early signs)	Any time post menarche or adrenarche
Scalp	Generally normal	Generally normal
Affected hairs	Miniaturization (finer, shorter hairs) and decreased hair density	Miniaturization not as uniform nor as profound in specific scalp areas as that in MPHL
Absolute baldness	Yes	No
Associated features	Higher incidence of coronary artery disease	Signs or symptoms of hyperandrogenism should he evaluated: Hirsuitism, moderate to severe or treatment-refractory acne, irregular menses, infertility, galactorrhea and canthosis nigricans
Hair pull	May be positive in active early hair loss in the central scalp but generally negative in longstanding hair loss	May be positive in active early hair loss in the central scalp but generally negative in longstanding hair loss

spontaneously reported or were questioned about painful sensations of the scalp. Pruritus was not considered, and specific dermatologic diseases of the scalp were excluded. Of 403 patients aged between 13 and 87 years (mean: 42 years), 311 were female (age range: 13–87 years; mean age: 46 years) and 92 were male (age range: 14–71; mean age: 31 years). Seventy of 403 patients (17%) suffered from trichodynia [65]. There was a significant relationship between the gender of patients and the complaint of trichodynia. Trichodynia preferably occurred in female patients with 62 of 311 female (20%) and only 8 of 92 male patients (9%), respectively (p = 0.0119 in Fisher's exact test) [65].

A higher prevalence of female patients might be connected to genderrelated differences in pain perception in relation to anxiety. The role of vasoactive neuropeptides in the interaction between the central nervous system and skin reactivity is discussed [65].

4.4.3 Other Diseases

Pattern hail loss is common in both genders but has ist special characteristics in each sex. In cicatricial alopecia, lichen planopilaris and chronic cutaneous lupus erythematosus occur more commonly in females while folliculitis decalvans and folliculitis keloidalis are more common in men. Acquired trichodystrophies and traction alopecia occur more commonly in women, given their tendency to uses cosmetic hair practices [61].

References

1. Dao H, Kazin RA. Gender differences in skin: a review of the literature. Gend Med. 2007;4(4):308–28.
2. Schlake T. Determination of hair structure and shape. Semin Cell Dev Biol. 2007;18(2):267–73.
3. Giacomoni PU, Mammone T, Teri M. Gender-linked differences in human skin. J Dermatol Sci. 2009;55(3):144–9.

4. Thornton MJ, Taylor AH, Mulligan K, Al-Azzawi F, Lyon CC, O'Driscoll J, et al. Oestrogen receptor beta is the predominant oestrogen receptor in human scalp skin. Exp Dermatol. 2003;12(2):181–90.

5. Pelletier G, Ren L. Localization of sex steroid receptors in human skin. Histol Histopathol. 2004;19(2):629–36.

6. Wehner G, Schweikert H-U. Estrone sulfate source of estrone and estradiol formation in isolated human hair roots: identification of a pathway linked to hair growth phase and subject to site-, gender-, and age-related modulations. J Clin Endocrinol Metab. 2014;99(4):1393–9.

7. Graham JD, Clarke CL. Physiological action of progesterone in target tissues. Endocr Rev. 1997;18(4):502–19.

8. Schmidt JB, Lindmaier A, Spona J. Hormone receptors in pubic skin of premenopausal and postmenopausal females. Gynecol Obstet Investig. 1990;30(2):97–100.

9. Dombovári J, Lajos P. Comparison of sample preparation methods for elemental analysis of human hair. Microchemistry. 1998;59(2):187–93.

10. Barbosa AC, Jardim W, Dórea JG, Fosberg B, Souza J. Hair mercury speciation as a function of gender, age, and body mass index in inhabitants of the Negro River basin, Amazon, Brazil. Arch Environ Contam Toxicol. 2001;40(3):439–44.

11. Takagi Y, Matsuda S, Imai S, Ohmori Y, Masuda T, Vinson JA, Mehra MC, Puri BK, Kaniewski A. Trace elements in human hair: an international comparison. Bull Environ Contam Toxicol. 1986;36(6):793–800.

12. Khalique A, Ahmad S, Anjum T, Jaffar M, Shah MH, Shaheen N, et al. A comparative study based on gender and age dependence of selected metals in scalp hair. Environ Monit Assess. 2005;104(1-3):45–57.

13. Tamburo E, Varrica D, Dongarrà G. Gender as a key factor in trace metal and metalloid content of human scalp hair. A multi-site study. Sci Total Environ. 2016;573:996–1002.

14. Dongarrà G, Lombardo M, Tamburo E, Varrica D, Cibella F, Cuttitta G. Concentration and reference interval of trace elements in human hair from students living in Palermo, Sicily (Italy). Environ Toxicol Pharmacol. 2011;32(1):27–34.

15. Senofonte O, Violante N, Caroli S. Assessment of reference values for elements in human hair of urban schoolboys. J Trace Elem Med Biol. 2000;14(1):6–13.

16. Skalny AV, Skalnaya MG, Tinkov AA, Serebryansky EP, Demidov VA, Lobanova YN, et al. Reference values of hair toxic trace elements content in occupationally non-exposed Russian population. Environ Toxicol Pharmacol. 2015;40(1):18–21.

17. Chojnacka K, Michalak I, Zielińska A, Górecka H, Górecki H. Inter-relationship between elements in human hair: the effect of gender. Ecotoxicol Environ Saf. 2010;73(8):2022–8.

18. Zaichick S, Zaichick V. The effect of age and gender on 37 chemical element contents in scalp hair of healthy humans. Biol Trace Elem Res. 2010;134(1):41–54.

19. Barman JM, Pecoraro V, Astore I. Method, technic and computations in the study of the trophic State of the human scalp hair. J Invest Dermatol. 1964;42:421–5.

20. Van Neste DJJ, Rushton DH. Gender differences in scalp hair growth rates are maintained but reduced in pattern hair loss compared to controls. Skin Res Technol. 2016;22(3):363–9.

21. Blume U, Ferracin J, Verschoore M, Czernielewski JM, Schaefer H. Physiology of the vellus hair follicle: hair growth and sebum excretion. Br J Dermatol. 1991;124(1):21–8.

22. Trüeb RM. Aging of hair. J Cosmet Dermatol. 2005;4(2):60–72.

23. Jo SJ, Paik SH, Choi JW, Lee JH, Cho S, Kim KH, et al. Hair graying pattern depends on gender, onset age and smoking habits. Acta Derm Venereol. 2012;92(2):160–1.

24. Foitzik K, Krause K, Conrad F, Nakamura M, Funk W, Paus R. Human scalp hair follicles are both a target and a source of prolactin, which serves as an autocrine and/or paracrine promoter of apoptosis-driven hair follicle regression. Am J Pathol. 2006;168(3):748–56.

25. Fabre N, Montastruc JL, Rascol O. Alopecia: an adverse effect of bromocriptine. Clin Neuropharmacol. 1993;16(3):266–8.

26. Langan EA, Ramot Y, Goffin V, Griffiths CEM, Foitzik K, Paus R. Mind the (gender) gap: does prolactin exert gender and/or site-specific effects on the human hair follicle? J Invest Dermatol. 2010;130(3):886–91.

27. Lu Z, Hasse S, Bodo E, Rose C, Funk W, Paus R. Towards the development of a simplified long-term organ culture method for human scalp skin and its appendages under serum-free conditions. Exp Dermatol. 2007;16(1):37–44.

28. Philpott MP, Green MR, Kealey T. Human hair growth in vitro. J Cell Sci. 1990;97(Pt 3):463–71.

29. Goffin V, Bernichtein S, Touraine P, Kelly PA. Development and potential clinical uses of human prolactin receptor antagonists. Endocr Rev. 2005;26(3):400–22.

30. Bernichtein S, Kayser C, Dillner K, Moulin S, Kopchick JJ, Martial JA, et al. J Biol Chem. 2003;278(38):35988–99.

31. Rippe RCA, Noppe G, Windhorst DA, Tiemeier H, van Rossum EFC, Jaddoe VWV, et al. Splitting hair for cortisol? Associations of socio-economic status, ethnicity, hair color, gender and other child characteristics with hair cortisol and cortisone. Psychoneuroendocrinology. 2016;66:56–64.

32. Manenschijn L, Schaap L, van Schoor NM, van der Pas S, Peeters GMEE, Lips P, et al. High long-term cortisol levels, measured in scalp hair, are associated with a history of cardiovascular disease. J Clin Endocrinol Metab. 2013;98(5):2078–83.

33. Spack NP. Management of transgenderism. JAMA. 2013;309(5):478–84.

34. Giltay EJ, Gooren LJ. Effects of sex steroid deprivation/administration on hair growth and skin sebum production in transsexual males and females. J Clin Endocrinol Metab. 2000;85(8):2913–21.

35. Stevenson MO, Wixon N, Safer JD. Scalp hair regrowth in hormone-treated transgender woman. Transgender Health. 2016;1(1):202–4.
36. Ginsberg BA. Dermatologic care of the transgender patient. Int J Womens Dermatol. 2017;3(1):65–7.
37. Capitán L, Simon D, Meyer T, Alcaide A, Wells A, Bailón C, et al. Facial feminization surgery: simultaneous hair transplant during forehead reconstruction. Plast Reconstr Surg. 2017;139(3):573–84.
38. Prahlow JA, Lantz PE, Cox-Jones K, Rao PN, Pettenati MJ. Gender identification of human hair using fluorescence in situ hybridization. J Forensic Sci. 1996;41(6):1035–7.
39. Singh H, Gorea R, Aggarwal O, Jasuja O. Determination of sex from hair. J Punjab Acad Forensic Med Toxicol. 2004;4(1):3–4.
40. McMichael AJ. Ethnic hair update: past and present. J Am Acad Dermatol. 2003;48(6 Suppl):S127–33.
41. Khumalo NP, Jessop S, Gumedze F, Ehrlich R. Hairdressing and the prevalence of scalp disease in African adults. Br J Dermatol. 2007;157(5):981–8.
42. Khumalo NP, Jessop S, Gumedze F, Ehrlich R. Hairdressing is associated with scalp disease in African schoolchildren. Br J Dermatol. 2007;157(1):106–10.
43. Camacho PM, Gharib H, Sizemore GW. Evidence-based endocrinology. Philadelphia: Lippincott Williams & Wilkins; 2007. 324p.
44. Dongarrà G, Varrica D, Tamburo E, D'Andrea D. Trace elements in scalp hair of children living in differing environmental contexts in Sicily (Italy). Environ Toxicol Pharmacol. 2012;34(2):160–9.
45. Blume-Peytavi U, Whiting DA, Trüeb RM. Hair growth and disorders, vol. XXVI. New York: Springer; 2008. p. 564.
46. Bencko V. Use of human hair as a biomarker in the assessment of exposure to pollutants in occupational and environmental settings. Toxicology. 1995;101(1-2):29–39.
47. Barbosa AC, Silva SR, Dórea JG. Concentration of mercury in hair of indigenous mothers and infants from the Amazon basin. Arch Environ Contam Toxicol. 1998;34(1):100–5.
48. Barbosa AC, Dórea JG. Indices of mercury contamination during breast feeding in the Amazon Basin. Environ Toxicol Pharmacol. 1998;6(2):71–9.
49. Chittleborough G. A chemist's view of the analysis of human hair for trace elements. Sci Total Environ. 1980;14(1):53–75.
50. Chojnacka K, Górecka H, Górecki H. The influence of living habits and family relationships on element concentrations in human hair. Sci Total Environ. 2006;366(2-3):612–20.
51. Huang L, Beauchemin D. Is it possible to identify gender and ethnicity via hair elements? Bioanalysis. 2014;6(22):2953–5.
52. Peña-Fernández A, Lobo-Bedmar MC, González-Muñoz MJ. Monitoring lead in hair of children and adolescents of Alcalá de Henares, Spain. A study by gender and residential areas. Environ Int. 2014;72:170–5.
53. Sanna E, Floris G, Vallascas E. Town and gender effects on hair lead levels in children from three Sardinian towns (Italy) with different environmental backgrounds. Biol Trace Elem Res. 2008;124(1):52–9.
54. Evrenoglou L, Partsinevelou SA, Stamatis P, Lazaris A, Patsouris E, Kotampasi C, et al. Children exposure to trace levels of heavy metals at the north zone of Kifissos River. Sci Total Environ. 2013;443:650–61.
55. Kozielec T, Pózniak J, Salacka A, Hornowska I, Kotkowiak L. Hair copper concentration in healthy children, teenagers, and adults living in Szczecin, Poland. Biol Trace Elem Res. 2003;93(1-3):47–54.
56. Pastorelli AA, Baldini M, Stacchini P, Baldini G, Morelli S, Sagratella E, et al. Human exposure to lead, cadmium and mercury through fish and seafood product consumption in Italy: a pilot evaluation. Food Addit Contam Part A Chem Anal Control Expo Risk Assess. 2012;29(12):1913–21.
57. Jones KL, Smith DW, Ulleland CN, Streissguth P. Pattern of malformation in offspring of chronic alcoholic mothers. Lancet. 1973;1(7815):1267–71.
58. Crunelle CL, Cappelle D, Covaci A, van Nuijs ALN, Maudens KE, Sabbe B, et al. Hair ethyl glucuronide as a biomarker of alcohol consumption in alcohol-dependent patients: role of gender differences. Drug Alcohol Depend. 2014;141:163–6.
59. Jones J, Jones M, Plate C, Lewis D, Fendrich M, Berger L, et al. Liquid chromatography-tandem mass spectrometry assay to detect ethyl glucuronide in human fingernail: comparison to hair and gender differences. Am J Anal Chem. 2012;3(1):83–91.
60. Morini L, Zucchella A, Polettini A, Politi L, Groppi A. Effect of bleaching on ethyl glucuronide in hair: an in vitro experiment. Forensic Sci Int. 2010;198(1-3):23–7.
61. Bergfield W, Harrison S. Hair disorders. In: Manuals of gender dermatology. Sudbury: Jones and Bartlett Learning; 2011. p. 121–31.
62. Olsen EA, Messenger AG, Shapiro J, Bergfeld WF, Hordinsky MK, Roberts JL, et al. Evaluation and treatment of male and female pattern hair loss. J Am Acad Dermatol. 2005;52(2):301–11.
63. Rebora A, Semino MT, Guarrera M. Trichodynia. Dermatology. 1996;192(3):292–3.
64. Grimalt R, Ferrando J, Grimalt F. Trichodynia. Dermatology. 1998;196(3):374.
65. Willimann B, Trüeb RM. Hair pain (trichodynia): frequency and relationship to hair loss and patient gender. Dermatology. 2002;205(4):374–7.

Nail Variations Related to Gender

Robert Baran and Doug Schoon

5.1 The Anatomy of the Nail Apparatus (Fig. 5.1)

The nail which grows throughout the life is a transparent, semi hard, oblong tablet with a long longitudinal axis in the hands, transverse in the feet. Its upper side is smooth and glossy. The nail plate sinks at an acute angle into a large deep groove, practically parallel to the cutaneous surface, the nail cul-de-sac (or posterior or proximal groove. The lateral nail grooves complete the bezel of the nail. They are lined by the lateral folds. The visible part of the nail ends with a free edge, which owes its whitish color to the underlying presence of air.

The nail bed's dorsal surface is characterized by longitudinal ridges, and a complementary set of ridges is also found on the underside of the nail plate contributing to adhesion between the nail plate and the nail bed.

The proximal nail fold (or dorsal or posterior) is an expansion of the epidermis of the dorsal aspect of the distal phalanx. Its ventral part constitutes the roof of the proximal nail groove, which covers, on approximately 0.5 cm, the thinned base of the nail that is loosely stuck to the matrix. The cuticle, is dead tissue which is detached from the eponychium and adheres strongly to the upper side of the plate and seals the virtual space that opens onto the nail cul-de-sac. The inner side of the lateral folds is also lined with a stratified epithelium and produces a soft keratin that does not flake off but tends to persist as a thin and rough membrane overflowing on the neighboring surface of the nail.

The nail matrix covers the floor of the cul-de-sac and rises on the posterior quarter of the roof of the proximal nail groove, the anterior three-quarters of which constitute the eponychium. The deep side of the matrix rests on the terminal osseous phalanx and forms a crescent with posteroinferior concavity.

The lunula, opaque white, with an anterior arc-shaped edge, corresponds to the distal and visible portion of the matrix. Particularly noticeable on the thumbs, it may be absent or covered by the proximal nail fold on the other fingers. The proximal portion of the matrix produces the upper third of the nail plate, its distal part the lower two-thirds.

The thickness of the nail (0.50–0.75 mm in the fingers, up to 1 mm in the toes) is proportional to the length of the matrix.

Ahead of the lunula, the pinkish area seen by transparency corresponds to the nail bed: the absence of fatty tissue puts the mesenchyme directly in contact with the bone. The hyponychium which contains the solenhorn

R. Baran (✉) · D. Schoon
Nail Disease Center, Cannes, France

Science and Technology, Creative Nail Design Inc., Vista, CA, USA

© Springer International Publishing AG, part of Springer Nature 2018
E. Tur, H. I. Maibach (eds.), *Gender and Dermatology*,
https://doi.org/10.1007/978-3-319-72156-9_5

Fig. 5.1 Nail unit
anatomy

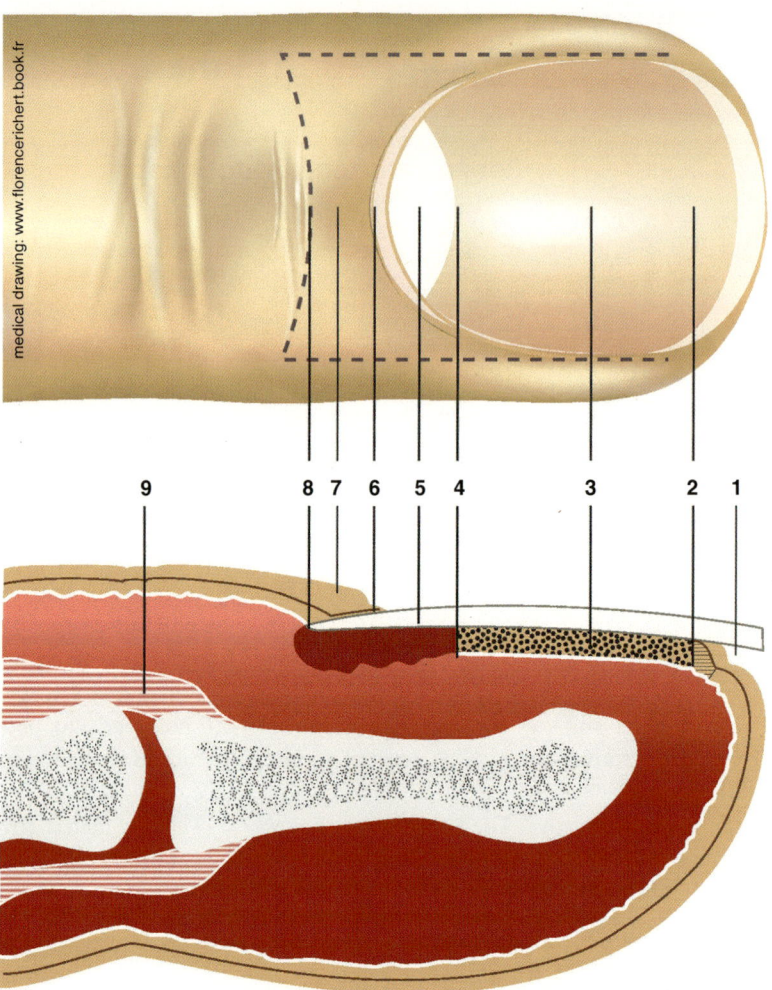

medical drawing: www.florencerichert.book.fr

1 - Distal groove
2 - Hyponychium
3 - Nail bed
4 - Distal border of the matrix
5 - Lunula
6 - Cuticle
7 - Proximal nail fold
8 - Proximal edge of the nail plate
9 - Extensor tendon

corresponds to the area where the nail plate loosens from the underlying tissue. Its horny substance accumulates physiologically in the distal groove, an arc-shaped furrow with anterior convexity. The distal groove marks the most distal boundary between the nail unit and the fingertip.

5.2 Physiological Factors and Nail Growth

Most studies concern fingernails [1]. Their rate of growth can vary between 1.9 and 4.4 mm month. A reasonable guide is 3 mm month or 0.1 mm day. Toenails are estimated to grow around 1 mm month. Population studies on nail growth have given the general findings that there is little marked seasonal change and nails are unaffected by mild intercurrent illnesses. The height or weight of the individual made no significant difference. Sex makes a small difference in early adulthood, with men having significantly (P < 0.001) faster linear nail growth up to the age of 19. They continue to do so with gradually diminishing significance levels, up to the age of 69, when there is a cross-over and women's nails grow faster than males'. There is rough agreement from Hillman in an earlier study [2], although he found that the crossover age was around 40. However, males continued to have a greater rate of nail growth throughout life if volume was measured, and not length. Children under 14 have faster growth than adults.

5.3   The Shape of the Nail

The shape of the nail depends on proportion and contour. The ratio of length to breadth is critical to its aesthetic appeal, and the two dimensions should be approximately equal, at least on the thumb. When the magic ratio differs from the ideal, the nail is less attractive. Polish, which enhances nail beauty, adds little in cosmetic improvement to a broad, short fingernail. Curiously, the racquet nail is three times more frequent in women than in men.

In the past, attractive nails were oval in shape, but today there is a tendency in women to cut the tip more or less squarely, although the basic nail shape may be round or almond-shaped.

Length creates the impression of thin, tapered, and graceful fingers. When too long, however, they may become unsightly. Excessive length may even interfere with the efficiency of hand performance [3]. Testing grip strength and dexterity with typing is one way of determining the effect of nail length on function. Jensen et al. demonstrated a significant loss of grip power and typing speed when extending nails from 0.5 cm at the free edge to 1 and 2 cm. In addition, a long nail may act as a lever and facilitate the rupture of the nail plate-nail bed attachment, a condition

called onycholysis. The form or style of the nail varies geographically. In some regions, nails tend to have shorter, almond-shaped free edges, intended to look natural, while in other areas individuals prefer longer nails with higher apex arches.

The nail plate's convex shape in both the longitudinal and transverse directions is thought to contribute to its mechanical rigidity, and overcurvature can be a symptom of local and/or systemic disorders. It is influenced by a person's gender, age, hand dominance and hand width. Thus, nails are flatter in the dominant hand, in men, in older individuals and in those with wider hands [4].

Transverse nail curvature was expressed as the radius of a circle whose curve most closely approximated the transverse curve of the nail plate. Thus, flatter nail plates have larger radii of curvature compared to curved ones. There are large differences in nail curvature of the five digits and between males and females. In contrast, hand side (right/left) and handedness were associated with much smaller differences in nail curvature. The multiple comparison Tukey test indicated that the mean curvature of the fingernails was significantly different from one another except for the index and middle fingernails which had similar curvature ($p = 0.3$ and 0.6 for males and females respectively).

Gender appears to influence nail curvature. General Linear Model was performed separately for the five fingernails to investigate the influence of gender as gender was shown to have a large influence on nail curvature.

The general linear models for the five digits' nail curvatures showed a highly significant influence of gender ($p < 0.05$), which explained between 26% and 33% of the total variance. Males have flatter fingernails. After controlling for gender, age, hand breadth and hand dominance explained a further 10–18% of the total variance, and were also significant factors ($p < 0.05$). The nails of the dominant hand are flatter, and older persons and those with wider hands have flatter nails. In contrast, hand length was not significantly associated with nail curvature ($p > 0.2$) [5]. According to Murdan [4], the nail plate's convex shape in both the longitudinal and transverse directions is thought to contribute to its mechanical rigidity, and overcurvature can be a symptom of local and/or systemic disorders. Although a number of methods to measure the longitudinal nail curvature have been proposed, evaluation of the transverse nail curvature has been largely limited to visual estimation of over curved nail plates.

Nail plate lipid composition varies with age and sex: the lipid composition of the fertile years shows distinct profiles compared that of childhood and old age, suggesting an influence of sex hormones on nail lipogenesis.

Age-dependent decrease in Cholesterol Sulfate (CS) levels might explain the previously observed higher incidence of brittle nails in women. Obviously, the metabolism of integral cholesterol (CH) and CS in fingernail and scalp hair differs between genders, and shows age-associated changes.

In women, a decrease in CS of nail plates is observed with age. As was shown in wool CS is important for structural stability. Interestingly, even healthy women suffer from nail brittleness much more frequently than men, with a ratio of men to women from 1:1.6 to 1.7 depending on age. Therefore, this nail symptom appears to be associated with reduced CS concentrations of nails [6].

Sertoli-Leydig cell tumor albeit rare, should be considered in post-menopausal women presenting virilization and elevated androgen levels in these patients. The nails looked most the flat with significant curved concave spoon shaped ends in 8 fingers. Importantly the fingernail changes started to gradually reverse after the curative tumor surgery and normalization of patient hormonal profile. The authors conclude that the nail signs were secondary to hyperandrogenemia [7].

Nail configuration is influenced by genetic factors, mechanical force, nutrition, neurogenic factors, blood flow, and factors that cause thinning and softening of nails. Of these factors, mechanical force may have a particularly pronounced effect on nail configuration and thus may be involved in the development of nail deformities. Carpenters, for example, had a sig-

nificantly higher mean pinch force and lower mean thumb nail curve index, which suggests that carpenters use a stronger pinch force in daily life and that the strength of the mechanical force affects nail morphology. The carpenters also had significantly thicker thumb nails. Repetitive pressure is an obvious cause of nail thickening due to subungual keratosis [8].

5.4   The Decoration of the Nail [9, 10]

For nails of equal length and corresponding contour, a painted nail is usually considered more attractive. Cosmetic procedures, especially artificial nails, may bring about reactions due to the cosmetics applied, encompassing reactions at the site of application and even secondarily at distance (Fig. 5.2) (ectopic contact dermatitis (Fig. 5.3), which is exceptional in men). Colorless nail polish dermatitis is of little significance in men. Only four cases have appeared in the literature between 1925 and 1993…

Nail cosmetic hazards may be occupational or accidental (especially in children). Individuals wearing artificial nails tend to wear their nails longer and should be more careful about them when washing their hands; therefore, the sanitary conditions for the wearing of artificial nails are paramount in preventing nail infections (Fig. 5.4).

Both women and men have long shown great interest in the care and adornment of the natural nail plate. Many implements, tools, products and services have been developed to enhance the attractiveness, improve the condition and maintain health of the nail unit as a whole. This innate desire existed in many ancient societies where nail beautification was an established practice.

5.5   Sculptured Nails ("Acrylic" Nails) [9, 10]

The original artificial nail enhancements were based on systems similar to orthodontic products which often utilized methacrylate monomers and polymers.

Fig. 5.2 Sites of origin and transfer of allergens (after C. Bonu)

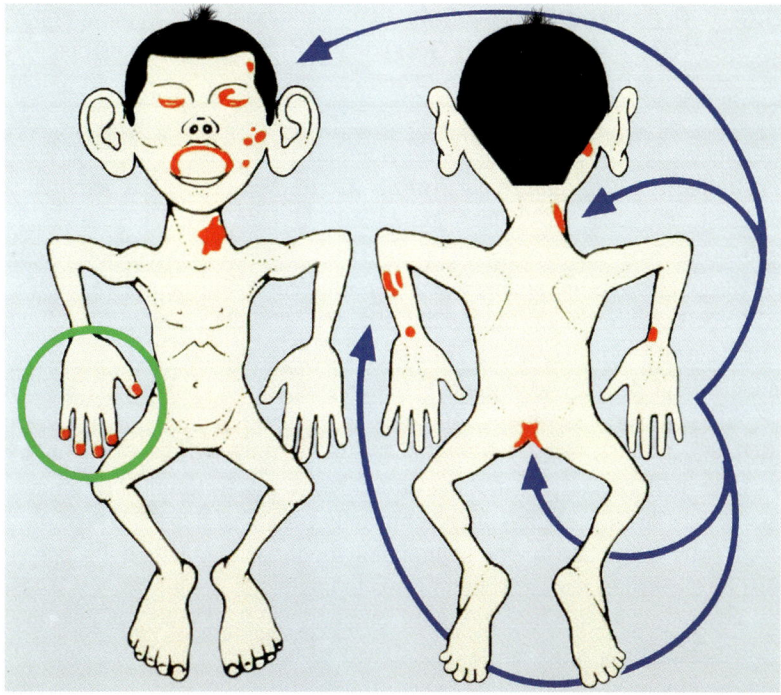

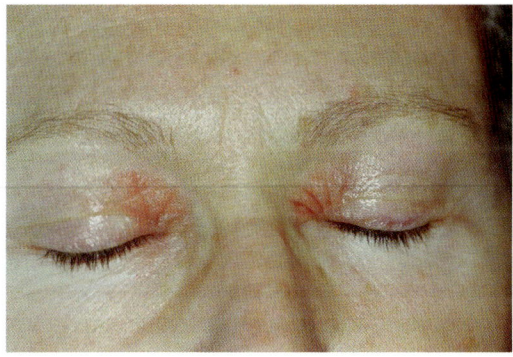

Fig. 5.3 Distant contact dermatitis

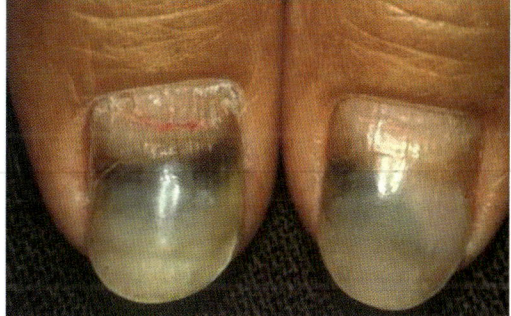

Fig. 5.4 Subungual nail infection associated with artificial nails

Methacrylate monomer-based artificial nail systems are among the most widely used artificial nails in the world.

Newer artificial nail formulations utilize monomers with significantly improved adhesion to the natural nail plate, so use of pretreatment factors called "primers" is now considered optional.

Artificial nail primers no longer utilize methacrylic acid since it may represent a corrosive hazard to young children and has led to severe injuries in the home.

To artificially extend the nail plate, a metalized paper-board template is first applied to the natural nail, before the liquid/powder slurry is applied. Each artificial nail must be refurbished (called rebalancing) every 2–3 weeks in order to make small repairs and fill in the area of new growth. Nail elongation is more commonly achieved by sticking a plastic preformed tip to the nail plate with CA monomer adhesive, then applying the liquid/powder slurry over the extension and allowing it to harden.

5.6 Premixed Acrylic Gels (Ultraviolet Cured Gels) [9, 10]

Certain types of artificial nail coatings cure under low-intensity UVA lights, typically 435–325 nm, to create artificial nails which are called "UV gels" (Fig. 5.5).

Ultraviolet gels are preblended and not mixed with another substance to initiate the polymerization (curing) process. These utilize primarily methacrylate or acrylate oligomers, but may also contain lesser amounts of methacrylate monomers.

Like their counterpart, *UV gel nail* enhancements may be clear, slightly tinted or heavily colored. Prior to application the natural nail should first be cleaned to remove contaminants to might contribute to adhesion loss and/or infection.

Ultraviolet gel artificial nails designed to be removed more easily are called "soak-off gels" or "soft gels". These products do not remove any faster than traditional liquid and powder products, typically 30 min soaking in an acetone-based product remover, but are more easily removed than traditional UV gel nails, which can only be removed by carefully filing with an abrasive.

5.7 UV LED Technology [9, 10]

Besides the use of traditional UV fluorescent bulbs, higher UV intensity obtainable by using light emitting diodes (LED) technology has been

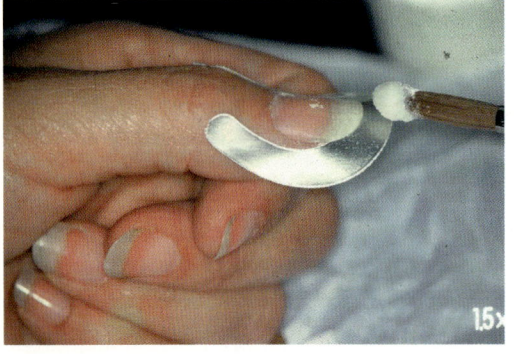

Fig. 5.5 Premixed acrylic gel

utilized to more rapidly and thoroughly cure UV gels. These nail lamps are more efficient because their output is focused in a narrower range, and thus they emit more of the nearly visible portion of the UVA spectrum needed by some photo initiators to drive polymerization reactions to completion. LED-style nail lamps have roughly one-third of the wattage of fluorescent-style nail lamps emit, yet emit more UVA. Therefore, it is not possible to estimate the UV output of a nail lamp by wattage, yet this is a commonly believed myth. Wattage describes power consumption of the nail lamp, not UV output. The UVA output is determined by a number of factors including the electronic of the unit, as well as distance from the hand to the UV emitters. Even some medical professionals don't appear to understand this technology, since some advice their clients to cure via LED and forego using UV nail lamps with fluorescent tubes, which clearly does not make scientific sense. The intensity of UVA emitted from the LED style nail lamps is much higher, however overall exposure to UV is about the same as traditional fluorescent-style nail lamps due to significantly shorter exposure typically 1 min versus 3 min, respectively. Dowdy and Sayre [11] characterize the UV exposure risks of both styles of nail lamps to be comparatively trivial, with 11–46 times less NMSC effective radiance when compared to overhead sunlight and vastly less hazardous than sunlamps. They also noted that the dorsum of the hands is naturally the most UV acclimatized, photo adapted, UV-resistant body site requiring four times more exposure to produce sunburns than the cheeks, chest or abdomen and about double the exposure to the dorsal or ventral arm. UVA cured nail polish coatings can last for at least 2 weeks without any signs of chipping, peeling or cracking. Typically, nail polish based on evaporation of solvents most often can be expected to last 3–4 days before it begins to dull, chip, crack and/or lose adhesion.

The recent development of nail salon-applied *UVA curing nail polish* can provide a viable solution to these issues. These new UVA curing nail polishes (aka UV gel manicure) can contain some volatile organic solvents or be 100% curable solids and are applied in the same fashion as traditional nail polish, but with an important difference: they have far superior adhesion, durability and crack resistance, therefore, they are much less likely to harbor pathogens than traditional nail polish.

5.8 "Dip" Nails

There has been a recent resurgence in the use of cyanoacrylates (CA) as nail coatings. In the 1990s, some salons began applying CA to the nail plate and sprinkling the uncured surface with methacrylate polymer powder designed for use in the so-called acrylic monomer and polymer nail systems. This was done to toughen the inherently weak CA coating, which are normally very susceptible to breakdown within about a week, if repeatedly exposed to water. The polymer powder increases both water and crack resistance, however, these systems remain inherently weaker, lasting only 2 weeks, so they eventually fell from favor only to resurface in 2016 and become widely used. Unlike other types of artificial nail systems, CA systems can only be used to elongate the nail and are not suitable for cosmetically altering the shape of the distorted plates. Rather than sprinkle powder over the surface of a CA coated nail plate, the new trend is to dip the fingertip and coated nail directly into a container filled with fine polymer powder that often ranges between 40 and 80 μ diameters. This can be unsanitary when performed in a salon setting, unless the unused portion of the polymer powder is discarded immediately and not subsequently reused on the next client. These types on nail coatings can last up to 2–3 weeks before they must be removed by soaking in an acetone based remover and replaced with a freshly applied CA/polymer coating.

5.9 "Press-on" Nail Art Coatings [9, 10]

Self-adherent colored plastic films (Fig. 5.6) are affixed to the nail plate to provide a nail polish-like color with even highly intricate and beauti-

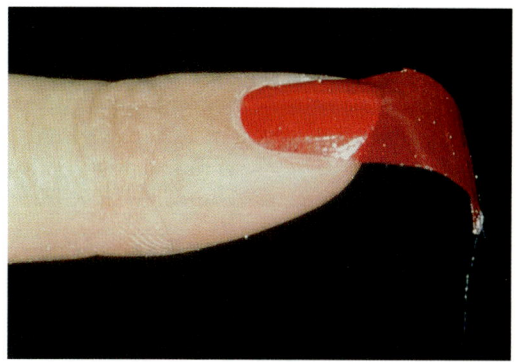

Fig. 5.6 Self-adherent colored plastic film

fully artistic designs. The cosmetic benefit is achieved quite quickly and easily. These newer type films wear moderately well on fingernails and have superior toenail adhesion. Problems can occur when these are forcible removed from the nail without using an appropriate remover solvent and allowing sufficient time for the adhesive backing to soften. Forcible removal can disrupt surface nails cells and the areas of damage can appear as whitish, irregular shaped patches. This is due to light-scattering from the surface roughness that is created by surface cell disruption.

5.10 Temporary/Press-on Artificial Nails [9, 10]

Preformed, plastic or gold plated prosthetic full nails (Fig. 5.7) may be used as temporary artificial nails, but are usually not worn for more than 48 h and are stuck into place with CA adhesives which may have accompanying hazards, especially when insufficient time or inadequate care is taken during removal.

5.11 Miscellaneous

It is easy to understand that women's nails are especially vulnerable due to daily chores, cosmetic procedures, and, on toenails, to repeated microtrauma, caused by improperly fitting shoes (too often, women wear shoes smaller than their feet). In addition, in 1999, a variant of the worn-

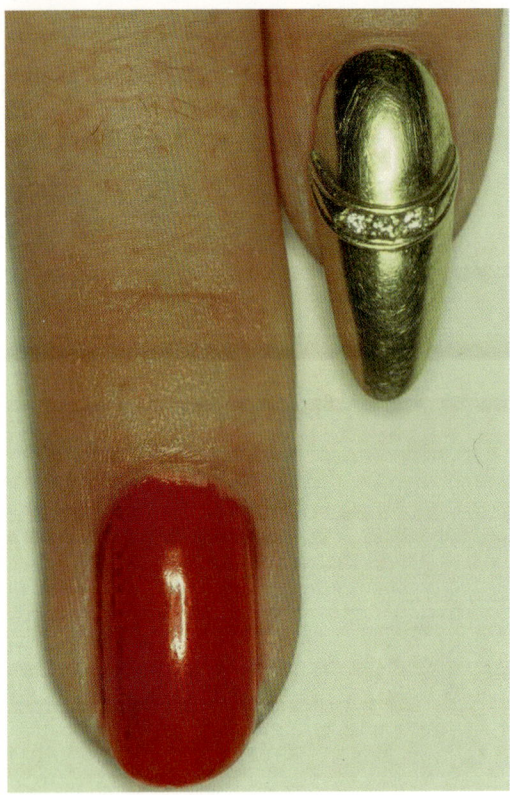

Fig. 5.7 Gold plated prosthetic full nail

down nail syndrome, the *bidet nail* was described [12]. This condition presents as a triangular defect with its base lying at the free edge of the nail plate and affecting the middle three fingers of the dominant hand. The patients are fastidious women in whom the desire for cleanliness verges on obsession; however, similar dystrophy has been reported more recently in tailors who rub their nails against cloth while sewing. The same result may be self-induced. For example, it can be caused by rubbing the nails against the anterior surface of the thigh when nervous or with other fingers, akin habit tic.

In Incontinentia Pigmenti, a woman's genetic condition, the subungual dyskeratotic tumors appear in young women, usually with multiple lesions and antecedents or signs of Incontinentia Pigmenti in themselves and/or in their family.

Physical damage and/or adverse skin reactions to the underside of the extended nail edge can cause the hyponychium to remained adhered to the ventral plate and become stretched and result in pain as the nail grows.

5.12 Nail Disorders Associated with Menstruation

Linear nail growth increases in the premenstrual phase [13]. Although nail disorders associated with menstruation are rarely observed, menstrual cycles may be associated with true transverse leukonychia [14]. Beau's lines have been associated with dysmenorrhea but they may also occur physiologically with each menstrual cycle [15].

5.13 Nail Disorders Related to the Contraceptive Pill

Rarely, finger nails may become firm, grow faster and no longer split or chip with the use of the contraceptive pill [16]. Adverse effects have also been reported: the contraceptive pill may produce estrogen-induced Porphyria Cutanea Tarda and variegata, and photo-onycholysis has been reported in some instances [17]. The pathogenesis of this type of porphyria is an inherited or acquired uroporphyrinogen-decarboxylase deficiency.

5.14 Pregnancy

The most commonly found nail change in pregnancy was leukonychia (24.4%). Ingrown toenail (9.0%) and onychoschizia (9.0%) represented the second most common nail changes. Rapid nail growth and subungual hyperkeratosis were observed in 6.7% and 4.2%, respectively, of subjects. When the alterations were evaluated according to gestational age, the most common nail pathology was leukonychia at both 14–28 weeks (16.3%) and 29–42 weeks (27.4%) of pregnancy. Onychoschizia, onycholysis, and brittle nail pathologies were also frequently observed at 29–42 weeks of pregnancy [18].

The increased adrenal and pituitary gland activity results in accelerated hair and nail growth during pregnancy while the latter slows down during lactation. Longitudinal melanonychia is rarely associated with hyperpigmentation, which is common in pregnancy [19]. Abnormal lifting of acrylic prostheses might be a possibility which could also appear in menopausal women.

We have intentionally left the risk of congenital drug-induced nail changes.

5.15 Nail Disorders Related to Daily Chores

The nail plate takes a minimum of 5 months to regenerate; however, it is vulnerable to daily insults. The nail may be damaged by repeated trauma or by chemical agents, such as detergents, alkalis, various solvents and, especially, hot water. The housewife is very susceptible. As in women the bridges between the nail corneocytes are possibly weaker than in males, accordingly frequent alternating periods of hydration and drying increase the incidence of brittle nails particularly in women [20]. The nail plate is reportedly 1000 times more permeable to water than is the skin [21, 22]. Water content of the nail plate has been previously reported to be 7–18%. One reason for this wide discrepancy is likely due to the effects of nail condition of water absorption and therefore water content is likely to be random. According to Kazlow Stern et al. [23] the mean water content for normal nails was 11.90% and for brittle nails 12.48%. There was no statistically significant difference between the two groups. The odds of having brittle nails was 3.23 greater among participants who received a professional manicure. Particularly at risk are the first three fingers of the dominant hand which may show four main types of brittle nails:

1. An isolated split at the free edge which sometimes extends proximally. This may result from onychorrhexis with shallow parallel furrows running in the superficial layer of the nail [9, 10].
2. Multiple, crenelated splitting which resembles the battlements of a castle. Triangular pieces may easily be torn away from the free margin;

3. Lamellar splitting into fine layers of the free edge of the nail. This may occur alone or associated with the other types; and
4. Transverse splitting and breaking of the lateral edge close to the distal margin.

Management of brittle nails requires preventive and protective measures to avoid quick nail plate dehydration. Affected individuals should wear cotton gloves beneath plastic gloves during household tasks, avoid repeated immersion in soap and water and keep their nails short. Frequent application of topical preparations containing hydrophilic substances may favor nail plate rehydration.

To conclude, as men have still not begun to wear high heels, are not yet addicted to cosmetic procedures, and, thus far, are not beset with domestic chores to any extent, it seems that their nails have good prospects for the future….

References

1. De Berker DAR, André J, Baran R. Nail biology and nail science. Int J Cosmest Sci. 2007;29:241–75.
2. Hilman R. Fingernail growth in the human subject. Hum Biol. 1955;27:247–83.
3. Jansen CW, Patterson R, Viegas SF. Effects on fingernail length on finger and hand performance. J Hand Ther. 2000;13:211–7.
4. Murdan S. Transverse fingernail curvature in adults: a quantitative evaluation and the influence of gender, age, and hand size and dominance. Int J Cosmet Sci. 2011;33:509–13.
5. Helmdach M, Thielitz A, Röpke EM, Gollnick H. Age and sex variation in lipid composition of human fingernail plates. Skin Pharmacol Appl Ski Physiol. 2000;13:111–9.
6. Brosche T, Dressler S, Platt D. Age-associated changes in integral cholesterol and cholesterol sulfate concentrations in human scalp hair and fingernail clippings. Aging Clin Exp Res. 2001;13:131–8.
7. Moghazy D, Sharan C, Nair M, et al. Sertoli-Leyding cell tumor with unique nail findings in a postmenopausal woman. J Ovarian Res. 2014;7:83.
8. Sano H, Shionoya K, Ogawa R. Fingernail configuration is influenced by mechanical forces on finger pads. J Dermatol. 2013;40:1056–7.
9. Baran R, Schoon D. Cosmetology for normal nails. In: Baran R, Maibach HI, editors. Textbook of cosmetic dermatology. London: Informa; 2017. p. 264–75.
10. Schoon D, Baran R. Cosmetics for abnormal and pathological nails. In: Baran R, Maibach HI, editors. Textbook of cosmetic dermatology. London: Informa; 2017. p. 276–86.

11. Dowdy JC, Sayre RM. Photobiological safety evaluation of UV nail lamps. Photochem Photobiol. 2013;89:961–7.
12. Baran R. The bidet nail: a French variant of the worn-down nail syndrome. Br J Dermatol. 1999;140:377.
13. Orentreich N, Markofsky J, Vogelman JH. The effect of aging on the rate of linear nail growth. J Invest Dermatol. 1979;73:120–30.
14. Daniel CR. Nail pigmentation abnormalities. Dermatol Clin. 1985;3:431–43.
15. Colver GB, Dawber RPR. Multiple Beau's lines due to dysmenorrhoea? Br J Dermatol. 1984;111:111–3.
16. Knight JF. Side benefits of the pill. Med J Aust. 1974;2:680.
17. Byrne JP, Boss JM, Dawber RP. Contraceptive pill induced porphyria cutanea tarda presenting with onycholysis of the finger nails. Postgrad Med. 1976;52:535–8.
18. Erpolat S, Eser A, Kaygusuz I, et al. Nail alterations during pregnancy: a clinical study. Int J Dermatol. 2016;55:1172–5.
19. Freyer JM, Werth VP. Pregnancy-associated hyperpigmentation associated with longitudinal melanonychia. J Am Acad Dermatol. 1992;26:493–4.
20. Lubach D, Beckers P. Wet working conditions increase brittleness of nails, but do not cause it. Dermatology. 1992;185:120–2.
21. Spruit D. Measurement of water vapor less through human nail in vivo. J Invest Dermatol. 1971;56:359–61.
22. Walters KA, Flynn GL, Marvel JR. Penetration of the human nail plate: the effects of vehicle pH on the permeation of homologous alcohols. J Pharm Pharmacol. 1985;37:4318–9.
23. Kazlow Stern D, Diamantis S, Smith E, et al. Water content and other aspects of brittle versus normal nails. J Am Acad Dermatol. 2007;57:31–6.

Cutaneous Autoimmune Connective Tissue Disorders

6

Wohl Yonit

6.1 Introduction

Over the last past years, the gender perspective on medical issues has gained popularity in an increasingly number of medical areas, focusing on gender differences in explaining the pathogenesis, the course and outcomes of diseases.

In the field of dermatology as well, enough data is gathering on different skin disorders especially collagen diseases that merits coining the name of "gender Dermatology "stressing the importance to use an unbiased gender approach in clinical practice, analyzing medical research and medical education [1].

Gender has a significant influence on the development of autoimmune diseases whereby in general, women are more susceptible than men. It also seems to play an important contributing factor in the complex puzzling picture of disease etiology, regulating the onset, severity and progression of the disorder.

Various types of organ and non-organ specific autoimmune diseases in both humans and experimental animals display a gender bias which can be modest such as in MS or strong as seen in SLE or Sjogren's syndrome.

Worldwide data highlight a very high (9:1) gender prevalence ratio toward females for SLE and Systemic Sclerosis occurring independent of country of assessment [2].

In addition to prevalence, the severity of the autoimmune disorder, pathological features such as the degree of inflammation and the survival can vary with gender.

Indeed, it is becoming increasingly clear that gender differences in disease manifestations are not due to a single cause, and etiologic factors can be found at many levels: genetic (X-chromosome inactivation or mosaicism), cellular (sex-specific receptor activity), organ (hormonal influences), gender, life stage (age), behavior (social activities, eating habits), life events (effects of pregnancy), socio-cultural, and environmental.

In attempt to spotlight Immunology, the area which was studied in depth in order to understand how gender may work Ngo et al. in their remarkable review elaborated on the possible underlying immuno-mechanisms which underlie the striking gender bias and are detailed below [3].

6.1.1 Differences in Immune System Components and Activity

In general, while the overall number of lymphocytes in male and females is the same, females as a gender group have better B-cell-mediated immunity than age-matched male counterparts.

W. Yonit
Maccabi Health Services, Tel Aviv, Israel

Ben Gurion University of the Negev,
Beer Sheva, Israel
e-mail: wohliy@012.net.il

© Springer International Publishing AG, part of Springer Nature 2018
E. Tur, H. I. Maibach (eds.), *Gender and Dermatology*,
https://doi.org/10.1007/978-3-319-72156-9_6

They have higher immunoglobulin levels, stronger antibody responses to various foreign antigens, and increased resistance to certain infections. Gender differences in T-cell-mediated immunity also exist, although the gender influences appear to be complex. Females have greater resistance to induced tolerance, increased ability to reject grafts, and increased CD4 to CD8 ratios. Also, females tend to secrete higher levels of interleukin (IL)-4,interferon-y (INF-y), and IL-1 [4]. Target organ vulnerability to damage is also different among genders as women have a better ability to tolerate cell and organ damage through their susceptibility to apoptosis, autophagy, mitochondrial function and biochemical pathways that promote survival such as the nf2 pathway [5].

6.1.2 The Impact of the Reproductive Role of the Female

Reproductive load has a significant impact on the initiation and progression of autoimmune disorders. The gender gap becomes even more prominent in women during the childbearing years, thus susceptibility to autoimmunity, particularly in females can alter dramatically in periods and life events such as puberty, pregnancy and menopause.

The effects of pregnancy on autoimmune diseases differ for inflammatory autoimmune diseases which tend to remit and antibody mediated autoimmune diseases where the effects are more variable for the different disorders and changing from woman to woman and from pregnancy to pregnancy in the same woman. For instance in MS and RA pregnancy is associated with the remission of symptoms although there could be a post partum flare. In contrast SLE is reported to worsen during pregnancy and scleroderma show no change in symptoms.

Because of the high incidence of many collagen diseases in women in their childbearing years special attention must be paid to contraception and pregnancy. Avoiding an unintended pregnancy in women with autoimmune collagen diseases, and trying to gain control over the disease before becoming pregnant, are extremely important.

Moreover, under the conditions of assisted pregnancy or ovarian hyper stimulation autoimmune diseases can appear, relapse or exacerbate.

Autoimmune disease during pregnancy can result in fetal manifestation of disease which is often transitory, due to placental transmission of autoantibodies. In more severe cases such as neonatal LE passively acquired autoimmunity can result in congenital heart block in neonates to mothers with SLE or other autoimmune disorders.

In attempt to spotlight the special hyper estrogenic immune-setting of pregnancy for instance, the theory seeing the fetus as an allograft to the immunologic reactive mother provides only partially explanations.

Updated concepts make a distinction between innate and adaptive immune system, and between Th1 and Th2 arms. A shift in Th1/Th2 activity in pregnancy favors increased Th2 related and reduced Th1 related activities which result in the improvement or even remission in Th1 mediated diseases such as Rheumatic Arthritis and the exacerbation of Th2 mediated disease such as SLE. This paradigm is an accepted marker of pregnancy success [6].

Lately, a novel paradigm emerged as regulatory T cells (Tregs) which mediate active immune tolerance to prevent ant maternal lymphocyte mediated damage were found to be elevated in normal pregnancies and to correlate with decreased activity of the Th1 arm.

Thus, the ratio of Treg/IL-17 is pivotal during pregnancy as its imbalance can lead to complications including recurrent pregnancy loss and preeclampsia [7].

Maternal michrochimerism, the persistence of cells in the fetus, is a possible source of graft versus host response in the offspring even in the adult life, underlie another mechanism in which pregnancy affects autoimmunity. Neonatal LE and Systemic Sclerosis are examples.

6.1.3 Sex Hormone Influences on the Immune System

Life cycle reproductive events impact on autoimmune diseases such as disease flares of SLE influenced by the age of onset of menarche, the use of oral contraceptives, the age of onset of menopause and hormonal treatments—all affected by the hormonal milieu of various sex hormones including estrogens, progesterone, androgens and prolactin.

In general, estrogen impacts immunity by modulating lymphocyte development and function and promoting cyto-protection. This could lead to a dual effect—the improvement of cell mediated disease on one hand or the worsening of antibody mediated disease on the other hand.

More complex, levels of exposure to estrogen greatly affects immunity, At high concentrations such as pregnancy estrogen inhibits Th-1 and pro-inflammatory pathways including TNF alpha, IL-1beta, IL-6 and stimulates Th2 anti-inflammatory pathways including IL-4, IL-10 and TGF beta.

Conversely, at low levels as seen after menopause estrogen stimulates pro- inflammatory arms including TNF alpha [8].

Also naturally exogenous estrogens (phyto/mico estrogens) and synthetic estrogen like compounds such as oral contraceptives and hormonal replacement therapy or environmental plastics, pesticides and industrial chemicals can accumulate in the adipose tissue and exert potent effects on immunity.

Progesterone and androgens exert anti- inflammatory and immunosuppressive effects which are beneficial in autoimmune disease while prolactin induces pro-inflammatory effects which tend to worsen autoimmune diseases.

While sex hormones alone are not responsible for the gender differences in the immune response and the development of autoimmune collagen diseases, they may provide fertile ground for other factors to trigger disease and influence its course.

6.1.4   The Influence of Genetic Factors on the Immune System

Genetic factors may contribute to differences between genders in autoimmunity on different levels.

As to susceptibility genes and the interaction of genes and gender the association between HLA genes and most autoimmune diseases shows a gender bias toward females. This was not yet clearly evaluated in case of the influence of polymorphism in non HLA genes on autoimmunity.

Chromosomal differences can explain gender dimorphism in autoimmunity. While the X chromosome contains a large number of genes that are involved in immunity the inactivation of one X chromosome and cellular mosaicism are mechanisms responsible for increased susceptibility for instance in SLE.

Epigenetic features that arise in autoimmune disease can be related to the sex of the parent via genomic imprinting. It is speculated that this process of imprinting micro RNAs which impact post transcriptional gene expression is regulated by different hormonal and chromosomal factors and thus can lead to sexual differences seen in autoimmune diseases [9].

6.1.5   Environmental Aspects

Environmental exposure to infectious agents, chemicals such as organic solvents or pesticides, ultraviolet light, different drugs and more- can interact with the genotype and can influence the prevalence and the risk of developing an autoimmune disease or its severity.

Certain ages of life (e.g., fetal, neonatal, or senescent stages of life) may be more susceptible to environmental chemical-induced autoimmunity.

Susceptibility to environmental chemical-induced autoimmunity may vary with the genetic background, gender, lifestyle, previous immune status, age and duration of exposure, and immune status at the time of contact with these agents. Chronic exposure (e.g., sustained low dose) may have more adverse effects than acute exposures.

Different exposure and response between genders to environmental factor might influence the risk of developing an autoimmune disease either thorough lifestyle behavior or DNA modification exerted by external stimuli such as tobacco smoke, sunlight and diet.

Examples for this gender bias are the exposure to cosmetics which is much greater in women speculating on the role of cosmetics in primary biliary cirrhosis which is more common in women, earlier adoption of smoking in men, increased unprotected exposure to sunlight in men and different dietary habits between genders [10].

More evidence for the environmental factor is seen in drug-induced systemic lupus erythematosus (SLE) and silica-induced scleroderma-like disease (predominant among men), and toxin-induced scleroderma-like disease (predominant among women).

6.2 Systemic Lupus Erythematosus (SLE)

SLE is a multisystem autoimmune condition with diverse clinical and immunological features. It is characterized serologically by auto-antibodies targeting self proteins, ANAs, which are present in all affected individuals. SLE can be life threatening due to the involvement of internal organs to varying degrees of severity: joints and muscles with arthritis and weakness; the nervous system with psychosis, seizures and organic brain syndrome; hematologic involvement with anemia, thrombocytopenia and development of thrombosis; and cardiopulmonary including pleuritis, pericarditis, myocarditis, and endocarditis.

Pathognomonic skin manifestations include the butterfly rash, photosensitivity, oral ulcers and alopecia.

The not yet completely understood pathogenesis involves the interaction of genetic, hormonal and environmental factors and is substantially more common in females of child bearing age with reported female: male ratio of 8–15:1. Prepubertal and postmenopausal ratios are much lower at 2–6:1 and 3–8:1, respectively.

This established striking predominance in females is related as described in depth previously to the complex interactions of sex hormones and the immune system. Other alternate genetic theories include the X-chromosome hypothesis as supported by the increased incidence of SLE in Klinefelter's syndrome, various somatic poly-

morphisms and disparities within the Toll-like receptor and interferon pathway. Despite that, there is limited evidence to suggest an altered hormonal milieu in men with lupus [11, 12].

Moreover, in their detailed review Murphy and Isenberg sought to clarify whether although males are protected in terms of incidence of disease, there is a distinct phenotype of male lupus and whether gender exerts an influence on the clinical presentation and outcome of SLE [13].

Data complicated by low patient numbers, cofounder factors such different ethnic groups, different disease duration or co morbidities and selection bias led to a suboptimal representation of clinical lupus phenotype in men.

Nevertheless there is consistent evidence that a number of clinical features are differently expressed in men with lupus.

Despite the apparently similar age of onset in male and female patients, males tend to display less of the typical mucocutaneous and musculoskeletal symptoms commonly present at diagnosis and subsequent disease course in women including arthralgia/arthritis, alopecia, oral ulcers, photosensitivity and Raynaud Phenomenon, with the suggestion of more prevalent serositis and discoid lupus [14, 15].

There seems to be an increased incidence of nephropathy, thrombotic episodes, neurologic disease, damage and augmented mortality risk in men with lupus [16, 17], but clear associations have not been consistently found in the literature and thus remain elusive.

In pediatric lupus erythematosus the ratio of women to men was reported 4.6:1, with no gender difference in the mean age of diagnosis. Except for a higher incidence of oral ulcers, alopecia and anti-single stranded antibodies in female pediatric patients, no further differences in clinical and laboratory features were found [18].

6.3 Cutaneous Lupus Erythematosus

Skin involvement occurs in 75–80% of patients with SLE. The cutaneous features of LE can be classified as specific or non specific. The specific skin features are further subject to Gillam's classification to acute cutaneous LE (ALE), subacute cutaneous LE (SCLE) and chronic cutaneous LE (CCLE) based on mainly clinical characteristics coupled with histologic and immunologic characteristics.

LE nonspecific skin lesions, are related to the immuno -pathogenic process but can be seen in other autoimmune diseases. Their identification in context with LE is very important since their presence may imply systemic involvement.

The commonest nonspecific skin lesions are vascular lesions such as leukocytoclastic vasculitis and livedo reticularis.

Although SLE epidemiology has been studied worldwide there is a gap of knowledge about CLE.

While numerous studies involving systemic lupus erythematosus (SLE) have attempted to identify gender differences in patients with lupus erythematosus only few reports on cutaneous lupus erythematous (CLE) have recognized gender differences.

Large-scale, population-based epidemiological studies reporting the incidence of isolated CLE are rare with very few reliable figures on the age- and gender-specific distribution of the incidence of CLE.

Among initial reports on isolated CLE Durosaro et al. analyzed a community-based population of patients with cutaneous LE from Olmsted County, Minnesota, over a 41-year period in aim to assess trends in the cutaneous variants of LE and to ascertain the incidence of CLE over decades.

A total of 156 patients with newly diagnosed CLE (100 females and 56 males) were identified between 1965 and 2005. The incidence rate (age and sex adjusted to the 2000 US white population) was 4.30 (95% confidence interval [CI], 3.62–4.98) per 100,000. Cutaneous LE had a female predominance during the last 3 decades of the study [19].

A more recent study has directly compared the incidence and prevalence of CLE with SLE in the same population and geographic area thereby assessing the role of similar genetic factors and possibly similar environmental agents in the path physiology of the conditions. The study assessed the incidence and prevalence of SLE and CLE from 1993 to 2005 in Olmsted County, Minnesota which provided a unique setting for such a study owing to resources of the Rochester Epidemiology Project.

The findings showed the age- and sex-adjusted incidence of SLE (2.9 per 100,000; 95% CI 2.0, 3.7) was similar to that of CLE (4.2 per 100,000; 95% CI 3.1, 5.2, p = 0.10). However, incidence of CLE was three times higher than SLE in males (2.4 versus 0.8 per 100,000, p = 0.009). The incidence of cutaneous lupus increases steadily with age [20].

A nationwide similar epidemiological study aimed to examine in a population-based cohort the incidence of CLE and its subsets in Sweden during 2005 to 2007 [21].

In this study the incidence of CLE was found to be 4.0/100,000; the female/male ratio was 3:1. Mean age at disease onset was 54 years. The most common subset was discoid lupus erythematosus (DLE) (80%, n = 868). A quarter of the patients (24%, n = 260) were already diagnosed with SLE at the time they were diagnosed with CLE. During the whole observation period (2005–2007), an additional 18% (n = 107) were diagnosed with SLE, average time to progression of about 8 years and the probability of receiving an additional SLE diagnosis being highest for the subacute CLE (SCLE) subset.

AS for skin specific manifestations Verra-Recabarren et al. retrospectively studied the medical records of 103 (33.4%) male and 205 (66.6%) female patients with CLE who were treated as inpatients or outpatients between January 1985 and December 2000. Female patients had a higher prevalence of Raynaud's phenomenon (P < 0.01), chilblain lupus (P = 0.005), arthralgias (P = 0.001) and SLE (P < 0.01).

Female patients were also more likely to have an increased erythrocyte sedimentation rate (P < 0.005), higher levels of antinuclear antibodies (P < 0.001) and decreased levels of C3 (P < 0.001), C4 (P < 0.01) and CH50 (P < 0.01). There was a higher prevalence of clinical and laboratory abnormalities in female patients who had both SLE and CLE than in male patients with both conditions [22].

6.3.1 Rheumatoid Arthritis

RA is a chronic multisystem disease of unknown etiology characterized by persistent inflammatory synovitis involving mainly the peripheral joints, and slow destruction of the joints leading to progressive disability. Both genetic and environmental factors have been implicated in the initiation of the disease and again, estrogens seem to play a central role.

Women are affected three times more often than men, with onset most often in the fourth and fifth decades of life. The ratio of women to men in women of childbearing age is 6:1 [23].

Moreover, it is a well-known phenomenon that during periods of estrogen deficiency, like menopause or postpartum, women have an increased risk of developing RA and show more severe progression of disease.

The likelihood of developing RA during pregnancy is decreased but increases thereafter, especially during the first 3 months after childbirth.

Analyses of RA differences include studies indicating higher disease activity and poorer functional status in women when compared with men.

Males sex was shown to be a major predictor of remission in early RA. Some studies have suggested that men have better responses to treatment with biologic agents than women. But on the other hand they have been shown to experience more adverse effects, particularly serious infections, during biologic treatments.

Gender differences in the phenotypes of RA were reported in a study from the Mayo Clinic. Involvement of large or axial joints was more common in men, with more and earlier radiographic damage compared with women. Although women evidenced a lower frequency of radiographic damage, they underwent more surgical procedures than men. In addition, the study described differences in extra-articular disease, with lung and pericardial disease more common in men, and eye disease more common in women [24].

6.3.2 Scleroderma

Scleroderma, systemic sclerosis, is an autoimmune systemic immune disorder whose predominant pathology is micro- vasculopathy, fibrotic destruction of the skin and internal organs, and the presence of antinuclear antibodies. Clinical manifestations include cutaneous edema followed by fibrosis of the skin, telangiectasias, calcinosis, Raynaud's phenomenon, accompanied by systemic involvement of the joints, gastrointestinal tract, respiratory and renal systems.

Older epidemiologic studies showed the gender balance to favor women, with an overall ratio of women to men of approximately 3:1 and a ratio of 5.7:1 and 12:1 for diffuse and limited scleroderma respectively.

This difference can reach a ratio of 15:1 in women during childbearing years [25].

Black women showed higher age-specific incidence rates than white women. Onset of disease in women occurred in their early 1940s, earlier than in men, and women displayed significantly longer survival rates than men in the limited scleroderma subtype [26].

More recent data from large randomized clinical trials in attempt to assess the course of clinical cutaneous and systemic features (modified Rodman skin score, HAQ- disability index and forced vital capacity) in 495 diffuse scleroderma patients during study period showed no difference in occurence between gender and three ethnicities [27].

6.3.3 Dermatomyositis

Dermatomyositis (DM) is a subset of idiopathic inflammatory myopathies (IIM), which are heterogeneous rheumatic disorders characterized by inflammation of skeletal muscle and progressive weakness.

Dermatomyositis is a rare disease with skeletal muscle damage by a predominantly inflammatory lymphocytic infiltration, accompanied by characteristic skin changes. These include a photodistributed erythema that becomes progressively poikilodermatous and indurated, periungual telangiectasias, the classic heliotrope rash on the face, pathognomonic Gottron's papules overlying the knuckles, and the Gottron's sign consisting of macules and plaques in the same distribution.

A significant and fundamental problem for conducting clinical trials is the inadequate classification criteria for IIM.

The ratio of women to men is reported to be 1.5:2.

Dermatomyositis both with and without malignancy predominantly affects white women, whereas dermatomyositis/polymyositis associated with connective tissue disease occurs in younger women, with a higher incidence in African Americans.

In some studies which investigated ethnic or gender differences in clinical manifestations in adult DM, juvenile DM (JDM) and amyopathic DM (ADM). Comparison between prevalence of skin manifestations for Caucasian and Asian ADM patients showed a higher prevalence for most skin variables in Caucasians, with the difference in prevalence of periungual erythema being most striking (p < 0.00001). No significant difference in autoantibody profile between the two groups was found.

Gender analyses for serology, muscle variables and skin manifestations revealed fewer differences compared to ethnic differences, and none remained statistically significant after correction for multiple testing [28, 29].

6.3.4 Sjögren's Syndrome

Sjögren's syndrome is an autoimmune disease and lymphoproliferative disorder in which lymphocytic destruction of salivary and lacrimal glands results in xerostomia and xerophthalmia.

The hallmark characteristic of SS is diminished secretory production from the primary exocrine gland and the lacrimal or salivary glands resulting in symptoms of dry eye and mouth.

The onset is greatest in the fourth and fifth decades of life, and it affects nine times more

women than men, a ratio that rises to 19:1 during childbearing years.

Although Sjögren's syndrome can occur in women during child-bearing years, most cases of SS occur soon after menopause around age 55–60. Clinical and animal model evidence indicates that estrogen and androgens like DHEA promote gland cell survival and protect against exocrine gland inflammation; and these hormone levels decline at menopause. Even though estrogen levels drop significantly prior to menopause and androgens gradually decrease, low levels of estrogen continue to drive autoantibody diversity.

The disease is believed to be mediated by an inflammatory and autoantibody response directed against salivary and lacrimal gland tissues. Overall, estrogen may increase the incidence of SS in women by increasing autoantibody production, even following menopause, leading to intracellular deposition, tissue damage, inflammasome activation, elevated IFNs, and exocrine gland dysfunction [30].

Gender-specific differences include significantly higher antinuclear antibody titers and erythrocyte sedimentation rate in the women. Clinically, women report more fatigue than do men. Because of other mucous membrane involvement, women may experience vaginal dryness, often noted before the onset of eye and oral disease.

Extraglandular manifestations of SS follow typical sex difference predominance with thyroiditis, Raynaud's phenomenon, depression, and fibromyalgia occurring more frequently in women than men, while lymphoma occurs more frequently in men.

6.4 Summary

In conclusion, since every individual has a gender and its influences will accompany him throughout the entire life, it is becoming mandatory to observe medical practice in a different light in order to provide better health care and offer more therapeutic strategies.

Table 6.1 Frequency ratios and illness course in different cutaneous collagen autoimmune diseases

Disease	Women overall	Women reproductive years	Childhood	Age of onset	Influence of pregnancy
SLE	3–8:1	8–15:1	4.6:1	Third to early fourth decade	Worsening
Cutaneous LE specific	3:1	.		Fifth decade	
Cutaneous LE non specific					
Scleroderma overall	3:1	15:1		Fifth to sixth decade	No effect
Diffuse cutaneous SS	5.7:1				
Limited cutaneous SS	12:1				
Rheumatoid arthritis	3:1	6:1	1.8:1	Fourth and fifth decade	Improving
Dermatomyositis	1.5:2		2.3:1	Fourth decade	Worsening
Sjögren's syndrome	9:1	19:1		Fourth and fifth decade	Worsening

While considerable progress has been made over the passing decade in research of main collagen disorders, there is still a lack of data in most cutaneous subgroups providing a challenging gap for future efforts.

The striking yet complex evidence of gender differences in cutaneous collagen autoimmune disease should dictate that future research and standard of care consider epidemiologic, clinical and potential therapeutic modalities in autoimmunity be stratified according to both gender and clinical diversity of the specific autoimmune skin disease (Table 6.1).

References

1. Brenner S, Wohl Y. Gender as a roadmap to dermatological diseases. Womens Health. 2007;3(2):127–9.
2. Eaton WW, Rose WR, et al. Epidemiology of autoimmune diseases in Denmark. J Autoimmun. 2007;29:1–9.
3. Ngo ST, Steyn FJ, McCombe PA. Gender differences in autoimmune disease. Front Neuroendocrinol. 2014;35:347–69.
4. Ansar Ahmed S, Hissong BD, Verthelyi D, Donner K, Becker K, Karpuzoglu-Sahin E. Gender and risk of autoimmune diseases: possible role of estrogenic compounds. Environ Health Perspect. 1999;107:681–6.
5. Si ML, Al-Sharafi B, Lai CC, Khandori R, Chang C, Su CY. Gender differences in cytoprotection induced by estrogen on female and male bovine aorthic endothelial cells. Endocrine. 2001;15:255–62.
6. Otensen M, Forgert F, Nelson JL, Schuhmacher A, Hebisch G, Villiger PM. Pregnancy in patients with rheumatic disease: anti-inflammatory cytokine increase in pregnancy and decrease post partum. Ann Rheum Dis. 2005;64:839–44.
7. Saito S, Nakashima A, Ito M, Shima T. Clinical implications of recent advances in our understanding of IL-17 and reproductive immunology. Expert Rev Clin Immunol. 2011;7:649–57.
8. Straub RH. The complex role of estrogens in inflammation. Endocr Rev. 2007;28:521–74.
9. Sharma S, Eghbali M. Influence of sex differences on micro RNA gene regulation in disease. Biol Sex Differ. 2014;5:3.
10. Chandran V, Raychaudhuri SP. Geo-epidemiology and environmental factors of psoriasis and psoriatic arthritis. J Autoimmun. 2010;34:314–21.
11. Mok CC, Lau CS. Profile of sex hormones in male patients with systemic lupus erythematosus. Lupus. 2000;9:252–7.
12. Chang DM, Chang CC, Kuo SY, et al. Hormonal profiles and immunological studies of male lupus in Taiwan. Clin Rheumatol. 1999;18:158–62.
13. Murphy G, Isenberg D. Effect of gender on clinical presentation in systemic lupus erythematosus. Rheumatology. 2013;52(12):2108–15.
14. Mok C, Lau C, Chan TS, et al. Clinical characteristics and outcome of southern Chinese males with systemic lupus erythematosus. Lupus. 1999;8:188–96.
15. Renau AI, Isenberg DA. A comparison of ethnicity, clinical features, serology and outcome over 30 year period. Lupus. 2012;21:1041–8.
16. Andrade R, Alacon G, Fernandez M, et al. Accelerated damage accrual among men with systemic lupus erythematosus. Results from a multi centric US cohort. Arthritis Rheum. 2007;56:622–30.
17. Tan TC, Fang H, Magder L, et al. Differences between male and female systemic lupus erythe-

matosus in a multi centric population. J Rheumatol. 2012;39:759–69.

18. Tamir E, Brenner S. Gender differences in collagen diseases. Skinmed. 2003;2(2):113.

19. Durosaro O, Davis MDP, Reed KB, et al. Incidence of cutaneous lupus erythematosus, 1965-2005. A population-based study. Arch Dermatol. 2009; 145(3):249–53.

20. Jarukitsopa S, Hoganson D, Crowson C, Sokumbi O, Davis MD, et al. Epidemiology of systemic lupus erythematosus and cutaneous lupus in a predominantly white population in the United States. Arthritis Care Res. 2015;26(6):817–28.

21. Grönhagen CM, Fored CM, Granath F, Nyberg F. Cutaneous lupus erythematosus and the association with systemic lupus erythematosus. A population-based cohort of 1088 patients in Sweden. Br J Dermatol. 2011;164(6):1335–41.

22. Vera-Recabarren M, Garcia-Carasaco M, Ramos-Casals M, Herrero C. Cutaneous lupus erythematosus: clinical and immunological study of 308 patients stratified by gender. Clin Exp Dermatol. 2009;35:729–35.

23. Ramsey-Goldman R, Mattai SA, Schilling E, et al. Increased risk of malignancy in patients with systemic lupus erythematosus. J Investig Med. 1998;46:217–22.

24. Weyland CM, Scmidt D, Wagner U, et al. The influence of sex on the phenotype of rheumatoid arthritis. Arthritis Rheum. 1998;41:817–22.

25. Schuna AA. Autoimmune rheumatic diseases in women. J Am Pharm Assoc. 2002;42:612–24.

26. Roberts-Thomson PJ, Jones M, Hakendorf P, et al. Scleroderma in South Australia: epidemiological observations of possible pathogenic significance. Intern Med J. 2001;31:220–9.

27. Nashid M, Khanna PP, Furst DE, Clements PJ, et al. Gender and ethnicity differences in patients with diffuse systemic sclerosis - analysis from three large randomized clinical trials. Rheumatology. 2011;50(2):335–42.

28. Tjarlund A, Rider TA, Mille L, Werth FW, Pilkington P, de Visser CA, Elin MF. Ethnic but not gender differences in disease manifestations in dermatomyositis patients. Arthritis Rheum. 2011;63:235.

29. Wohl Y, Heyman R, Shemesh P, Brenner S. Dermatomyositis illustrating the gender gap: a retrospective analysis of a series. Cutis. 2008;82(2):137–9.

30. Brandt JE, Priori R, Valesini G, Fairweather D. Sex differences in Sjögren's syndrome: a comprehensive review of immune mechanisms. Biol Sex Differ. 2015;6:19.

Gender Differences in Psoriasis

Sivan Sheffer Levi and Yuval Ramot

7.1 Introduction

Psoriasis is a common chronic inflammatory immune-mediated skin disease, which is estimated to affect 2–4% of the population in Western countries [1–3]. It is characterized by increased proliferation and abnormal differentiation of keratinocytes, resulting in the psoriatic plaques. The pathogenesis is multi-factorial and only partially understood, with the immune system playing a key role [4]. Psoriasis has a significant negative impact on the patients' physical, emotional and psychosocial well-being [5], and imposes a high economic burden [6, 7].

There are interesting gender-specific differences in the epidemiology, severity, comorbidities and treatment adherence and utilization in psoriasis. These differences may stem from several complex mechanisms. A brief review on gender medicine and psoriasis was recently published and provided hints for the presence of sex differences in various aspects of the disease [8]. The differences may be influenced by changes in skin anatomy and physiology between the sexes, sex hormones, genetics and epigenetic effects, but may also be affected by social, cultural, ethnic and environmental factors. Despite the growing interest in gender medicine and the high prevalence of psoriasis, the available data connecting the two is sparse. This chapter will review the current literature regarding gender differences in various aspects of psoriasis and discuss possible explanations.

7.2 Epidemiology

7.2.1 Prevalence

In a large number of studies, equal prevalence of psoriasis among Caucasian males and females has been reported [9–13]. Nevertheless, several studies have shown differences between the genders. A retrospective population-based study from the United States, which examined trends in the incidence of adult-onset psoriasis between 1970 and 2000, showed that the overall age-adjusted incidence in males was higher than in females (85.5 vs. 73.2 per 100,000; p = 0.003), except for the sixth decade of life where a peak in incidence among females was observed (90.7 per 100,000) [14]. Male preponderance was also reported in other populations, including Mongoloids [15], Japanese [16], Chinese [17], Indians [18], Taiwanese [19] and Koreans [20]. In a study of elderly patients (60 years and older) with psoriasis in the Cote d'lvore (mostly black population), the sex ratio was 1.9 in favor of men [21]. In contrast, studies in Turkey and the Helsinki area demonstrated slightly higher prevalence of psoriasis in females [22, 23].

S. S. Levi · Y. Ramot (✉)
Department of Dermatology, Hadassah - Hebrew University Medical Center, Jerusalem, Israel
e-mail: yramot@gmail.com

© Springer International Publishing AG, part of Springer Nature 2018
E. Tur, H. I. Maibach (eds.), *Gender and Dermatology*,
https://doi.org/10.1007/978-3-319-72156-9_7

7.2.2 Age of Onset

Psoriasis may appear for the first time at any age, with two reported peaks: 15–20 and 55–60 years [5]. Information gained from several studies suggests that the age of psoriasis onset is lower in females than in males. This has been shown in women from different ethnicities, including Caucasian, Indian, Japanese and Korean [16, 20, 23, 24]. An interesting population-based historical cohort in Norwegian twins aged 19–31 years examined the occurrence of psoriasis by age and sex [25]. While no sex differences in the overall prevalence rates were found, a significantly higher point prevalence emerged in females in the teenage-year intervals. Additionally, a linear increase in incidence rates by every 4-year age-interval peaked at a lower age in females. The mean age at onset was also significantly lower in females (14.8 years) than in males (17.3 years). The absolute risk of developing psoriasis was higher for females across the entire age range but was minimized in the older age groups so that by the age of 31, the cumulative risk of developing psoriasis was almost similar in females and males.

These findings suggest a role for sex hormones in the pathogenesis of psoriasis, as females reach puberty at an earlier age than males. Additionally, a peak in incidence of adult-onset psoriasis among females in the sixth decade of life, which corresponds to the postmenopausal period, was demonstrated in the Olmsted County population-based study [14]. This may also be attributed to hormonal effects. Another possible explanation for sex differences in the age of onset of psoriasis is the existence of sex-specific genetic effects, as demonstrated by a differential association of HLA haplotypes according to sex [26, 27].

7.3 Pathogenesis

The pathogenesis of psoriasis is complex, and thought to be triggered by different environmental factors in genetically-predisposed individuals.

7.3.1 Genetics and Epigenetics

The fact that psoriasis has a strong genetic basis has been known for many years [28], based on epidemiological studies, including twin pairs and siblings studies [29–31]. Despite that, only about a third of psoriatic patients have an affected first-degree relative [32], suggesting that environmental factors play a strong role in its pathogenesis. The frequency of family history was reported to be only slightly higher in female patients (27%) than male patients (24%) in a Korean study [20], while other studies did not address this issue.

Several putative susceptible loci were identified through genome-wide-linkage scans with psoriasis susceptibility (PSOR) 1 being the most consistent [33]. It is located in the MHC region (chromosome 6p21.3), which contains the HLA genes. HLA-Cw6 was found to be the most relevant risk allele and demonstrated the highest relative risk for psoriasis in white populations as well as an earlier age of onset [34, 35]. In a study from Iceland, 369 psoriasis patients from 73 families were investigated in order to assess differences between Cw6-positive and Cw6-negative patients. Their finding confirmed previous reports of an earlier age of onset among Cw6-positive patients, but interestingly, also observed a gender difference. Cw6-positive females had an earlier disease onset than Cw6-positive males (p = 0.02), but such a difference was not observed for the Cw6-negative patients [36]. Differential association of HLA according to sex was demonstrated in two additional studies [26, 27], suggesting that an interaction between gender and immunogenetics participates in determining the susceptibility to psoriasis.

A non-Mendelian mode of transmission, referred to as genomic imprinting, has also been proposed for psoriasis [37]. This epigenetic effect causes differential gene expression depending on the sex of the transmitting parent. As an example for such an effect, the birth weight of children born to parents with psoriasis was found to be influenced by the sex of the psoriatic parent, with offsprings of psoriatic fathers weighing 270 g more than the offsprings of psoriatic mothers [38]. Another interesting parent-of-origin effect is a higher penetrance of psoriasis with an affected father than an affected mother, shown for both psoriasis and psoriatic arthritis [39, 40].

7.3.2   Triggering Factors

Psoriasis can be precipitated by multiple factors, both exogenous and endogenous. Exogenous factors include, for example, trauma (in the context of Koebner phenomenon), infections, drugs, smoking, alcohol consumption and psychogenic stress. Endogenous factors include allergies and hormonal effects. Several gender differences have been described with relation to the triggering factors in psoriasis.

7.3.2.1 Alcohol Consumption

Alcohol consumption was suggested as a triggering or precipitating factor for psoriasis, although the relation between the two remains controversial. A number of studies support the role of ethanol and its metabolites as triggering factors of psoriasis and a drinking habit appears to exacerbate a preexisting psoriasis. The magnitude of alcohol consumption may be related to both higher incidence and greater severity of psoriasis [41].

Since drinking habits are different between men and women due to social, cultural and environmental effects, the effect of alcohol on psoriasis may be influenced by gender. Nevertheless, controversial data exist regarding the effect of gender on this trigger.

An Italian multicenter case–control study pointed to a moderate association with alcohol misuse in psoriatic men, but this association was not significant in psoriatic women [42]. In a more recent multicenter study from Germany, involving 1203 in-patients with different subtypes of psoriasis, disease severity correlated with alcohol consumption only in female patients [43]. Similar findings were found in a small Swedish study. The authors concluded that females might be more prone to alcohol-induced exacerbation of psoriasis [44]. Another study investigated the effect of alcohol on treatment outcome and showed a less favorable response to treatment in

male, but not female, patients who consumed more than 80 g of ethanol per day [45].

A tendency for patients, especially women with psoriasis, to drink more following diagnosis, which probably reflects the negative impact of psoriasis on lifestyle was also suggested [46]. Differences between the male and female immune system, with different responses to alcohol intake, may be responsible in part for the above-mentioned gender differences.

7.3.2.2 Smoking

Smoking is a well-established environmental risk factor for psoriasis. There is a positive association between smoking and psoriasis prevalence and severity [47].

A combined analysis from the United States highlighted the role of smoking as an independent risk factor for psoriasis in both men and women [48]. In a meta-analysis of case-control studies published in 2011, strong evidence of a positive association between smoking and the risk of psoriasis was observed, and gender did not seem to markedly influence the results. However, a stronger association in women is suspected according to a number of studies. Smoking was found to be associated with clinical severity of psoriasis in a hospital-based cross-sectional study from Italy [49]. Separate analyses for men and women showed that the effect of cigarette-years on psoriasis severity was stronger for women than for men. The results were consistent with previous studies that showed increased risk of psoriasis in women, but not in men [50, 51]. Another Italian, multi-center, case-control study involving 318 men and 242 women with newly diagnosed psoriasis and 690 controls reported that while there was a significant association for male past smokers but not females, for current smokers, the risk was higher in women than in men [52]. An earlier Italian study also showed that the relation with smoking was stronger and more consistent among women when compared to men. Also in this study, a significant association was restricted to the ex-smoker status in men [42].

On the other hand, other studies identified a stronger association in men. A Chinese study showed that smoking is a risk factor for psoriasis only among men [53]. A Polish study examined the association between smoking and the metabolic syndrome in psoriasis patients aged 30–49 years. The authors reported that patients with psoriasis are more likely to be smokers and the frequency of smoking in men is approximately 25% higher than in men from the control group. A statistically significant difference was not found among women [54].

In conclusion, there is some disagreement with regard to gender, but overall the association between smoking and psoriasis seems stronger in women.

7.3.2.3 Psychogenic Stress

Influence of stressful life events on psoriasis onset and exacerbation has been suspected for a long time with some controversy found in the literature. Most studies, though, support the role of psychogenic factors as an important risk factor [55–60]. In regards to gender differences, the association seems to be more evident for women.

In an Italian case-control study, an association emerged between psoriasis and stressful life events in the year preceding the diagnosis. When men and women were considered separately, the trend in risk was evident only for women [52]. In a case-control study from Romania, women with psoriasis vulgaris and men with guttate psoriasis seemed to be more sensitive to stress [61]. A retrospective study from Italy examined the role of family stress events in psoriatic patients. Women reported higher values in the scales assessing anxiety and depression than men [62].

7.3.2.4 Hormones

Several hormones have been suggested to play a role in the pathogenesis of psoriasis, with sex hormones and prolactin being the major candidates [63], mandating gender differences. The role of sex hormones is implicated from their influence on the course of the disease with a peak during puberty, postpartum, and menopause, and improvement during pregnancy [64, 65]. Also the severity of psoriasis in female patients may fluctuate with hormonal changes [66]. A cross-sectional study from Turkey examined the sex hormone profile in male psoriasis patients and evaluated their correlation with the severity of psoriasis [67]. Their results showed significantly increased estradiol levels among psoriasis patients relative to controls and an inverse correlation with psoriasis severity. In addition, serum testosterone levels were significantly lower among psoriasis patients relative to control patients. The authors suggested a role for estrogen in the pathogenesis of psoriasis, potentially inhibiting inflammation and immunological activity at high doses. Sex-specific effects on the immune system have been reported [68, 69], and may explain the connection between sex hormones and psoriasis.

7.4 Clinical Characteristics

In general, there are no differences in lesion morphology between male and female patients with psoriasis [10]. Nevertheless, some reports indicate that the disease tends to be more severe in males than in females. For example, Na et al. reported that higher proportions of moderate (5–30% body involvement) and severe cases (>30% body involvement) were observed in male patients when compared to females (46% vs 43.5% and 17.4% vs 12.4%, respectively) [20], confirming previous reports [70]. The same study also showed that male patients seem to have moderate to severe disease activity more commonly when compared to female patients (56.1% vs 51.7%) [20].

Palmoplantar pustulosis (PPP), which is strongly associated with psoriasis and regarded by some authors as a variant of palmoplantar psoriasis [71], is characterized by the appearance of sterile pustules on the palms and soles. It is much more common in women than in men, with percentages varying between 64% and 92% [72–81]. In contrast to PPP, palmoplantar plaque psoriasis affects men and women equally [82].

Generalized pustular psoriasis (GPP) is a rare and severe variant of psoriasis, which can be life-threatening [83]. There is a clear female predominance in GPP, with most studies reporting a male:female ratio in the range of 0.70–0.77 [83–86]. A more recent study even showed a female to male ratio of 2:1 [87]. In children, however, it seems that there is no difference between males and females [88]. Only one small study reported a slight male predominance (61% males out of 34 patients) [89].

7.5   Psoriatic Arthritis

One of the more common comorbidities in psoriasis is psoriatic arthritis (PsA), affecting approximately 30% of the patients with psoriasis [90]. Classically, five types of PsA have been described: distal interphalangeal (DIP) arthritis, asymmetric oligoarthritis, polyarthritis, arthritis mutilans, and spondylitis [91]. Generally, PsA is thought to have an equal distribution between men and women [40, 92], a fact that has been documented in a large number of studies worldwide [93–96]. Nevertheless, there are several studies that showed male predominance [97–103]. Only a small number of studies reported women predominance of PsA [104, 105].

A recent large study compared the clinical and radiographic characteristics between males and females with PsA. This was a cross-sectional study evaluating 345 men and 245 women [106]. In this study, a positive family history, either for PsA or psoriasis, was reported more often in women than in men [106]. The same study also found that men tended to have a more severe axial disease than women. This finding was in agreement with previous, smaller studies [107, 108]. The more severe axial disease is accompanied by more severe radiographic damage to the peripheral joints and higher proportion of erosive disease in men than in women [106]. The pattern of arthritis at diagnosis was also different between men and women, as men had oligoarthritis as the main common pattern, while women presented more commonly with polyarticular involvement, a finding that was confirmed by a recent Spanish study [109].

Although the radiographic damage is more severe in men, women with PsA tend to have a worse quality of life, a higher degree of disability in daily function and more severe fatigue [106, 109–111]. The higher fatigue scores do not correlate with disease activity, but are rather related to physical limitations, mental dysfunction and fibromyalgia [111].

The underlying factors responsible for the gender differences in PsA are not entirely known. Possible factors include sex hormones, occupational activity and different treatment regimens between men and women [106]. Genetic factors are also thought to play a role, as a close correlation was found between male sex, HLA-B27 positivity and the risk for psoriatic spondyloarthropathy [112–114]. Nevertheless, the large study by Eder et al. did not find a difference between genders in HLA-B27 positivity, but rather a higher frequency of HLA-Cw6 in women compared to men. This finding was suggested to underlie the earlier onset of PsA that was also observed in women in this study [106].

Treatment of PsA is also affected by sex, and may be influenced by the different clinical manifestations between the genders. For example, disease modifying antirheumatic drugs (DMARDs), which are used more frequently for the polyarticular pattern of disease, were used more frequently in women [106]. Nevertheless, anti-tumor necrosis factor (TNF) agents were used comparably by men and women, although men had a higher proportion of an axial disease [106]. Retention rate is an indirect way to measure treatment efficacy. The retention rate of different treatment modalities between men and women with PsA was recently evaluated in a systematic literature review [115]. No difference was found in methotrexate retention rates between the sexes [116], but women demonstrated lower retention rates with anti-TNFs [117–120].

7.6   Comorbidities

Psoriasis does not involve only the skin and joints. Associated comorbidities include cardiovascular disease, diabetes, dyslipidemia, obesity, metabolic syndrome, nonalcoholic fatty liver, other immune mediated diseases such as Crohn's disease, and psychiatric disorders, mostly depression and anxiety [121]. According to the recently proposed concept of the psoriatic march, systemic inflammation results in insulin resistance and endothelial dysfunction, finally increasing the cardiovascular risk in psoriasis [122, 123].

There is paucity of information regarding gender-specific differences in comorbidities associated with psoriasis. In a few studies, different prevalence rates of comorbid conditions were demonstrated among men and women. Increased rates of osteoporosis [124], masked hypertension [125], hepatitis C infection [126, 127] and migratory glossitis [128] were reported in men and increased rates of metabolic syndrome [129–133], diabetes [134–136], obesity [134, 137–139] and psychological comorbidities [140–146] were reported in women. In addition, an increased risk of malignancies was demonstrated mostly in male patients [147–152]. Here we will provide more details regarding the differences between male and female psoriasis patients in the associated comorbidities.

7.6.1 Masked Hypertension

A study from Turkey investigated the prevalence of masked hypertension (normal office blood pressure with elevated ambulatory blood pressure) among psoriasis patients versus controls. The authors indicated that male sex was identified as an independent predictor for masked hypertension, together with waist circumference and diffuse psoriatic involvement [125].

7.6.2 Obesity

In a study of inpatients in Sweden, the association with obesity was considerably stronger in psoriatic women than men. Actually, no significant association was found in men alone [134]. A significant difference in body mass index (BMI) between patients with psoriasis and the same-gender full sibling control was seen for women, but not for men, in a study that was conducted in Texas [137]. A small study from Brazil indicated that women with psoriasis were more likely to have central obesity and dyslipidemia than men with psoriasis [138]. A hospital-based retrospective case-control

study from Japan reported an association between BMI and psoriasis that varied between men and women. The age brackets with significantly larger BMI were 40s to 70s for men and 20s, 30s and 70s for women. The BMI ratio was higher in women than in men, with the largest BMI ratio observed in women in their 30s. The authors of this study concluded that younger women were less likely to acquire psoriasis unless they had a high BMI, while men were more likely to develop psoriasis in middle or older age with a milder degree of obesity [139]. The relationship between obesity and psoriasis has been suggested to result from chronic inflammation, as adipose tissue is a source for pro-inflammatory mediators [153]. The gender differences may be partially explained by gender-related differences in body composition, body fat distribution and complex interactions with sex hormones.

7.6.3 Diabetes

Psoriasis was associated with diabetes only in female patients in a study from Sweden [134]. A cross-sectional study from India reported that within psoriatic patients, the prevalence of diabetes in women was significantly higher than in men, and concluded that psoriasis is a risk factor for diabetes, especially in women [135]. Another population-based, cross-sectional study from Israel assessed the association between PsA and diabetes. According to this study, female patients with PsA were more likely to be diagnosed with diabetes than age- and sex-matched patients without psoriasis. The association remained statistically significant after controlling for potential confounders, including obesity. An association between PsA and diabetes was not found among males [154]. However, other authors reported an association between psoriasis and diabetes, independent of age and gender [136].

7.6.4 Metabolic Syndrome

The metabolic syndrome is a cluster of common pathologies, including central obesity, dyslipidemia, hypertension and glucose intolerance, and is considered a strong predictor of cardiovascular disease. Its association with psoriasis has been reported by many studies [155–157], but inconclusive data exist regarding the influence of gender.

A population-based study from Norway showed that the association between psoriasis and the metabolic syndrome was influenced by age and sex. The strongest association was found in young women with almost fourfold increased odds [129]. Other studies from the United States and the United Kingdom also suggested a stronger association between psoriasis and the metabolic syndrome among women [130, 131]. A case-control Tunisian study reported a significantly higher prevalence of the metabolic syndrome only in psoriatic women, which was mainly attributed to decreased HDL-cholesterol and central obesity [132]. Additional studies from India and Turkey also supported higher prevalence of the metabolic syndrome in female psoriatic patients [133, 158]. However, other studies demonstrated that an association between metabolic syndrome and psoriasis exists without gender differences [155, 159–161].

7.6.5   Psychological Comorbidities

Many studies have indicated that women with psoriasis might incur a higher risk for psychological comorbidities than men. In an Italian cross-sectional study, the psychological status of women was found to be worse than that of men, independent from the extension of psoriasis. The authors concluded that female gender was the most important predictive factor for psychological distress in patients with psoriasis [140]. An Italian cross-sectional study reported that shame, worry and annoyance were more frequent in women than in men with psoriasis [141]. In a multi-center study from Spain, assessing the impact of psoriasis severity on mood and anxiety disorders, a sex-specific effect was noted; women were more likely to have anxiety and depression problems than men [142]. In a prospective study investigating the temperament profile of psoriasis patients in Tunisia, no significant differences were found between psoriasis patients and healthy controls. However, significant gender differences were noted, with women scoring higher in depressive and anxious temperaments [143]. In a study examining the prevalence of depression and anxiety in patients with PsA and psoriasis without PsA, female sex was associated with a higher likelihood of anxiety, but not depression [144].

In a case-control study from Poland, female gender was found to be an important risk factor for depressive symptoms. For women, the risk for depression was more than double than that for men. The extent of psoriasis was unrelated to the risk of depression in women, and was a statistically significant determinant, although weak, of depressive symptoms in men [145]. Female sex was found to be an independent risk factor for depression and insomnia in a nationwide cohort study from Taiwan [146].

7.6.6   Malignancies

Several studies have shown that patients with psoriasis have an increased risk of malignancy. Incident rates of various malignancies differed according to gender in different studies. A Danish follow-up study confirmed an increased risk of cancer in psoriasis patients, mainly due to skin and lung cancer in both sexes and cancer of the pharynx and larynx in men. Women exhibited the highest risk for basal cell carcinoma in the age range of 20–40 years, while men in the age range of 30–60 years had a particularly high risk for squamous cell carcinoma (SCC) [147].

In a Swedish cohort of patients treated with psoralen and ultraviolet A radiation (PUVA), comprising mostly psoriasis patients, an increased incidence of cutaneous SCC was found in both sexes with a relative risk of 5.6 in men and 3.6 in women. A significant increase was also noted in the incidence of respiratory cancer in both sexes and of kidney cancer in women [148]. In a cohort study from the United States, measuring the incidence of cancer in psoriatic patients, lymphoma and skin cancer risk was greater in men than in women [149]. Another population-based study using a large United Kingdom database found an increased overall risk of incident cancer (mainly lymphohematopoietic and pancreatic cancers) in psoriasis patients that was most prominent in males [150]. Two studies from Taiwan investigated the risk for cancer development in association with psoriasis. A retrospective population-based study reported a higher cancer risk in male patients. In this study, cutaneous malignant melanoma, lymphoma, leukemia, and cancers of the urinary bladder, lung, liver and gallbladder were significantly associated with male psoriatic patients, while colorectal cancer was associated with female patients [151]. The second study from Taiwan showed that the most common cancer was nonmelanoma skin cancer, which was more frequent in female patients [152].

7.6.7 Other Comorbidities

An association between psoriasis and osteoporosis was observed among males, but not females, in an Israeli population-based case-control study [124]. However, a population-based analysis from Taiwan found a significant association between osteoporosis and a previous diagnosis of psoriasis in both sexes [162].

An association between psoriasis and hepatitis C infection was reported recently in Japan, with a male predominance [126, 127]. Migratory glossitis among psoriasis patients was reported to be more prevalent in males compared to females [128].

7.7 Quality of Life

Psoriasis has a significant negative impact on patients' quality of life (QoL), comparable to other major illnesses, including diabetes, heart disease and cancer [5, 163, 164]. Means of measure such as the Dermatology Life Quality Index (DLQI) and non-specific QoL scales are widely used to assess the severity of this aspect of the disease. The role of gender is inconclusive and controversial data have been published over the years. Most studies found a relation between

female gender and a poorer QoL or health-related quality of life (HRQoL) [165–174], while others found no gender differences [175–177] or even greater impact in male patients [178, 179]. We will present a short review of the main studies on the subject in a chronological order.

In an early report, male gender was associated with lower psychosocial morbidity. The authors discuss that society tends to place a lesser importance on the appearance of men than women lessening the psychosocial morbidity resulting from the effect of psoriasis upon appearance and socialization [165]. In 1995, Gupta et al. reported a greater work-related stress among male patients with psoriasis, but no gender differences in regards to stigmatization. The authors proposed that social norms have changed over the years, with impact of appearance becoming equally important for both sexes [178].

In a large follow up cohort of psoriasis patients previously treated with PUVA in 16 centers in the United States, women were more likely than men to report impairment in QoL dimensions [166]. In a study investigating psoriasis-related QoL in a large cohort of Nordic psoriasis patients, gender was not found to be a predictor of QoL. However, women generally reported greater disease severity and affected area than men, while men had greater Psoriasis Assessment Severity Index (PASI) scores than women. In addition, women experienced more disease-related stressful events than men. Another interesting finding was a significant interaction between sex and marital status. Although both men and women living alone scored higher in scales measuring the impact of psoriasis on aspects of daily living and subjective stress related to psoriasis than married men and women, the differences were greater for men than for women [175]. Another study from the United States describing the determinants of QoL in patients with psoriasis reported that the extent of skin involvement had the strongest association with decrement in QoL, but younger patients and female patients had also statistically significant reductions. Female patients had greater impairment in QoL than male patients, despite having a similar self-reported extent of psoriasis [167].

In 2004, a systematic literature review on QoL in patients with psoriasis was published by De Korte. A total of 17 studies were included with eight of them presenting data on the relationship between age, sex, and QoL and/or disability. Associations between sex and QoL and/or disability were very weak, inconsistent, or absent. Few correlation coefficients were presented, all being very low (0.00–0.15). The authors concluded that sex and QoL were unrelated [176].

A German study focusing on the stigmatization experience in psoriasis patients reported a significantly more intensive feeling of discrimination in women than in men, but only in men the somatic course of the psoriasis had a significant influence on their stigmatization experience [180].

A hospital-based study from Italy investigated the impairment in QoL in psoriasis patients according to age, gender, psychosocial distress, disease severity and duration. Women had consistently worse QoL than men, especially older women with anxiety or depression. The authors discussed the difference to be due to gender differences in body image and investment in appearance [168]. A study from Japan also reported a worse QoL in female patients and concluded that QoL assessment may play a greater role in females than in males, when assessing the severity of psoriasis [181]. A study from Germany explored the relationship between gender (among other factors) and QoL in psoriasis patients. They reported no differences in the perceptions of symptom severity between men and women, but women reported a higher discomfort level, a higher reduction in self-esteem, and felt less able to maintain composure in social situations. The different experience of stigmatization between genders did not seem to alter the ultimate difference for QoL. The authors concluded that women bear a higher psychosocial burden, including lower mental health, because of psoriasis [182].

In contrary, a Polish study demonstrated no gender difference in terms of HRQoL and optimism among psoriatic patients. Both men and women declared comparable levels of the psychological variables [177].

A cross-sectional observational study from Spain aiming to establish a correlation between HRQoL and associated comorbidities in psoriasis found that women were more affected in the mental health component than men [183]. In a study from the United States assessing the relationship between psoriasis severity and QoL using the Short Form-12 (SF-12) (a shorter version of the SF-36, a generic QoL instrument), men scored higher on both mental and physical components than women [169]. In a large sample study from Sweden women reported a significantly lower HRQoL than men, but men had more severe psoriasis (higher PASI) [184].

A multi-center study from Italy evaluated the impact of psoriasis on work-related problems via questionnaires. The authors reported that work limitations were strongly associated with female sex [185]. This was in contrast to the study by Gupta, previously mentioned. A potential explanation presented by the author was the fact that women have adopted a more important role with regard to socioeconomic status in Italy in recent years and the high importance given by the society to physical appearance of women.

A cross-sectional observational study from the Netherlands investigated the impact of fingernail psoriasis on patients' QoL using validated questionnaires. Fingernail disease is highly visible, presumably leading to a greater impact on QoL. Results revealed a greater impairment in QoL among women [170]. Similar results were obtained in other studies; a study from France using a new questionnaire specifically for nail psoriasis [171] and an epidemiologic study on nail psoriasis in Germany [172].

Female gender was found to be associated with a greater impairment of QoL in psoriasis patients in an observational study from Spain [173]. A study from Hungary reported that female gender was associated with a lower HRQoL but higher expectations regarding improvement and life expectancy [174]. A Greek study on QoL and psychosocial aspects in psoriasis patients showed no statistically significant differences in DLQI across gender, but female patients presented with lower self-esteem than male patients [186].

A recent review summarizing data from the European literature over the past 5 years regarding HRQoL in psoriasis patients mentioned eight publications in which the relationship between gender and HRQoL was studied. In six of them, women presented with poorer HRQoL compared with men and two did not find any correlation between gender and HRQoL [187].

A recent Polish study reported a significant difference in general QoL between psoriatic men and women. When testing for different dimensions of QoL (psychological, physical, environmental and social), a significant difference emerged only for the social life dimension, with a worse QoL declared by men [179].

Additional possible gender differences in psoriasis related to QoL include coping mechanisms and social support more utilized by women [188] and a greater sexual distress and sexual dysfunction experienced by women [189, 190].

7.8   Treatment

There are many options for the treatment of psoriasis, starting from topical medications, through phototherapy and traditional systemic medications, to the newer biologic drugs. These treatments allow symptom relief and control of clinical manifestations, but not cure. The choice of treatment depends on many variables, including disease severity, patients' characteristics, previous therapy and impact of the disease on patients' quality of life. Gender also plays a role in choosing the adequate treatment option, in part due to the teratogenic risk of some of the medications (e.g. methotrexate, retinoids).

In studies performed before the introduction of the biologic agents, some significant sex-specific differences were noted in the treatment of psoriasis. In a study from the United States, male patients were more likely to receive systemic treatments for severe psoriasis [191]. A questionnaire-based study assessing the treatment of psoriasis in 5739 Nordic patients, reported a higher rate of use of topical treatments among women and a higher rate of use of systemic treatments among men [192]. Other studies also demonstrated a higher proportion of psoriatic men receiving systemic treatments [193–196]. Possible explanations for the differences

include different disease severity, different treatment preferences, physician bias and the teratogenic potential of some of the systemic medications. A retrospective analysis from Sweden has shown substantial differences in the treatment costs for women and men with psoriasis, with men requesting more assistance in applying ointments and receiving a greater number of ultraviolet treatments. Women were more likely than men to administer self-care at home [194]. The authors assumed that gender differences in treatment compliance with self-care may be a contributing factor.

There are limited data regarding gender differences in treatment efficacy. A study from India comparing the outcomes of conventional drug therapy of plaque psoriasis found female sex to be negatively associated with response to treatment [197]. Phototherapy using narrow-band ultraviolet B (UVB) irradiation was shown to be more efficacious in female patients in another study [198]. A cross-sectional survey from the United States found that female patients were more likely to seek care or see a physician for their psoriasis compared with male patients [199].

Gender differences in the treatment of immune-mediated chronic inflammatory diseases were analyzed in an observational study from the Netherlands [200]. Patients' characteristics were analyzed at the start of systemic (biologic or non-biologic) treatment. Women with rheumatoid arthritis or psoriasis scored significantly higher than men on subjective, but not objective, disease activity measures. A similar trend was seen for patients with inflammatory bowel disease. This indicates that all three diseases have a greater effect on women than on men at the same level of treatment. These findings might suggest that in all three diseases, subjective measures are discounted to some extent in the therapeutic decision-making process, which could indicate under-treatment in female patients.

The biologic therapies have revolutionized the treatment of moderate to severe psoriasis. Many studies assessed the relationship between gender and response to biologic treatments. No association was found between gender and treatment outcomes in most studies [201–203], although some controversies exist. Male sex was associated with a diminished response to treatment with ustekinumab in a Spanish cohort study [204] but with a greater likelihood of response to anti-tumor necrosis factor α (TNFα) agents in a study from Italy [205]. Treatment with anti-TNFα agents for psoriasis was associated with a reduced risk of myocardial infarction, and gender did not significantly impact this effect [206]. A few studies showed that men were much more likely to receive biologic treatments than women [200, 202, 207, 208]. A population-based cohort study using data from a nationwide registry of psoriasis patients in Sweden concluded that the male dominance probably reflected the differing disease activity between the sexes, with men suffering from more severe disease [208].

Adherence to treatment and patients' satisfaction are important factors in psoriasis care due to its chronicity requiring a long-term approach. In a prospective study from England, adherence to topical and oral therapies for psoriasis was higher in women [209]. A gender perspective on patients' views on care and treatment for psoriasis was explored through questionnaires and interviews in the setting of an outpatient dermatology ward in Sweden [195]. The main results included a different gender-related approach to patient information and education, a different attitude towards greasing and less phototherapy treatments prescribed for women. Another report of a gender perspective on psoriasis care consumption and expectations reported differences in utilization of psoriasis care due to diversities in income and gender roles [210]. Men visited a dermatologist more often, while women visited a general practitioner and treated themselves topically more frequently. Adherence to treatment with the biologic agents (also referred to as 'drug survival') is becoming a popular outcome measure as an indicator for treatment success in psoriasis. It reflects a long-term therapeutic performance in a real-life setting. Biologic therapies seem to lose their efficacy over time, and many studies were performed to assess the predictors of drug survival. A consistent finding in many studies is that male patients treated with different biologic therapies (anti-TNF agents

and ustekinumab) show a longer drug survival compared to women [207, 211–215]. Female sex was found to be a consistent predictor for discontinuation of biologic therapies due to side effects in two studies from the Netherlands [213, 216]. A shorter drug survival in women treated with different biologic agents was also reported for psoriatic arthritis and rheumatoid arthritis [118, 119, 217–220]. The reasons for this trend are still unknown. A possible explanation is difference in compliance between males and females, but genetic or hormonal factors may also play a role. The observation across different indications and different biologic agents is in favor of a biological rather that psychological explanation.

Possible gender-related treatment safety profile concerns include a higher risk for hepatic damage from methotrexate or infliximab in female patients [221, 222], and a higher risk for weight gain with anti-TNFα treatment in male patients [223]. Also, the induction or exacerbation of psoriasis by anti-TNFα agents was described more frequently in females in some reports [224–227].

Conclusion

Despite the growing interest in gender medicine and the high prevalence of psoriasis, the information regarding the effect of gender on psoriasis is sparse and inconclusive. When reviewing the literature, some interesting gender-specific differences are highlighted as mentioned in this chapter. These differences may be influenced by an interplay between genetic predisposition, hormonal factors, environmental triggers and socio-cultural background. More research is warranted in order to explore the gender-specific characteristics in psoriasis and gather practical implications regarding prognosis and management.

References

1. Stern RS, Nijsten T, Feldman SR, Margolis DJ, Rolstad T. Psoriasis is common, carries a substantial burden even when not extensive, and is associated with widespread treatment dissatisfaction. J Investig Dermatol Symp Proc. 2004;9(2):136–9.

2. Gelfand JM, Weinstein R, Porter SB, Neimann AL, Berlin JA, Margolis DJ. Prevalence and treatment of psoriasis in the United Kingdom: a population-based study. Arch Dermatol. 2005;141(12):1537–41.

3. Kurd SK, Gelfand JM. The prevalence of previously diagnosed and undiagnosed psoriasis in US adults: results from NHANES 2003-2004. J Am Acad Dermatol. 2009;60(2):218–24.

4. Krueger J, Bowcock A. Psoriasis pathophysiology: current concepts of pathogenesis. Ann Rheum Dis. 2005;64(Suppl 2):ii30–6.

5. Langley RG, Krueger GG, Griffiths CE. Psoriasis: epidemiology, clinical features, and quality of life. Ann Rheum Dis. 2005;64(Suppl 2):ii18–23; discussion ii4-5.

6. Sander HM, Morris LF, Phillips CM, Harrison PE, Menter A. The annual cost of psoriasis. J Am Acad Dermatol. 1993;28(3):422–5.

7. Javitz HS, Ward MM, Farber E, Nail L, Vallow SG. The direct cost of care for psoriasis and psoriatic arthritis in the United States. J Am Acad Dermatol. 2002;46(6):850–60.

8. Colombo D, Cassano N, Bellia G, Vena GA. Gender medicine and psoriasis. World J Dermatol. 2014;3(3):36–44.

9. Christophers E. Psoriasis: epidemiology and clinical spectrum. Clin Exp Dermatol. 2001;26(4):314–20.

10. Gudjonsson JE, Elder JT. Psoriasis: epidemiology. Clin Dermatol. 2007;25(6):535–46.

11. Farber EM, Nall L. Epidemiology in psoriasis research. Hawaii Med J. 1982;41(11):430–42.

12. Tollefson MM, Crowson CS, McEvoy MT, Kremers HM. Incidence of psoriasis in children: a population-based study. J Am Acad Dermatol. 2010;62(6):979–87.

13. Bell LM, Sedlack R, Beard CM, Perry HO, Michet CJ, Kurland LT. Incidence of psoriasis in Rochester, Minn, 1980-1983. Arch Dermatol. 1991;127(8):1184–7.

14. Icen M, Crowson CS, McEvoy MT, Dann FJ, Gabriel SE, Kremers HM. Trends in incidence of adult-onset psoriasis over three decades: a population-based study. J Am Acad Dermatol. 2009;60(3):394–401.

15. Yip SY. The prevalence of psoriasis in the mongoloid race. J Am Acad Dermatol. 1984;10(6):965–8.

16. Takahashi H, Nakamura K, Kaneko F, Nakagawa H, Iizuka H. Analysis of psoriasis patients registered with the Japanese Society for Psoriasis Research from 2002-2008. J Dermatol. 2011;38(12):1125–9.

17. Zhang X, Wang H, Te-Shao H, Yang S, Chen S. The genetic epidemiology of psoriasis vulgaris in Chinese Han. Int J Dermatol. 2002;41(10):663–9.

18. Bedi TR. Psoriasis in North India. Geographical variations. Dermatologica. 1977;155(5):310–4.

19. Tsai TF, Wang TS, Hung ST, Tsai PI, Schenkel B, Zhang M, et al. Epidemiology and comorbidities of psoriasis patients in a national database in Taiwan. J Dermatol Sci. 2011;63(1):40–6.

20. Na SJ, Jo SJ, Youn JI. Clinical study on psoriasis patients for past 30 years (1982-2012) in Seoul National University Hospital Psoriasis Clinic. J Dermatol. 2013;40(9):731–5.

21. Kassi K, Djeha D, Gbery IP, Kouame K, Sangare A. Psoriasis in elderly patients in the Cote d'Ivoire: socio-demographic, clinical, and therapeutic aspects, and follow-up. Int J Dermatol. 2016;55(2):e83–6.

22. Könönen M, Torppa J, Lassus A. An epidemiological survey of psoriasis in the greater Helsinki area. Acta Derm Venereol Suppl. 1985;124:1–10.

23. Kundakci N, Tursen U, Babiker MO, Gurgey E. The evaluation of the sociodemographic and clinical features of Turkish psoriasis patients. Int J Dermatol. 2002;41(4):220–4.

24. Kaur I, Handa S, Kumar B. Natural history of psoriasis: a study from the Indian subcontinent. J Dermatol. 1997;24(4):230–4.

25. Olsen AO, Grjibovski A, Magnus P, Tambs K, Harris JR. Psoriasis in Norway as observed in a population-based Norwegian twin panel. Br J Dermatol. 2005;153(2):346–51.

26. Mallon E, Bunce M, Wojnarowska F, Welsh K. HLA-CW*0602 is a susceptibility factor in type I psoriasis, and evidence Ala-73 is increased in male type I psoriatics. J Invest Dermatol. 1997;109(2):183–6.

27. Kim TG, Lee HJ, Youn JI, Kim TY, Han H. The association of psoriasis with human leukocyte antigens in Korean population and the influence of age of onset and sex. J Invest Dermatol. 2000;114(2):309–13.

28. Hoede K. The problem of heredity of soriasis. Hautartz. 1957;8(10):433–8.

29. Lomholt G, Anna L. Psoriasis. Prevalence, spontaneous course, and genetics. A census study on the prevalence of skin diseases on the Faroe Islands (Translated by Anna la Cour) [A Thesis]. Copenhagen: G.E.C. Gad; 1963.

30. Hansen HE. Psoriasis in monozygotic twins: variations in expression in individuals with identical genetic constitution. Acta Derm Venereol. 1982;62:229–36.

31. Duffy D, Spelman L, Martin N. Psoriasis in Australian twins. J Am Acad Dermatol. 1993;29(3):428–34.

32. Farber E, Nall M. The natural history of psoriasis in 5,600 patients. Dermatology. 1974;148(1):1–18.

33. Sagoo GS, Cork MJ, Patel R, Tazi-Ahnini R. Genome-wide studies of psoriasis susceptibility loci: a review. J Dermatol Sci. 2004;35(3):171–9.

34. Tiilikainen A, Lassus A, Karvonen J, Vartiainen P, Julin M. Psoriasis and HLA-Cw6. Br J Dermatol. 1980;102(2):179–84.

35. Henseler T, Christophers E. Psoriasis of early and late onset: characterization of two types of psoriasis vulgaris. J Am Acad Dermatol. 1985;13(3):450–6.

36. Guðjónsson JE, Karason A, Antonsdottir AA, Rúnarsdottir EH, Gulcher JR, Stefansson K, et al. HLA-Cw6-positive and HLA-Cw6-negative patients with psoriasis vulgaris have distinct clinical features. J Invest Dermatol. 2002;118(2):362–5.

37. Nguyen CM, Liao W. Genomic imprinting in psoriasis and atopic dermatitis: a review. J Dermatol Sci. 2015;80(2):89–93.

38. Gelfand JM, Gladman DD, Mease PJ, Smith N, Margolis DJ, Nijsten T, et al. Epidemiology of psoriatic arthritis in the population of the United States. J Am Acad Dermatol. 2005;53(4):573.

39. Buntin DM, Skinner RB Jr, Rosenberg EW. Onset of psoriasis at age 108. J Am Acad Dermatol. 1983;9(2):276–7.

40. Shbeeb M, Uramoto KM, Gibson LE, O'Fallon WM, Gabriel SE. The epidemiology of psoriatic arthritis in Olmsted County, Minnesota, USA, 1982-1991. J Rheumatol. 2000;27(5):1247–50.

41. Cassano N, Vestita M, Apruzzi D, Vena GA. Alcohol, psoriasis, liver disease, and anti-psoriasis drugs. Int J Dermatol. 2011;50(11):1323–31.

42. Naldi L, Peli L, Parazzini F. Association of early-stage psoriasis with smoking and male alcohol consumption: evidence from an Italian case-control study. Arch Dermatol. 1999;135(12):1479–84.

43. Gerdes S, Zahl V, Weichenthal M, Mrowietz U. Smoking and alcohol intake in severely affected patients with psoriasis in Germany. Dermatology. 2009;220(1):38–43.

44. Zou L, Lonne-Rahm S-B, Helander A, Stokkeland K, Franck J, Nordlind K. Alcohol intake measured by phosphatidylethanol in blood and the lifetime drinking history interview are correlated with the extent of psoriasis. Dermatology. 2015;230(4):375–80.

45. Gupta MA, Schork NJ, Gupta AK, Ellis CN. Alcohol intake and treatment responsiveness of psoriasis: a prospective study. J Am Acad Dermatol. 1993;28(5):730–2.

46. Higgins E. Alcohol, smoking and psoriasis. Clin Exp Dermatol. 2000;25(2):107–10.

47. Richer V, Roubille C, Fleming P, Starnino T, McCourt C, McFarlane A, et al. Psoriasis and smoking a systematic literature review and meta-analysis with qualitative analysis of effect of smoking on psoriasis severity. J Cutan Med Surg. 2016. https://doi.org/10.1177/1203475415616073.

48. Li W, Han J, Choi HK, Qureshi AA. Smoking and risk of incident psoriasis among women and men in the United States: a combined analysis. Am J Epidemiol. 2012;175(5):402–13.

49. Fortes C, Mastroeni S, Leffondré K, Sampogna F, Melchi F, Mazzotti E, et al. Relationship between smoking and the clinical severity of psoriasis. Arch Dermatol. 2005;141(12):1580–4.

50. Poikolainen K, Reunala T, Karvonen J, Lauharanta J, Kärkkäinen P. Alcohol intake: a risk factor for psoriasis in young and middle aged men? Br Med J. 1990;300(6727):780–3.

51. Poikolainen K, Reunala T, Karvonen J. Smoking, alcohol and life events related to psoriasis among women. Br J Dermatol. 1994;130(4):473–7.

52. Naldi L, Chatenoud L, Linder D, Fortina AB, Peserico A, Virgili AR, et al. Cigarette smoking, body mass index, and stressful life events as risk factors for psoriasis: results from an Italian case–control study. J Invest Dermatol. 2005;125(1):61–7.

53. Nakanishi N, Takatorige T, Suzuki K. Cigarette smoking and the risk of the metabolic syndrome in middle-aged Japanese male office workers. Ind Health. 2005;43(2):295–301.

54. Owczarczyk-Saczonek AB, Nowicki R. The association between smoking and the prevalence of metabolic syndrome and its components in patients with psoriasis aged 30 to 49 years. Postepy Dermatol Alergol. 2015;32:331–6.

55. Naldi L. Epidemiology of psoriasis. Curr Drug Targets Inflamm Allergy. 2004;3(2):121–8.

56. Naldi L, Peli L, Parazzini F, Carrel CF, Psoriasis Study Group of the Italian Group for Epidemiological Research in Dermatology. Family history of psoriasis, stressful life events, and recent infectious disease are risk factors for a first episode of acute guttate psoriasis: results of a case-control study. J Am Acad Dermatol. 2001;44(3):433–8.

57. Seville R. Psoriasis and stress. Br J Dermatol. 1977;97(3):297–302.

58. Park BS, Youn JI. Factors influencing psoriasis: an analysis based upon the extent of involvement and clinical type. J Dermatol. 1998;25(2):97–102.

59. Picardi A, Mazzotti E, Gaetano P, Cattaruzza M, Baliva G, Melchi C, et al. Stress, social support, emotional regulation, and exacerbation of diffuse plaque psoriasis. Psychosomatics. 2005;46(6):556–64.

60. Gupta M, Gupta A, Grob J, Stern R, Mackie R, Weinstock W. Psychological factors and psoriasis. In: Epidemiology, causes and prevention of skin diseases. Oxford: Blackwell Science; 1997. p. 129–41.

61. Manolache L, Petrescu-Seceleanu D, Benea V. Life events involvement in psoriasis onset/recurrence. Int J Dermatol. 2010;49(6):636–41.

62. Campolmi E, Zanieri F, Santosuosso U, D'Erme A, Betti S, Lotti T, et al. The importance of stressful family events in psoriatic patients: a retrospective study. J Eur Acad Dermatol Venereol. 2012;26(10):1236–9.

63. Roman II, Constantin AM, Marina ME, Orasan RI. The role of hormones in the pathogenesis of psoriasis vulgaris. Clujul Med. 2016;89(1):11–8.

64. Murase JE, Chan KK, Garite TJ, Cooper DM, Weinstein GD. Hormonal effect on psoriasis in pregnancy and post partum. Arch Dermatol. 2005;141(5):601–6.

65. Wheeler D, Grandinetti L. Psoriasis: evolving treatment for a complex disease. Cleve Clin J Med. 2012;79(6):413.

66. Ceovic R, Mance M, Bukvic Mokos Z, Svetec M, Kostovic K, Stulhofer Buzina D. Psoriasis: female skin changes in various hormonal stages throughout life—puberty, pregnancy, and menopause. Biomed Res Int. 2013;2013:571912.

67. Cemil BC, Cengiz FP, Atas H, Ozturk G, Canpolat F. Sex hormones in male psoriasis patients and their correlation with the psoriasis area and severity index. J Dermatol. 2015;42(5):500–3.

68. Bouman A, Heineman MJ, Faas MM. Sex hormones and the immune response in humans. Hum Reprod Update. 2005;11(4):411–23.

69. Whitacre CC, Reingold SC, O'Looney PA, Blankenhorn E, Brinley F, Collier E, et al.

A gender gap in autoimmunity. Science. 1999;283(5406):1277–8.

70. Farber EM, Nall ML. The natural history of psoriasis in 5,600 patients. Dermatologica. 1974;148(1):1–18.

71. Farley E, Masrour S, McKey J, Menter A. Palmoplantar psoriasis: a phenotypical and clinical review with introduction of a new quality-of-life assessment tool. J Am Acad Dermatol. 2009;60(6):1024–31.

72. Asumalahti K, Ameen M, Suomela S, Hagforsen E, Michaelsson G, Evans J, et al. Genetic analysis of PSORS1 distinguishes guttate psoriasis and palmoplantar pustulosis. J Invest Dermatol. 2003;120(4):627–32.

73. de Waal AC, van de Kerkhof PC. Pustulosis palmoplantaris is a disease distinct from psoriasis. J Dermatol Treat. 2011;22(2):102–5.

74. Eriksson MO, Hagforsen E, Lundin IP, Michaelsson G. Palmoplantar pustulosis: a clinical and immunohistological study. Br J Dermatol. 1998;138(3):390–8.

75. Hellgren L, Mobacken H. Pustulosis palmaris et plantaris. Prevalence, clinical observations and prognosis. Acta Derm Venereol. 1971;51(4):284–8.

76. Brunasso AM, Puntoni M, Aberer W, Delfino C, Fancelli L, Massone C. Clinical and epidemiological comparison of patients affected by palmoplantar plaque psoriasis and palmoplantar pustulosis: a case series study. Br J Dermatol. 2013;168(6):1243–51.

77. Adisen E, Tekin O, Gulekon A, Gurer MA. A retrospective analysis of treatment responses of palmoplantar psoriasis in 114 patients. J Eur Acad Dermatol Venereol. 2009;23(7):814–9.

78. Enfors W, Molin L. Pustulosis palmaris et plantaris. A follow-up study of a ten-year material. Acta Derm Venereol. 1971;51(4):289–94.

79. Gimenez-Garcia R, Sanchez-Ramon S, Cuellar-Olmedo LA. Palmoplantar pustulosis: a clinico-epidemiological study. The relationship between tobacco use and thyroid function. J Eur Acad Dermatol Venereol. 2003;17(3):276–9.

80. Miot HA, Miot LD, Lopes PS, Haddad GR, Marques SA. Association between palmoplantar pustulosis and cigarette smoking in Brazil: a case-control study. J Eur Acad Dermatol Venereol. 2009;23(10):1173–7.

81. Michaelsson G, Kristjansson G, Pihl Lundin I, Hagforsen E. Palmoplantar pustulosis and gluten sensitivity: a study of serum antibodies against gliadin and tissue transglutaminase, the duodenal mucosa and effects of gluten-free diet. Br J Dermatol. 2007;156(4):659–66.

82. Kumar B, Saraswat A, Kaur I. Palmoplantar lesions in psoriasis: a study of 3065 patients. Acta Derm Venereol. 2002;82(3):192–5.

83. Baker H, Ryan TJ. Generalized pustular psoriasis. A clinical and epidemiological study of 104 cases. Br J Dermatol. 1968;80(12):771–93.

84. Augey F, Renaudier P, Nicolas JF. Generalized pustular psoriasis (Zumbusch): a French epidemiological survey. Eur J Dermatol. 2006;16(6):669–73.

85. Ohkawara A, Yasuda H, Kobayashi H, Inaba Y, Ogawa H, Hashimoto I, et al. Generalized pustular psoriasis in Japan: two distinct groups formed by differences in symptoms and genetic background. Acta Derm Venereol. 1996;76(1):68–71.

86. Tay YK, Tham SN. The profile and outcome of pustular psoriasis in Singapore: a report of 28 cases. Int J Dermatol. 1997;36(4):266–71.

87. Choon SE, Lai NM, Mohammad NA, Nanu NM, Tey KE, Chew SF. Clinical profile, morbidity, and outcome of adult-onset generalized pustular psoriasis: analysis of 102 cases seen in a tertiary hospital in Johor, Malaysia. Int J Dermatol. 2014;53(6):676–84.

88. Zelickson BD, Muller SA. Generalized pustular psoriasis in childhood. Report of thirteen cases. J Am Acad Dermatol. 1991;24(2 Pt 1):186–94.

89. Borges-Costa J, Silva R, Goncalves L, Filipe P, Soares de Almeida L, Marques Gomes M. Clinical and laboratory features in acute generalized pustular psoriasis: a retrospective study of 34 patients. Am J Clin Dermatol. 2011;12(4):271–6.

90. Ritchlin CT, Kavanaugh A, Gladman DD, Mease PJ, Helliwell P, Boehncke WH, et al. Treatment recommendations for psoriatic arthritis. Ann Rheum Dis. 2009;68(9):1387–94.

91. Moll JM, Wright V. Psoriatic arthritis. Semin Arthritis Rheum. 1973;3(1):55–78.

92. Gladman DD, Antoni C, Mease P, Clegg DO, Nash P. Psoriatic arthritis: epidemiology, clinical features, course, and outcome. Ann Rheum Dis. 2005;64(Suppl 2):ii14–7.

93. Jamshidi F, Bouzari N, Seirafi H, Farnaghi F, Firooz A. The prevalence of psoriatic arthritis in psoriatic patients in Tehran, Iran. Arch Iran Med. 2008;11(2):162–5.

94. Tam LS, Tomlinson B, Chu TT, Li M, Leung YY, Kwok LW, et al. Cardiovascular risk profile of patients with psoriatic arthritis compared to controls – the role of inflammation. Rheumatology. 2008;47(5):718–23.

95. Thumboo J, Tham SN, Tay YK, Chee T, Mow B, Chia HP, et al. Patterns of psoriatic arthritis in Orientals. J Rheumatol. 1997;24(10):1949–53.

96. Yamamoto T, Yokozeki H, Nishioka K. Clinical analysis of 21 patients with psoriasis arthropathy. J Dermatol. 2005;32(2):84–90.

97. Baek HJ, Yoo CD, Shin KC, Lee YJ, Kang SW, Lee EB, et al. Spondylitis is the most common pattern of psoriatic arthritis in Korea. Rheumatol Int. 2000;19(3):89–94.

98. Deesomchok U, Tumrasvin T. Clinical comparison of patients with ankylosing spondylitis, Reiter's syndrome and psoriatic arthritis. J Med Assoc Thail. 1993;76(2):61–70.

99. Elkayam O, Segal R, Caspi D. Human leukocyte antigen distribution in Israeli patients with psoriatic arthritis. Rheumatol Int. 2004;24(2):93–7.

100. Prasad PV, Bikku B, Kaviarasan PK, Senthilnathan A. A clinical study of psoriatic arthropathy. Indian J Dermatol Venereol Leprol. 2007;73(3):166–70.

101. Rajendran CP, Ledge SG, Rani KP, Madhavan R. Psoriatic arthritis. J Assoc Physicians India. 2003;51:1065–8.

102. Tsai YG, Chang DM, Kuo SY, Wang WM, Chen YC, Lai JH. Relationship between human lymphocyte antigen-B27 and clinical features of psoriatic arthritis. J Microbiol Immunol Infect. 2003;36(2):101–4.

103. Nossent JC, Gran JT. Epidemiological and clinical characteristics of psoriatic arthritis in northern Norway. Scand J Rheumatol. 2009;38(4):251–5.

104. Al-Awadhi AM, Hasan EA, Sharma PN, Haider MZ, Al-Saeid K. Angiotensin-converting enzyme gene polymorphism in patients with psoriatic arthritis. Rheumatol Int. 2007;27(12):1119–23.

105. Alenius GM, Jidell E, Nordmark L, Rantapaa Dahlqvist S. Disease manifestations and HLA antigens in psoriatic arthritis in northern Sweden. J Clin Rheumatol. 2002;21(5):357–62.

106. Eder L, Thavaneswaran A, Chandran V, Gladman DD. Gender difference in disease expression, radiographic damage and disability among patients with psoriatic arthritis. Ann Rheum Dis. 2013;72(4):578–82.

107. Gladman DD, Brubacher B, Buskila D, Langevitz P, Farewell VT. Psoriatic spondyloarthropathy in men and women: a clinical, radiographic, and HLA study. Clin Invest Med. 1992;15(4):371–5.

108. Queiro R, Sarasqueta C, Torre JC, Tinture T, Lopez-Lagunas I. Comparative analysis of psoriatic spondyloarthropathy between men and women. Rheumatol Int. 2001;21(2):66–8.

109. Queiro R, Tejon P, Coto P, Alonso S, Alperi M, Sarasqueta C, et al. Clinical differences between men and women with psoriatic arthritis: relevance of the analysis of genes and polymorphisms in the major histocompatibility complex region and of the age at onset of psoriasis. Clin Dev Immunol. 2013;2013:482691.

110. Husted JA, Tom BD, Farewell VT, Schentag CT, Gladman DD. A longitudinal study of the effect of disease activity and clinical damage on physical function over the course of psoriatic arthritis: does the effect change over time? Arthritis Rheum. 2007;56(3):840–9.

111. Husted JA, Tom BD, Schentag CT, Farewell VT, Gladman DD. Occurrence and correlates of fatigue in psoriatic arthritis. Ann Rheum Dis. 2009;68(10):1553–8.

112. Queiro R, Alperi M, Lopez A, Sarasqueta C, Riestra JL, Ballina J. Clinical expression, but not disease outcome, may vary according to age at disease onset in psoriatic spondylitis. Joint Bone Spine. 2008;75(5):544–7.

113. Queiro R, Sarasqueta C, Belzunegui J, Gonzalez C, Figueroa M, Torre-Alonso JC. Psoriatic spondyloarthropathy: a comparative study between HLA-B27 positive and HLA-B27 negative disease. Semin Arthritis Rheum. 2002;31(6):413–8.

114. Ruiz DG, Azevedo MN, Lupi O. HLA-B27 frequency in a group of patients with psoriatic arthritis. An Bras Dermatol. 2012;87(6):847–50.

115. Generali E, Scire CA, Cantarini L, Selmi C. Sex differences in the treatment of psoriatic arthritis: a systematic literature review. Isr Med Assoc J. 2016;18(3-4):203–8.

116. Lie E, van der Heijde D, Uhlig T, Heiberg MS, Koldingsnes W, Rodevand E, et al. Effectiveness and retention rates of methotrexate in psoriatic arthritis in comparison with methotrexate-treated patients with rheumatoid arthritis. Ann Rheum Dis. 2010;69(4):671–6.

117. Fabbroni M, Cantarini L, Caso F, Costa L, Pagano VA, Frediani B, et al. Drug retention rates and treatment discontinuation among anti-TNF-alpha agents in psoriatic arthritis and ankylosing spondylitis in clinical practice. Mediat Inflamm. 2014;2014:862969.

118. Glintborg B, Ostergaard M, Dreyer L, Krogh NS, Tarp U, Hansen MS, et al. Treatment response, drug survival, and predictors thereof in 764 patients with psoriatic arthritis treated with anti-tumor necrosis factor alpha therapy: results from the nationwide Danish DANBIO registry. Arthritis Rheum. 2011;63(2):382–90.

119. Glintborg B, Ostergaard M, Krogh NS, Andersen MD, Tarp U, Loft AG, et al. Clinical response, drug survival, and predictors thereof among 548 patients with psoriatic arthritis who switched tumor necrosis factor alpha inhibitor therapy: results from the Danish Nationwide DANBIO Registry. Arthritis Rheum. 2013;65(5):1213–23.

120. Heiberg MS, Koldingsnes W, Mikkelsen K, Rodevand E, Kaufmann C, Mowinckel P, et al. The comparative one-year performance of anti-tumor necrosis factor alpha drugs in patients with rheumatoid arthritis, psoriatic arthritis, and ankylosing spondylitis: results from a longitudinal, observational, multicenter study. Arthritis Rheum. 2008;59(2):234–40.

121. Kimball AB, Gladman D, Gelfand JM, Gordon K, Horn EJ, Korman NJ, et al. National Psoriasis Foundation clinical consensus on psoriasis comorbidities and recommendations for screening. J Am Acad Dermatol. 2008;58(6):1031–42.

122. Boehncke WH, Boehncke S, Tobin AM, Kirby B. The 'psoriatic march': a concept of how severe psoriasis may drive cardiovascular comorbidity. Exp Dermatol. 2011;20(4):303–7.

123. Davidovici BB, Sattar N, Jörg PC, Puig L, Emery P, Barker JN, et al. Psoriasis and systemic inflammatory diseases: potential mechanistic links between skin disease and co-morbid conditions. J Investig Dermatol. 2010;130(7):1785–96.

124. Dreiher J, Weitzman D, Cohen AD. Psoriasis and osteoporosis: a sex-specific association. J Invest Dermatol. 2009;129(7):1643–9.

125. Bacaksiz A, Erdogan E, Sonmez O, Sevgili E, Tasal A, Onsun N, et al. Ambulatory blood pressure monitoring can unmask hypertension in patients with psoriasis vulgaris. Med Sci Monit. 2013;19:501–9.

126. Imafuku S, Naito R, Nakayama J. Possible association of hepatitis C virus infection with late-onset

psoriasis: a hospital-based observational study. J Dermatol. 2013;40(10):813–8.

127. Imafuku S, Nakayama J. Profile of patients with psoriasis associated with hepatitis C virus infection. J Dermatol. 2013;40(6):428–33.

128. Singh S, Nivash S, Mann BK. Matched case-control study to examine association of psoriasis and migratory glossitis in India. Indian J Dermatol Venereol Leprol. 2013;79(1):59.

129. Danielsen K, Wilsgaard T, Olsen AO, Eggen AE, Olsen K, Cassano PA, et al. Elevated odds of metabolic syndrome in psoriasis: a population-based study of age and sex differences. Br J Dermatol. 2015;172(2):419–27.

130. Love TJ, Qureshi AA, Karlson EW, Gelfand JM, Choi HK. Prevalence of the metabolic syndrome in psoriasis: results from the National Health and Nutrition Examination Survey, 2003-2006. Arch Dermatol. 2011;147(4):419–24.

131. Langan SM, Seminara NM, Shin DB, Troxel AB, Kimmel SE, Mehta NN, et al. Prevalence of metabolic syndrome in patients with psoriasis: a population-based study in the United Kingdom. J Invest Dermatol. 2012;132(3):556–62.

132. Mebazaa A, El Asmi M, Zidi W, Zayani Y, Cheikh Rouhou R, El Ounifi S, et al. Metabolic syndrome in Tunisian psoriatic patients: prevalence and determinants. J Eur Acad Dermatol Venereol. 2011;25(6):705–9.

133. Lakshmi S, Nath AK, Udayashankar C. Metabolic syndrome in patients with psoriasis: a comparative study. Indian Dermatol Online J. 2014;5(2):132–7.

134. Lindegård B. Diseases associated with psoriasis in a general population of 159,200 middle-aged, urban, native Swedes. Dermatology. 1986;172(6):298–304.

135. Ghiasi M, Nouri M, Abbasi A, Hatami P, Abbasi MA, Nourijelyani K. Psoriasis and increased prevalence of hypertension and diabetes mellitus. Indian J Dermatol. 2011;56(5):533.

136. Cohen A, Dreiher J, Shapiro Y, Vidavsky L, Vardy D, Davidovici B, et al. Psoriasis and diabetes: a population-based cross-sectional study. J Eur Acad Dermatol Venereol. 2008;22(5):585–9.

137. Murray M, Bergstresser P, Adams-Huet B, Cohen J. Relationship of psoriasis severity to obesity using same-gender siblings as controls for obesity. Clin Exp Dermatol. 2009;34(2):140–4.

138. Santos M, Fonseca HM, Jalkh AP, Gomes GP, Cavalcante Ade S. Obesity and dyslipidemia in patients with psoriasis treated at a dermatologic clinic in Manaus. An Bras Dermatol. 2013;88(6):913–6.

139. Naito R, Imafuku S. Distinguishing features of body mass index and psoriasis in men and women in Japan: a hospital-based case-control study. J Dermatol. 2016;43:1406.

140. Finzi A, Colombo D, Caputo A, Andreassi L, Chimenti S, Vena G, et al. Psychological distress and coping strategies in patients with psoriasis: the PSYCHAE study. J Eur Acad Dermatol Venereol. 2007;21(9):1161–9.

141. Sampogna F, Tabolli S, Abeni D. Living with psoriasis: prevalence of shame, anger, worry, and problems in daily activities and social life. Acta Derm Venereol. 2012;92(3):299–303.

142. Pujol R, Puig L, Daudén E, Sánchez-Carazo J, Toribio J, Vanaclocha F, et al. Mental health self-assessment in patients with moderate to severe psoriasis: an observational, multicenter study of 1164 patients in Spain (the VACAP study). Actas Dermosifiliogr. 2013;104(10):897–903.

143. Litaiem N, Youssef S, Jabeur K, Dhaoui MR, Doss N. Affective temperament profile in psoriasis patients in Tunisia using TEMPS-A. J Affect Disord. 2013;151(1):321–4.

144. McDonough E, Ayearst R, Eder L, Chandran V, Rosen CF, Thavaneswaran A, et al. Depression and anxiety in psoriatic disease: prevalence and associated factors. J Rheumatol. 2014;41(5):887–96.

145. Wojtyna E, Lakuta P, Marcinkiewicz K, Bergler-Czop B, Brzezinska-Wcislo L. Gender, body image and social support: biopsychosocial deter-minants of depression among patients with psoriasis. Acta Derm Venereol. 2017;97:91.

146. Wu CY, Chang YT, Juan CK, Shen JL, Lin YP, Shieh JJ, et al. Depression and insomnia in patients with psoriasis and psoriatic arthritis taking tumor necrosis factor antagonists. Medicine (Baltimore). 2016;95(22):e3816.

147. Frentz G, Olsen J. Malignant tumours and psoriasis: a follow-up study. Br J Dermatol. 1999;140:237–42.

148. Lindelöf B, Sigurgeirsson B, Tegner E, Larkö O, Johannesson A, Ljunggren B, et al. PUVA and cancer risk: the Swedish follow-up study. Br J Dermatol. 1999;141:108–12.

149. Margolis D, Bilker W, Hennessy S, Vittorio C, Santanna J, Strom BL. The risk of malignancy associated with psoriasis. Arch Dermatol. 2001;137(6):778–83.

150. Brauchli YB, Jick SS, Miret M, Meier CR. Psoriasis and risk of incident cancer: an inception cohort study with a nested case–control analysis. J Invest Dermatol. 2009;129(11):2604–12.

151. Chen Y-J, Wu C-Y, Chen T-J, Shen J-L, Chu S-Y, Wang C-B, et al. The risk of cancer in patients with psoriasis: a population-based cohort study in Taiwan. J Am Acad Dermatol. 2011;65(1):84–91.

152. Lee MS, Lin RY, Chang YT, Lai MS. The risk of developing non-melanoma skin cancer, lymphoma and melanoma in patients with psoriasis in Taiwan: a 10-year, population-based cohort study. Int J Dermatol. 2012;51(12):1454–60.

153. Sterry W, Strober B, Menter A. Obesity in psoriasis: the metabolic, clinical and therapeutic implications. Report of an interdisciplinary conference and review. Br J Dermatol. 2007;157(4):649–55.

154. Dreiher J, Freud T, Cohen AD. Psoriatic arthritis and diabetes: a population-based cross-sectional study. Dermatol Res Pract. 2013;2013:580404.

155. Gisondi P, Tessari G, Conti A, Piaserico S, Schianchi S, Peserico A, et al. Prevalence of metabolic syndrome

in patients with psoriasis: a hospital-based case–control study. Br J Dermatol. 2007;157(1):68–73.

156. Sommer DM, Jenisch S, Suchan M, Christophers E, Weichenthal M. Increased prevalence of the metabolic syndrome in patients with moderate to severe psoriasis. Arch Dermatol Res. 2007;298(7):321–8.

157. Armstrong AW, Harskamp CT, Armstrong EJ. Psoriasis and metabolic syndrome: a systematic review and meta-analysis of observational studies. J Am Acad Dermatol. 2013;68(4):654–62.

158. Zindancı I, Albayrak O, Kavala M, Kocaturk E, Can B, Sudogan S, et al. Prevalence of metabolic syndrome in patients with psoriasis. Scientific World J. 2012;2012:1.

159. Meziane M, Kelati A, Najdi A, Berraho A, Nejjari C, Mernissi FZ. Metabolic syndrome in Moroccan patients with psoriasis. Int J Dermatol. 2015;55:396.

160. Nisa N, Qazi MA. Prevalence of metabolic syndrome in patients with psoriasis. Indian J Dermatol Venereol Leprol. 2010;76(6):662.

161. Kim G-W, Park H-J, Kim H-S, Kim S-H, Ko H-C, Kim B-S, et al. Analysis of cardiovascular risk factors and metabolic syndrome in Korean patients with psoriasis. Ann Dermatol. 2012;24(1):11–5.

162. Keller JJ, Kang J-H, Lin H-C. Association between osteoporosis and psoriasis: results from the Longitudinal Health Insurance Database in Taiwan. Osteoporos Int. 2013;24(6):1835–41.

163. Rapp SR, Feldman SR, Exum ML, Fleischer AB, Reboussin DM. Psoriasis causes as much disability as other major medical diseases. J Am Acad Dermatol. 1999;41(3):401–7.

164. Bhosle MJ, Kulkarni A, Feldman SR, Balkrishnan R. Quality of life in patients with psoriasis. Health Qual Life Outcomes. 2006;4(1):1.

165. Roenigk RK, Roenigk H Jr. Sex differences in the psychological effects of psoriasis. Cutis. 1978;21(4):529–33.

166. McKenna K, Stern R. The impact of psoriasis on the quality of life of patients from the 16-center PUVA follow-up cohort. J Am Acad Dermatol. 1997;36(3):388–94.

167. Gelfand JM, Feldman SR, Stern RS, Thomas J, Rolstad T, Margolis DJ. Determinants of quality of life in patients with psoriasis: a study from the US population. J Am Acad Dermatol. 2004;51(5):704–8.

168. Sampogna F, Chren M, Melchi C, Pasquini P, Tabolli S, Abeni D. Age, gender, quality of life and psychological distress in patients hospitalized with psoriasis. Br J Dermatol. 2006;154(2):325–31.

169. Grozdev I, Kast D, Cao L, Carlson D, Pujari P, Schmotzer B, et al. Physical and mental impact of psoriasis severity as measured by the compact Short Form-12 Health Survey (SF-12) quality of life tool. J Invest Dermatol. 2012;132(4):1111–6.

170. van der Velden HM, Klaassen KM, van de Kerkhof PC, Pasch MC. The impact of fingernail psoriasis on patients' health-related and disease-specific quality of life. Dermatology. 2014;229(2):76–82.

171. Ortonne J, Baran R, Corvest M, Schmitt C, Voisard J, Taieb C. Development and validation of nail psoriasis quality of life scale (NPQ10). J Eur Acad Dermatol Venereol. 2010;24(1):22–7.

172. Augustin M, Reich K, Blome C, Schäfer I, Laass A, Radtke M. Nail psoriasis in Germany: epidemiology and burden of disease. Br J Dermatol. 2010;163(3):580–5.

173. Fernandez-Torres RM, Pita-Fernandez S, Fonseca E. Quality of life and related factors in a cohort of plaque-type psoriasis patients in La Coruna, Spain. Int J Dermatol. 2014;53(11):e507–11.

174. Rencz F, Holló P, Kárpáti S, Péntek M, Remenyik É, Szegedi A, et al. Moderate to severe psoriasis patients' subjective future expectations regarding health-related quality of life and longevity. J Eur Acad Dermatol Venereol. 2015;29(7):1398–405.

175. Zachariae R, Zachariae H, Blomqvist K, Davidsson S, Molin L, Mørk C, et al. Quality of life in 6497 Nordic patients with psoriasis. Br J Dermatol. 2002;146(6):1006–16.

176. De Korte J, Mombers FM, Bos JD, Sprangers MA. Quality of life in patients with psoriasis: a systematic literature review. J Investig Dermatol Symp Proc. 2004;9:140.

177. Miniszewska J, Chodkiewicz J, Ograczyk A, Zalewska-Janowska A. Optimism as a predictor of health-related quality of life in psoriatics. Postepy Dermatol Alergol. 2013;30:91.

178. Gupta MA, Gupta AK. Age and gender differences in the impact of psoriasis on quality of life. Int J Dermatol. 1995;34(10):700–3.

179. Owczarek K, Jaworski M. Quality of life and severity of skin changes in the dynamics of psoriasis. Postepy Dermatol Alergol. 2016;33(2):102–8.

180. Schmid-Ott G, Kunsebeck H-W, Jager B, Sittig U, Hofste N, Ott R, et al. Significance of the stigmatization experience of psoriasis patients: a 1-year follow-up of the illness and its psychosocial consequences in men and women. Acta Derm Venereol. 2005;85(1):27–32.

181. Mabuchi T, Yamaoka H, Kojima T, Ikoma N, Akasaka E, Ozawa A. Psoriasis affects patient's quality of life more seriously in female than in male in Japan. Tokai J Exp Clin Med. 2012;37(3):84–8.

182. Bohm D, Stock Gissendanner S, Bangemann K, Snitjer I, Werfel T, Weyergraf A, et al. Perceived relationships between severity of psoriasis symptoms, gender, stigmatization and quality of life. J Eur Acad Dermatol Venereol. 2013;27(2):220–6.

183. Sanchez-Carazo JL, Lopez-Estebaranz JL, Guisado C. Comorbidities and health-related quality of life in Spanish patients with moderate to severe psoriasis: a cross-sectional study (Arizona study). J Dermatol. 2014;41(8):673–8.

184. Norlin JM, Steen Carlsson K, Persson U, Schmitt-Egenolf M. Analysis of three outcome measures in moderate to severe psoriasis: a registry-based study of 2450 patients. Br J Dermatol. 2012;166(4):797–802.

185. Ayala F, Sampogna F, Romano GV, Merolla R, Guida G, Gualberti G, et al. The impact of psoriasis on work-related problems: a multicenter

cross-sectional survey. J Eur Acad Dermatol Venereol. 2014;28(12):1623–32.

186. Kouris A, Christodoulou C, Stefanaki C, Livaditis M, Tsatovidou R, Kouskoukis C, et al. Quality of life and psychosocial aspects in Greek patients with psoriasis: a cross-sectional study. An Bras Dermatol. 2015;90(6):841–5.

187. Obradors M, Blanch C, Comellas M, Figueras M, Lizan L. Health-related quality of life in patients with psoriasis: a systematic review of the European literature. Qual Life Res. 2016;25:2739.

188. Žarković Palijan T, Kovačević D, Koić E, Ružić K, Dervinja F. The impact of psoriasis on the quality of life and psychological characteristics of persons suffering from psoriasis. Coll Antropol. 2011;35(2):81–5.

189. Meeuwis K, De Hullu J, Van de Nieuwenhof H, Evers A, Massuger L, Van de Kerkhof P, et al. Quality of life and sexual health in patients with genital psoriasis. Br J Dermatol. 2011;164(6):1247–55.

190. Türel Ermertcan A, Temeltaş G, Deveci A, Dinç G, Gueler HB, Öztürkcan S. Sexual dysfunction in patients with psoriasis. J Dermatol. 2006;33(11):772–8.

191. Hotard RS, Feldman SR, Fleischer AB. Sex-specific differences in the treatment of severe psoriasis. J Am Acad Dermatol. 2000;42(4):620–3.

192. Zachariae H, Zachariae R, Blomqvist K, Davidsson S, Molin L, Mørk C, et al. Treatment of psoriasis in the nordic countries: a questionnaire survey from 5739 members of the psoriasis associations. Acta Derm Venereol. 2001;81:116–21.

193. White D, O'Shea S, Rogers S. Do men have more severe psoriasis than women? J Eur Acad Dermatol Venereol. 2012;26(1):126–7.

194. Nyberg F, Osika I, Evengård B. "The Laundry Bag Project"–unequal distribution of dermatological healthcare resources for male and female psoriatic patients in Sweden. Int J Dermatol. 2008;47(2):144–9.

195. Waernulf L, Moberg C, Henriksson EW, Evengard B, Nyberg F. Patients' views on care and treatment after phototherapy for psoriasis and atopic eczema including a gender perspective. J Dermatolog Treat. 2008;19(4):233–40.

196. Ormerod A, Augustin M, Baker C, Chosidow O, Cohen A, Dam T, et al. Challenges for synthesising data in a network of registries for systemic psoriasis therapies. Dermatology. 2012;224(3):236–43.

197. Gupta AK, Pandey SS, Pandey BL. Effectiveness of conventional drug therapy of plaque psoriasis in the context of consensus guidelines: a prospective observational study in 150 patients. Ann Dermatol. 2013;25(2):156–62.

198. Al Robaee AA. The usefulness of narrowband UVB as a monotherapy for the treatment of chronic plaque psoriasis. J Drugs Dermatol. 2010;9(8):989–91.

199. Bhutani T, Wong JW, Bebo BF, Armstrong AW. Access to health care in patients with psoriasis and psoriatic arthritis: data from National Psoriasis Foundation survey panels. JAMA Dermatol. 2013;149(6):717–21.

200. Lesuis N, Befrits R, Nyberg F, van Vollenhoven RF. Gender and the treatment of immune-mediated chronic inflammatory diseases: rheumatoid arthritis, inflammatory bowel disease and psoriasis: an observational study. BMC Med. 2012;10:82.

201. Edson-Heredia E, Sterling KL, Alatorre CI, Cuyun Carter G, Paczkowski R, Zarotsky V, et al. Heterogeneity of response to biologic treatment: perspective for psoriasis. J Invest Dermatol. 2014;134(1):18–23.

202. Salah LA, Gillstedt M, Osmancevic A. A retrospective study of patients with psoriasis treated with biologics: relation to body mass index and gender. Acta Derm Venereol. 2016;96:974.

203. Giunta A, Babino G, Manetta S, Mazzotta A, Chimenti S, Esposito M. Clinical markers predictive of primary inefficacy: a "real life" retrospective study in psoriatic patients treated with etanercept. Drug Dev Res. 2014;75(Suppl 1):S27–30.

204. Puig L, Ruiz-Salas V. Long-term efficacy, safety and drug survival of ustekinumab in a Spanish cohort of patients with moderate to severe plaque psoriasis. Dermatology. 2015;230(1):46–54.

205. De Simone C, Caldarola G, Maiorino A, Tassone F, Campana I, Sollena P, et al. Clinical predictors of nonresponse to anti-TNF-alpha agents in psoriatic patients: a retrospective study. Dermatol Ther. 2016;29:372.

206. Wu JJ, Poon KY. Association of gender, tumor necrosis factor inhibitor therapy, and myocardial infarction risk in patients with psoriasis. J Am Acad Dermatol. 2013;69(4):650–1.

207. Gniadecki R, Kragballe K, Dam T, Skov L. Comparison of drug survival rates for adalimumab, etanercept and infliximab in patients with psoriasis vulgaris. Br J Dermatol. 2011;164(5):1091–6.

208. Hagg D, Eriksson M, Sundstrom A, Schmitt-Egenolf M. The higher proportion of men with psoriasis treated with biologics may be explained by more severe disease in men. PLoS One. 2013;8(5):e63619.

209. Zaghloul SS, Goodfield MJD. Objective assessment of compliance with psoriasis treatment. Arch Dermatol. 2004;140(4):408–14.

210. Uttjek M, Dufaker M, Nygren L, Stenberg B. Psoriasis care consumption and expectations from a gender perspective in a psoriasis population in northern Sweden. Acta Derm Venereol. 2005;85(6):503–8.

211. Esposito M, Gisondi P, Cassano N, Ferrucci G, Del Giglio M, Loconsole F, et al. Survival rate of antitumour necrosis factor-alpha treatments for psoriasis in routine dermatological practice: a multicentre observational study. Br J Dermatol. 2013;169(3):666–72.

212. van den Reek JM, van Lumig PP, Driessen RJ, van de Kerkhof PC, Seyger MM, Kievit W, et al. Determinants of drug survival for etanercept in a

long-term daily practice cohort of patients with psoriasis. Br J Dermatol. 2014;170(2):415–24.

213. van den Reek JM, Tummers M, Zweegers J, Seyger MM, van Lumig PP, Driessen RJ, et al. Predictors of adalimumab drug survival in psoriasis differ by reason for discontinuation: long-term results from the Bio-CAPTURE registry. J Eur Acad Dermatol Venereol. 2015;29(3):560–5.

214. Gniadecki R, Bang B, Bryld L, Iversen L, Lasthein S, Skov L. Comparison of long-term drug survival and safety of biologic agents in patients with psoriasis vulgaris. Br J Dermatol. 2015;172(1):244–52.

215. Warren RB, Smith CH, Yiu ZZ, Ashcroft DM, Barker JN, Burden AD, et al. Differential drug survival of biologic therapies for the treatment of psoriasis: a prospective observational cohort study from the British Association of Dermatologists Biologic Interventions Register (BADBIR). J Invest Dermatol. 2015;135(11):2632–40.

216. Zweegers J, van den Reek JM, van de Kerkhof PC, Otero ME, Kuijpers AL, Koetsier MI, et al. Body mass index predicts discontinuation due to ineffectiveness and female sex predicts discontinuation due to side-effects in psoriasis patients treated with adalimumab, etanercept or ustekinumab in daily practice. A prospective, comparative, long-term drug survival study from the BioCAPTURE registry. Br J Dermatol. 2016;175:340.

217. Hetland ML, Christensen IJ, Tarp U, Dreyer L, Hansen A, Hansen IT, et al. Direct comparison of treatment responses, remission rates, and drug adherence in patients with rheumatoid arthritis treated with adalimumab, etanercept, or infliximab: results from eight years of surveillance of clinical practice in the nationwide Danish DANBIO registry. Arthritis Rheum. 2010;62(1):22–32.

218. Saad AA, Ashcroft DM, Watson KD, Hyrich KL, Noyce PR, Symmons DP. Persistence with anti-tumour necrosis factor therapies in patients with psoriatic arthritis: observational study from the British Society of Rheumatology Biologics Register. Arthritis Res Ther. 2009;11(2):1.

219. Iannone F, Lopriore S, Bucci R, Scioscia C, Anelli MG, Notarnicola A, et al. Two-year survival rates of anti-TNF-alpha therapy in psoriatic arthritis (PsA) patients with either polyarticular or oligoarticular PsA. Scand J Rheumatol. 2015;44(3):192–9.

220. Generali E. Sex differences in the treatment of psoriatic arthritis: a systematic literature review. Isr Med Assoc J. 2016;18:203.

221. Amital H, Arnson Y, Chodick G, Shalev V. Hepatotoxicity rates do not differ in patients with rheumatoid arthritis and psoriasis treated with methotrexate. Rheumatology. 2009;48(9):1107–10.

222. Mancini S, Amorotti E, Vecchio S, de Leon MP, Roncucci L. Infliximab-related hepatitis: discussion of a case and review of the literature. Intern Emerg Med. 2010;5(3):193–200.

223. Mahé E, Reguiai Z, Barthelemy H, Quiles-Tsimaratos N, Chaby G, Girard C, et al. Evaluation of risk factors for body weight increment in psoriatic patients on infliximab: a multicentre, cross-sectional study. J Eur Acad Dermatol Venereol. 2014;28(2):151–9.

224. Wollina U, Hansel G, Koch A, Schönlebe J, Köstler E, Haroske G. Tumor necrosis factor-α inhibitor-induced psoriasis or psoriasiform exanthemata. Am J Clin Dermatol. 2008;9(1):1–14.

225. Ko JM, Gottlieb AB, Kerbleski JF. Induction and exacerbation of psoriasis with TNF-blockade therapy: a review and analysis of 127 cases. J Dermatol Treat. 2009;20(2):100–8.

226. Cullen G, Kroshinsky D, Cheifetz A, Korzenik J. Psoriasis associated with anti-tumour necrosis factor therapy in inflammatory bowel disease: a new series and a review of 120 cases from the literature. Aliment Pharmacol Ther. 2011;34(11–12):1318–27.

227. Shmidt E, Wetter DA, Ferguson SB, Pittelkow MR. Psoriasis and palmoplantar pustulosis associated with tumor necrosis factor-α inhibitors: the Mayo Clinic experience, 1998 to 2010. J Am Acad Dermatol. 2012;67(5):e179–e85.

Gender Dermatology: Pigmentation Disorders

8

Mor Pavlovsky

8.1 Introduction

The fact that men and women are genetically different goes without saying. How does this factor affect various aspects of skin pigmentation is an extensive area of study.

The skin is one of the many organs capable of metabolizing hormones, and many of the sexual dimorphisms can be attributed to the effect of distinctive sexual milieus between the sexes.

But in addition to obvious hormonal differences, variations in environmental and occupational exposures might influence different skin characteristics between the two sexes, including skin tone.

Better understanding of gender differences in skin pigmentation can shed a new light on the pathogenesis of pigmentation disorders and aid in discovering of more effective treatments.

This chapter will focus on gender influence on skin pigmentation in health and disease.

8.2 Gender Differences in Health

8.2.1 Melanocyte Biology and Melanogenesis

The melanocyte is a neural crest-derived cell, and during embryogenesis precursor cells (melanoblasts) migrate along a dorsolateral pathway via the mesenchyme to reach the epidermis and hair follicles.

The major determinant of normal skin color is the activity of the melanocytes, i.e. the quantity and quality of pigment production, process known as melanogenesis.

Melanogenesis is influenced by the number of melanocytes in the basal layer of the epidermis, the size and number of melanosomes, melanin synthesis in the melanosomes, dendricity of the melanocytes, transport of melanosomes from melanocytes to keratinocytes, and proliferation and thickening of the epidermis and stratum corneum. There are a large number of melanogenic stimuli, including ultraviolet B [1], cAMP-elevating agents, such as melanocyte stimulating hormone (MSH) [2, 3], and estrogen [4].

Melanocytes express estrogen receptors (ER) [5] which are involved in estrogen induced melanogenesis, because the inhibition of ER by its antagonist leads to reduction in melanogenesis [6].

Estrogens are considered to stimulate melanogenesis in cultured human melanocytes by inducing synthesis of melanogenic enzymes such

M. Pavlovsky
Department of Dermatology, Tel Aviv Sourasky
Medical Center, Tel Aviv, Israel

© Springer International Publishing AG, part of Springer Nature 2018
E. Tur, H. I. Maibach (eds.), *Gender and Dermatology*,
https://doi.org/10.1007/978-3-319-72156-9_8

as tyrosinase, TRP-1, TRP-2, and MITF [6–8]. In addition, estrogen-induced melanogenesis could be associated with the activation of the cAMP-PKA pathway, because estrogens enhance cAMP levels and upregulation of tyrosinase and MITF attenuation by blocking the PKA pathway [7]. On the other hand there are evidence of inhibitory effect of progesterone on proliferation of human melanocytes, which may counteract the stimulatory effects of estrogen [9].

Androgens may also modulate tyrosinase activity at the posttranslational level through the cell membrane signaling pathway [10].

In summary, sex hormones play an important role in melanocyte homeostasis and melanogenesis and this may partially explain sexual dimorphism in skin color and pigmentary skin disease.

8.2.2   Skin Tone

Normal skin colour is determined by a number of chromophores, the most important of which is melanin. Besides melanin, haemoglobin (in both the oxygenated and reduced state) and carotenoids both contribute significantly to skin colour. Melanin is synthetized in melanocytes, dendritic cells located on the basal layer of the epidermis, each one injecting melanosomes into 24–36 keratinocytes. Melanocytes are differently distributed, varying from 17–8 per mm of histology section on the shoulders, to 12–7 per mm on legs and arms, to 3–2 per mm on the anterior part of the trunk [11]. No gender-linked difference has been reported for melanocyte distribution [12].

Two types of melanin pigmentation occur in humans. The first is constitutive skin colour, which is the amount of melanin pigmentation that is genetically determined in the absence of sun exposure. Constitutive pigmentation has been regarded classically as the colour of the buttock skin. Facultative skin colour is associated with exposure to sunlight, and denotes the pigmentation of exposed skin.

Studies from Iran [13], India [14], Korea [15] and Australia [16] have demonstrated women within individual ethnic group have lighter constitutive pigmentation than men. Men on the other hand have darker and less reflective complexions [17, 18].

It has been suggested that this is the consequence of men having a more vascularized upper dermis [19] and more melanin [13, 14]. These differences could have hormonal causes because they arise during puberty and also increase with age [20].

Men undergo a more intense facultative pigmentation after sun exposure and retain it for longer time than women [21] and women's skin lightens faster than men's skin [16].

8.3   Gender Differences in Disease

Pigmentation disorders include a large number of heterogeneous conditions that are usually characterized by altered melanocyte density, melanin concentration, or both, and result in altered pigmentation of the skin.

There are three categories of pigmentation abnormalities: hypopigmenatation, hyperpigmentations caused by accumulation of or a disorder of the distribution of normal pigment in the skin, and hyperpigmentations resulting from the abnormal presence in the skin of a pigment, originating either exogenously or endogenously [22].

Leukoderma and hypopigmentation are general terms used to designate disorders characterized by lightening of the skin. Hypomelanosis is a more specific term that denotes an absence or reduction of melanin within the skin; amelanosis signifies the total absence of melanin. Depigmentation usually implies a total loss of skin color, most commonly due to disappearance of preexisting melanin pigmentation, as in vitiligo.

In the following chapter, acquired pigmentation disorders that are not a manifestation of a known dermatologic condition will be addressed.

8.4   Vitiligo and Other Acquired Disorders of Hypopigmentation

8.4.1   Vitiligo

Vitiligo is an autoimmune disease [23] characterized by circumscribed depigmented macules and patches that result from a progressive loss of functional melanocytes. Three different forms are classified according to the distribution of lesions; namely non-segmental, segmental and mixed vitiligo.

Vitiligo affects approximately 0.5–2.0% of the general population worldwide and may appear at any age.

Although there is known "autoimmunity" predilection for women [24] and genome wide association studies have linked vitiligo to other autoimmune diseases [25], no female predominance was found in vitiligo prevalence in the literature [26, 27].

This might be explained by the multifactorial nature of this disease, with other nongenetic factors playing another important role in its pathogenesis.

In a cross-sectional analysis of clinicoepidemiological features of vitiligo performed in India, no significant differences between the mean ages of males and females was detected but males were found to have a longer duration of disease when seeking medical advice and were significantly more likely to report a positive family history of vitiligo [28].

Vitiligo is not life threatening or physically incapacitating, but it can considerably influence the psychological well-being of patients [29]. The quality of life impairment in women affected with vitiligo is greater than that in men with same disease severity [30, 31]. This discrepancy between the genders may be implicated in the different attributions that women and men give to health and illness. This also stands in line with the fact that women are more likely to seek medical help for cosmetic problems [32].

In summary, vitiligo is a disease that demonstrates that although no epidemiologic differences are found between the genders there is a great difference in disease interpretation that has a tremendous influence on quality of life.

8.4.2 Other Acquired Disorders of Hypopigmentation
(Table 8.1)

Table 8.1 Gender differences in other disorders of hypopigmentation

Disease	Gender related epidemiology
Post inflammatory hypopigmentation	There is no gender difference in the incidence [33]
Pityriasis alba	The role of sex in the incidence has not been established [34], although there is a tendency for male predominance [35]
Progressive macular hypomelanosis	A tendency toward female predominance. In some case series a 7:1 female-to-male ratio was noted [36]
Idiopathic guttate hypomelanosis	No gender preference [37]. Earlier age of onset in women [38]

8.5 Melasma and Other Acquired Disorders of Hyperpigmentation

8.5.1 Melasma

Melasma is a common acquired disorder characterized by symmetric, hyperpigmented irregular light to dark brown macules and patches on sun-exposed areas of the skin.

When talking about gender differences in dermatology, melasma is one of the first conditions to be discussed because of its much higher prevalence among women [39].

There are some features of melasma in men that seem to differ from those seen in women. These features will be the focus of the following discussion.

8.5.1.1 Epidemiology
In women, the overall prevalence of melasma varies by geography and population between 1.5% and 33.3% [40, 41]. While there is a considerable amount of data on the prevalence of melasma in women, the data regarding the prevalence of melasma in men are limited. Men form between 10% [42] and 25% [43] of the total melasma patients. A recent population-based survey by Pichardo et al. [44] showed the prevalence of 14.5% among male Latino migrant workers in the United States.

8.5.1.2 Etiology

While the exact underlying etiology for melasma remains a mystery, several well known risk factors exist. Melasma is more common in darker skin types, particularly Fitzpatrick skin types III and IV. Other reported risk factors include genetic predisposition, exposure to ultraviolet light, pregnancy, and exogenous hormones (i.e., oral contraceptives and hormone replacement therapy) [45]. However, these associated factors are mostly reported in women. Little is known about the etiology of melasma in men.

Among the aggravating factors, men with melasma are more likely to have a positive family history and chronic sun exposure than women [46].

Hormonal influences are known to be a cause of melasma in women. A recent multicenter survey of females from nine countries found that 41% of women surveyed had onset of disease after pregnancy but before menopause [47]. Importantly, only 8% noted spontaneous remission. Only 25% of patients taking oral contraceptives had an onset of melasma after starting their contraceptive. While melasma was thought to be a pregnancy- and contraceptive-related disorder in the past, recent studies show that in many patients it is a chronic disorder that may last for decades [45]. The relatively high prevalence of melasma in men of color also supports this hypothesis.

Hormonal changes, although different from women, may analogously play a role in the development of melasma in men. When compared with age matched control men, the circulating LH was significantly higher and testosterone was markedly lower in the melasmic men, which may point to subtle testicular resistance in men with melasma [48].

8.5.1.3 Clinical Presentation

Three clinical patterns of melasma have been described: the centrofacial, the malar and the mandibular pattern.

In men, the malar pattern, representing 44.1–61% of patients, is more common than the centrofacial and mandibular patterns whereas in women, the centrofacial pattern is the most common [49].

8.5.1.4 Histologic Findings

There are two basic patterns of melasma: an epidermal form that featured melanin deposition mainly in the basal and suprabasal layers and melanocytes that were highly dendritic and full of pigment, and a dermal form with superficial and deep perivascular melanophages in the dermis with noticeably less prominent epidermal pigmentation [50, 51].

In comparison between male and female melasma increased vascularity was found in the lesion of male melasma. In addition, there was a significant increase of stem cell factor and c-kit expression. The lesion to nonlesion ratio of stem cell factor was increased in male melasma compared with female melasma [52]. These results suggest that chronic UV radiation associated with signaling of paracrine cytokines play an important role in the mechanism of melasma in male patients [49].

8.5.1.5 Management

Although the treatment options for melasma in both genders are similar, some considerations should be taken into account when treating melasma in men as opposed to women.

Men want to see immediate visible improvement [53]. Unfortunately, since the management of melasma is challenging, there is still no such treatment modality for this entity to date.

The most widely used treatment modalities are Hydroquinone formulations and laser therapy.

Regarding the formulation, men generally prefer using a solution rather than cream or ointment [54].

In addition, the products should not be heavily fragranced or have overly feminine packaging [49].

8.5.1.6 Quality of Life

Melasma has a negative impact on the quality of life in both genders [44, 55].

It can be a source of embarrassment in men because of its unsightly appearance and the social stigma of being categorized as a disease in pregnant women [49].

Table 8.2 Gender differences in other disorders of hyperpigmentation

Disease	Gender related epidemiology
Post inflammatory hyperpigmentation	No gender preference [56]
Erythema dyschromicum perstans	May be a slight female predominanace [57]
Confluent and reticulated papillomatosis (CARP)	No gender preference [58]
Prurigo pigmentosa	Women are twice as likely to be affected as men. Mostly of Japanese origin [59]

8.5.2 Other Acquired Disorders of Hyperpigmentation (Table 8.2)

References

1. Friedmann PS, Gilchrest BA. Ultraviolet radiation directly induces pigment production by cultured human melanocytes. J Cell Physiol. 1987;133(1):88–94.
2. Pears JS, Jung RT, Bartlett W, Browning MC, Kenicer K, Thody AJ. A case of skin hyperpigmentation due to alpha-MSH hypersecretion. Br J Dermatol. 1992;126(3):286–9.
3. Ranson M, Posen S, Mason RS. Human melanocytes as a target tissue for hormones: in vitro studies with 1 alpha-25, dihydroxyvitamin D3, alpha-melanocyte stimulating hormone, and beta-estradiol. J Invest Dermatol. 1988;91(6):593–8.
4. McLeod SD, Ranson M, Mason RS. Effects of estrogens on human melanocytes in vitro. J Steroid Biochem Mol Biol. 1994;49(1):9–14.
5. Jee SH, Lee SY, Chiu HC, Chang CC, Chen TJ. Effects of estrogen and estrogen receptor in normal human melanocytes. Biochem Biophys Res Commun. 1994;199(3):1407–12.
6. Kim NH, Cheong KA, Lee TR, Lee AY. PDZK1 upregulation in estrogen-related hyperpigmentation in melasma. J Invest Dermatol. 2012;132(11):2622–31.
7. Jian D, Jiang D, Su J, Chen W, Hu X, Kuang Y, et al. Diethylstilbestrol enhances melanogenesis via cAMP-PKA-mediating up-regulation of tyrosinase and MITF in mouse B16 melanoma cells. Steroids. 2011;76(12):1297–304.
8. Kippenberger S, Loitsch S, Solano F, Bernd A, Kaufmann R. Quantification of tyrosinase, TRP-1, and Trp-2 transcripts in human melanocytes by reverse transcriptase-competitive multiplex PCR—regulation by steroid hormones. J Invest Dermatol. 1998;110(4):364–7.
9. Wiedemann C, Nagele U, Schramm G, Berking C. Inhibitory effects of progestogens on the estrogen stimulation of melanocytes in vitro. Contraception. 2009;80(3):292–8.
10. Tadokoro T, Rouzaud F, Itami S, Hearing VJ, Yoshikawa K. The inhibitory effect of androgen and sex-hormone-binding globulin on the intracellular cAMP level and tyrosinase activity of normal human melanocytes. Pigment Cell Res. 2003;16(3):190–7.
11. Whiteman DC, Parsons PG, Green AC. Determinants of melanocyte density in adult human skin. Arch Dermatol Res. 1999;291(9):511–6.
12. Giacomoni PU, Mammone T, Teri M. Gender-linked differences in human skin. J Dermatol Sci. 2009;55(3):144–9.
13. Mehrai H, Sunderland E. Skin colour data from Nowshahr City, northern Iran. Ann Hum Biol. 1990;17(2):115–20.
14. Banerjee S. Pigmentary fluctuation and hormonal changes. J Genet Hum. 1984;32(5):345–9.
15. Roh K, Kim D, Ha S, Ro Y, Kim J, Lee H. Pigmentation in Koreans: study of the differences from caucasians in age, gender and seasonal variations. Br J Dermatol. 2001;144(1):94–9.
16. Green A, Martin NG. Measurement and perception of skin colour in a skin cancer survey. Br J Dermatol. 1990;123(1):77–84.
17. Kalla AK, Tiwari SC. Sex differences in skin colour in man. Acta Genet Med Gemellol. 1970;19(3):472–6.
18. Kalla AK. Ageing and sex differences in human skin pigmentation. Z Morphol Anthropol. 1973;65(1):29–33.
19. Tur E. Physiology of the skin—differences between women and men. Clin Dermatol. 1997;15(1):5–16.
20. Kelly RI, Pearse R, Bull RH, Leveque JL, de Rigal J, Mortimer PS. The effects of aging on the cutaneous microvasculature. J Am Acad Dermatol. 1995;33(5 Pt 1):749–56.
21. Frost P. Human skin color: a possible relationship between its sexual dimorphism and its social perception. Perspect Biol Med. 1988;32(1):38–58.
22. Ortonne JP. Normal and abnormal skin color. Ann Dermatol Venereol. 2012;139(Suppl 4):S125–9.
23. Picardo M, Dell'Anna ML, Ezzedine K, Hamzavi I, Harris JE, Parsad D, et al. Vitiligo. Nat Rev Dis Primers. 2015;1:15011.
24. Ngo ST, Steyn FJ, McCombe PA. Gender differences in autoimmune disease. Front Neuroendocrinol. 2014;35(3):347–69.
25. Jin Y, Andersen G, Yorgov D, Ferrara TM, Ben S, Brownson KM, et al. Genome-wide association studies of autoimmune vitiligo identify 23 new risk loci and highlight key pathways and regulatory variants. Nat Genet. 2016;48(11):1418–24.
26. Howitz J, Brodthagen H, Schwartz M, Thomsen K. Prevalence of vitiligo. Epidemiological survey on the Isle of Bornholm, Denmark. Arch Dermatol. 1977;113(1):47–52.
27. Kyriakis KP, Palamaras I, Tsele E, Michailides C, Terzoudi S. Case detection rates of vitiligo by gender and age. Int J Dermatol. 2009;48(3):328–9.

28. Patil S, Gautam M, Nadkarni N, Saboo N, Godse K, Setia MS. Gender differences in clinicoepidemiological features of vitiligo: a cross-sectional analysis. ISRN Dermatol. 2014;2014:186197.

29. Talsania N, Lamb B, Bewley A. Vitiligo is more than skin deep: a survey of members of the Vitiligo Society. Clin Exp Dermatol. 2010;35(7):736–9.

30. Ongenae K, Van Geel N, De Schepper S, Naeyaert JM. Effect of vitiligo on self-reported health-related quality of life. Br J Dermatol. 2005;152(6):1165–72.

31. Borimnejad L, Parsa Yekta Z, Nikbakht-Nasrabadi A, Firooz A. Quality of life with vitiligo: comparison of male and female muslim patients in Iran. Gend Med. 2006;3(2):124–30.

32. Kleck RE, Christopher Strenta A. Gender and responses to disfigurement in self and others. J Soc Clin Psychol. 1985;3(3):257–67.

33. Vachiramon V, Thadanipon K. Postinflammatory hypopigmentation. Clin Exp Dermatol. 2011; 36(7):708–14.

34. Miazek N, Michalek I, Pawlowska-Kisiel M, Olszewska M, Rudnicka L. Pityriasis alba—common disease, enigmatic entity: up-to-date review of the literature. Pediatr Dermatol. 2015;32(6):786–91.

35. Blessmann Weber M, Sponchiado de Avila LG, Albaneze R, Magalhaes de Oliveira OL, Sudhaus BD, Cestari TF. Pityriasis alba: a study of pathogenic factors. J Eur Acad Dermatol Venereol. 2002;16(5):463–8.

36. Relyveld GN, Menke HE, Westerhof W. Progressive macular hypomelanosis: an overview. Am J Clin Dermatol. 2007;8(1):13–9.

37. Juntongjin P, Laosakul K. Idiopathic guttate hypomelanosis: a review of its etiology, pathogenesis, findings, and treatments. Am J Clin Dermatol. 2016;17(4):403–11.

38. Kim SK, Kim EH, Kang HY, Lee ES, Sohn S, Kim YC. Comprehensive understanding of idiopathic guttate hypomelanosis: clinical and histopathological correlation. Int J Dermatol. 2010;49(2):162–6.

39. Grimes PE. Melasma. Etiologic and therapeutic considerations. Arch Dermatol. 1995;131(12):1453–7.

40. Hiletework M. Skin diseases seen in Kazanchis health center. Ethiop Med J. 1998;36(4):245–54.

41. Werlinger KD, Guevara IL, Gonzalez CM, Rincon ET, Caetano R, Haley RW, et al. Prevalence of self-diagnosed melasma among premenopausal Latino women in Dallas and Fort Worth, Tex. Arch Dermatol. 2007;143(3):424–5.

42. Vazquez M, Maldonado H, Benmaman C, Sanchez JL. Melasma in men. A clinical and histologic study. Int J Dermatol. 1988;27(1):25–7.

43. Sarkar R, Jain RK, Puri P. Melasma in Indian males. Dermatol Surg. 2003;29(2):204.

44. Pichardo R, Vallejos Q, Feldman SR, Schulz MR, Verma A, Quandt SA, et al. The prevalence of melasma and its association with quality of life in adult male Latino migrant workers. Int J Dermatol. 2009;48(1):22–6.

45. Sheth VM, Pandya AG. Melasma: a comprehensive update: part I. J Am Acad Dermatol. 2011;65(4):689–97; quiz 98.

46. Sarkar R, Puri P, Jain RK, Singh A, Desai A. Melasma in men: a clinical, aetiological and histological study. J Eur Acad Dermatol Venereol. 2010;24(7):768–72.

47. El-Essawi D, Musial JL, Hammad A, Lim HW. A survey of skin disease and skin-related issues in Arab Americans. J Am Acad Dermatol. 2007;56(6):933–8.

48. Sialy R, Hassan I, Kaur I, Dash RJ. Melasma in men: a hormonal profile. J Dermatol. 2000;27(1):64–5.

49. Vachiramon V, Suchonwanit P, Thadanipon K. Melasma in men. J Cosmet Dermatol. 2012;11(2):151–7.

50. Sanchez NP, Pathak MA, Sato S, Fitzpatrick TB, Sanchez JL, Mihm MC Jr. Melasma: a clinical, light microscopic, ultrastructural, and immunofluorescence study. J Am Acad Dermatol. 1981;4(6):698–710.

51. Kang WH, Yoon KH, Lee ES, Kim J, Lee KB, Yim H, et al. Melasma: histopathological characteristics in 56 Korean patients. Br J Dermatol. 2002;146(2):228–37.

52. Jang YH, Sim JH, Kang HY, Kim YC, Lee ES. The histopathological characteristics of male melasma: comparison with female melasma and lentigo. J Am Acad Dermatol. 2012;66(4):642–9.

53. Fried RG. Esthetic treatment modalities in men: psychologic aspects of male cosmetic patients. Dermatol Ther. 2007;20(6):379–84.

54. Keeling J, Cardona L, Benitez A, Epstein R, Rendon M. Mequinol 2%/tretinoin 0.01% topical solution for the treatment of melasma in men: a case series and review of the literature. Cutis. 2008;81(2):179–83.

55. Ikino JK, Nunes DH, Silva VP, Frode TS, Sens MM. Melasma and assessment of the quality of life in Brazilian women. An Bras Dermatol. 2015;90(2):196–200.

56. Callender VD, St Surin-Lord S, Davis EC, Maclin M. Postinflammatory hyperpigmentation: etiologic and therapeutic considerations. Am J Clin Dermatol. 2011;12(2):87–99.

57. Combemale P, Faisant M, Guennoc B, Dupin M, Heyraud JD. Erythema dyschromicum perstans: report of a new case and critical review of the literature. J Dermatol. 1998;25(11):747–53.

58. Tamraz H, Raffoul M, Kurban M, Kibbi AG, Abbas O. Confluent and reticulated papillomatosis: clinical and histopathological study of 10 cases from Lebanon. J Eur Acad Dermatol Venereol. 2013;27(1):e119–23.

59. Boer A, Misago N, Wolter M, Kiryu H, Wang XD, Ackerman AB. Prurigo pigmentosa: a distinctive inflammatory disease of the skin. Am J Dermatopathol. 2003;25(2):117–29.

Gender and Genodermatoses

9

Sivan Sheffer Levi and Vered Molho-Pessach

9.1 Introduction

Genodermatoses are a large and growing group of inherited skin disorders, with hundreds of genes recognized to be associated with cutaneous phenotypes over the years. Advances in molecular research and technology, as well as expanding genetic knowledge and sequencing methods have led to better understanding of the molecular basis of this diverse group of disorders [1, 2]. New classification systems have emerged based on the integration of molecular and clinical data [3, 4]. As with other inherited disorders, genodermatoses have different modes of inheritance, with the X-linked inheritance pattern causing gender-specific expression. X-linked genodermatoses include different groups of diseases; among them are ichthyoses, enzyme deficiencies, ectodermal dysplasias, disorders of pigmentation and disorders associated with immunodeficiency.

Due to the difference in karyotype, (normally 46,XX for women and 46,XY for men), women have a double dose of the X chromosome in comparison with men. However, only one X chromosome is active in every cell (except for the pseudoautosomal region). The mechanism responsible for this dosage compensation is called lyonization [5, 6]. It is a random, irreversible, stably inherited inactivation of one of the two X chromosomes that occurs in each cell, via an epigenetic mechanism during early embryonic development (Fig. 9.1). All cells derived from the progenitor cell will have the same inactivated X chromosome. The inactivation of the X chromosome represents a functional form of mosaicism and can result in skin lesions that follow Blaschko's lines (Fig. 9.2) or other mosaic distribution patterns, if an X chromosome gene is mutated. When one of the alleles of an X-linked gene contains a disease-causing mutation, the phenotype will depend on the proportion of the cells expressing the mutated allele. On average, each allele of an X-linked gene will be expressed in half of the cells in a woman. This proportion may change, as in the case of nonrandom or skewed X inactivation, suggesting a negative selection against cells with the mutation.

Since males have only one X chromosome and females undergo variable X inactivation, X-linked inherited genodermatoses exhibit gender specific expression. Disorders with an X-linked recessive mode of inheritance typically affect males. Females may be asymptomatic or present with variable clinical manifestations which are usually mild. X-linked dominant genodermatoses are usually lethal in male embryos and thus are seen almost exclusively in female heterozygotes, usually presenting with skin involvement in a mosaic distribution.

S. S. Levi · V. Molho-Pessach (✉)
Department of Dermatology, Hadassah-Hebrew University Medical Center, Jerusalem, Israel

© Springer International Publishing AG, part of Springer Nature 2018
E. Tur, H. I. Maibach (eds.), *Gender and Dermatology*,
https://doi.org/10.1007/978-3-319-72156-9_9

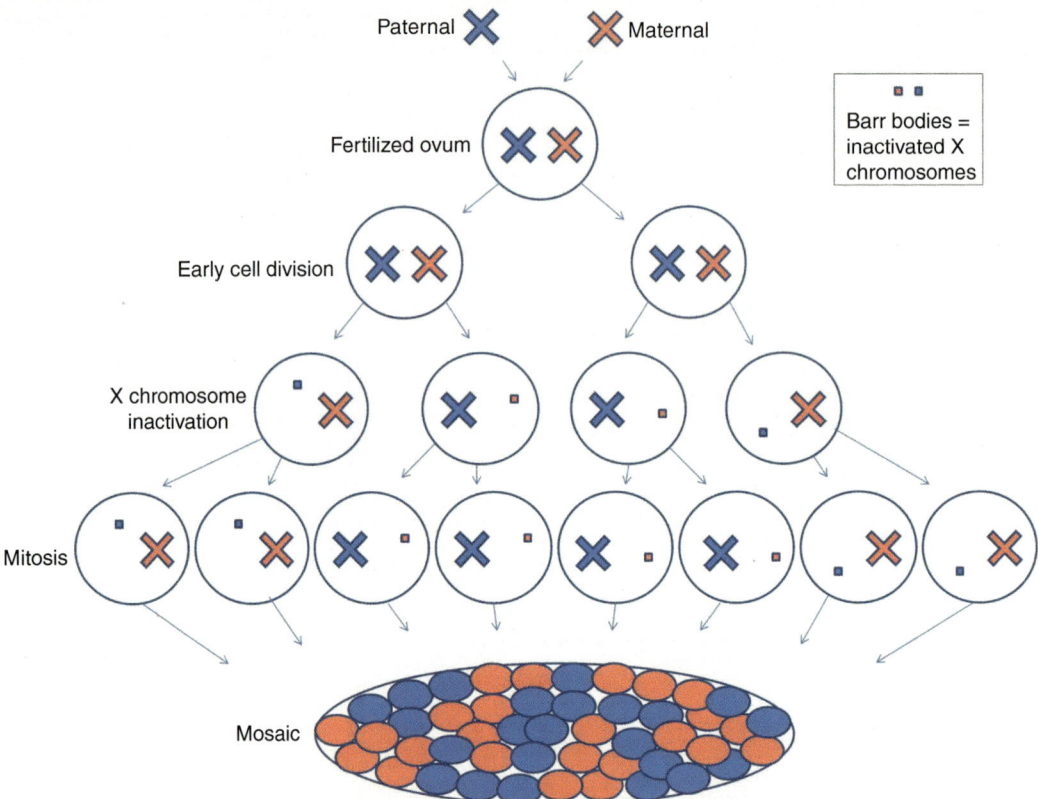

Fig. 9.1 X inactivation in a female embryo. Both X chromosomes are transcribed until about the 20-cell stage. At this point, one X chromosome is randomly inactivated by condensation of the DNA into heterochromatin (the Barr body). The same X chromosome remains inactivated in all daughter cells

9.2   X-Linked Recessive Genodermatoses

Patients are typically male, while female "carriers" may be asymptomatic or present with variable milder phenotypes due to lyonization. An affected father will not transmit the mutated allele to any of his sons, since they receive his Y chromosome. Thus, male-to-male transmission cannot occur. Daughters of an affected father are obligate carriers, who will later transmit the mutated allele to 50% of their children. X-linked recessive genodermatoses are presented in Table 9.1. Several of these disorders are reviewed in detail ahead.

9.2.1   Steroid Sulfatase Deficiency/ X-Linked Ichthyosis

Steroid sulfatase deficiency, also known as X-linked ichthyosis, was first described as a distinct type of ichthyosis in 1965 [7]. It is the second most common type of ichthyosis, with a worldwide incidence of between 1 in 2000 to 1 in 9500, affecting almost exclusively males. Deficiency of the enzyme steroid sulfatase causes impaired hydrolysis of cholesterol sulfate and dehydroepiandrosterone with subsequent accumulation of cholesterol 3-sulfate in the epidermis [8]. Cholesterol sulfate is thought to play a role in membrane integrity and normal desquamation,

Fig. 9.2 The lines of Blaschko. Blaschko's lines represent pathways of epidermal cell migration and proliferation during development. Functional mosaicism occurring in females due to normal X inactivation, results in Blachko-linear distribution of X linked genodermatoses in females

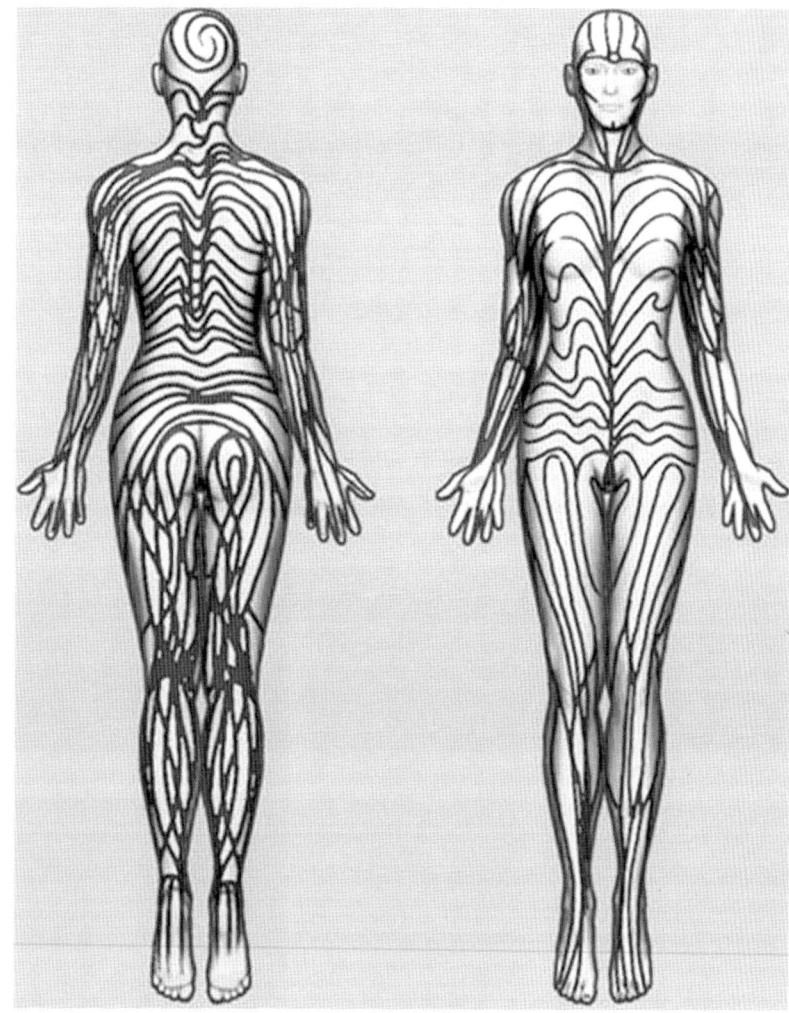

and its' excess results in this inherited disorder of cutaneous keratinization with possible extracutaneous manifestations [9]. The disorder is caused by a deletion of the entire STS gene (mapped to Xp22.31) in 90% of the patients, and inactivating mutations in others [10, 11]. The STS gene escapes lyonization and has a double expression in females compared with males. For this reason, female carriers do not develop this condition through functional mosaicism [12]. A family of three homozygous women, daughters of an affected male and a female carrier of X-linked ichthyosis has been described [13].

9.2.1.1 Clinical Features in Males

During the neonatal period, most affected males will present with mild erythroderma and generalized peeling with exfoliating large translucent scales [14]. Later, during infancy, symmetrically distributed large polygonal dark-brown adherent scales develop on the extremities, trunk and neck. The neck is almost always involved while palms, soles and face are spared.

Extracutaneous manifestations include asymptomatic corneal opacities that can be seen in 10–50% of patients [15]. Another extracutaneous finding is cryptorchidism, occurring in

Table 9.1 X-linked recessive genodermatoses

Disorder	Gene / Gene product / Chromosomal location	Mechanism	Incidence	Onset	Mucocutaneous features
Steroid sulfatase deficiency (X-linked recessive ichthyosis)	STS / Steroid sulfatase / Xp22.31	A deletion of the entire STS gene in 90% of the patients is responsible for diminution or complete absence of steroid sulfatase causing impaired hydrolysis of cholesterol sulfate and dehydroepiandrosterone. Subsequent accumulation of cholesterol 3-sulfate in the epidermis inhibits transglutaminase-1	1:2000–1:9500 male births	Neonatal period	*Neonatal period*—mild erythroderma and generalized peeling, often with exfoliation of large, translucent scales *Infancy*—fine to large, dark adherent scales on extremities, trunk, neck and lateral face; typical polygonal dark-brown adherent scale The neck is almost invariably involved ("dirty-neck disease") *Early childhood*—fine scaling of the scalp, diminished over time —characteristically sparing of the palms, soles and face with the exception of the preauricular area
Fabry disease (Anderson-Fabry disease, alpha-galactosidase A deficiency)	GLA / α-Galactosidase A / Xq22.1	Deficient activity of lysosomal alpha-galactosidase A results in accumulation of globotriaosylceramide (Gb3) within lysosomes, believed to trigger a cascade of cellular events	1:40,000 men	First two to three decades of life	Angiokeratomas of the skin and mucous membranes, tend to be clustered between the umbilicus and the knees but can present anywhere, hypohidrosis
Ichthyosis follicularis, atrichia and photophobia (IFAP) syndrome	MBTPS2 / Membrane-bound transcription factor peptidasesite 2 / Xp22.12-p22.11	A zinc metalloprotease with roles in cholesterol homeostasis and the ER stress response		Neonatal period	Congenital atrichia with absence of eyebrows and eyelashes, follicular keratoses ("nutmeg grater" skin), psoriasiform plaques. Occasionally lamellar scaling or hyperkeratosis of the palms and soles, nail dystrophy Increased susceptibility to mucocutaneous bacterial and fungal infections

Keratosis follicularis spinulosa decalvans (KFSD)	MBTPS2 Membrane-bound transcription factor peptidasesite 2 Xp22.12-p22.11	Keratinization defect		Childhood	Erythematous follicular papules with central keratotic plugs involving the face, scalp, limbs and trunk and eventuating in follicular atrophy. Scarring alopecia of the scalp, eyebrows and eyelashes. Associated keratosis pilaris on the extremities and trunk, palmoplantar keratoderma. Facial erythema
Hypohidrotic ectodermal dysplasia (anhidrotic ectodermal dysplasia, Chris–Siemens–Touraine syndrome)	EDA Ectodysplain A Xq12-q13.1	The genetic defect affects the ectodysplasin signal transduction pathway resulting in aplasia, hypoplasia or dysplasia of teeth, hair follicles and eccrine glands	1:10,000 live born boys	Neonatal period	Affected newborns may present with a collodion-like membrane or marked skin scaling. Sparse to absent scalp hair, often lighty pigmented in children, markedly decreased sweating, hypodontia, conical teeth, normal nails, smooth skin (due to absence of eccrine pores). Eczema—commo, periorbital wrinkling and hyperpigmentation, sebaceous hyperplasia of the face
Hypohidrotic ectodermal dysplasia—immune deficiency	NEMO NF-κB essential modulator Xq28	Mutations in the NEMO gene that encodes a subunit of a regulatory kinase that activates NF-κB downstream in the ectodysplasin and tumor necrosis factor-α (TNF-α) pathways	Rare		Sparse scalp hair, hypotrichosis. Hypodontia, conical teeth. Mildly decreased sweating. Normal nails. Extensive intertrigo, seborrheic or atopic-like dermatitis that develops into erythroderma. Reticulated hyperpigmentation

(continued)

Table 9.1 (continued)

Disorder	Gene Gene product Chromosomal location	Mechanism	Incidence	Onset	Mucocutaneous features
Menkes disease (kinky hair disease, trichopoliodystrophy, Menkes steely hair disease)	ATP7A A copper transporting P-type ATPase Xq21.1	An inherited form of copper deficiency. Defective copper absorption with low levels in blood, liver and hair causing decreased activity of several enzymes, including cytochrome C oxidase (brain), lysil oxidase (connective tissue and blood vesssels) and ascorbic acid oxidase (bones)	1:100,000 (1:50,000–1:360,000)	2–3 months	Alopecia with abnormal hair shafts, pili torti, monilethrix and trichorrhexis. Hair may appear light in color, sparse, fragile and kinky. Patients may have diffuse cutaneous pigmentary dilution
Congenital generalized hypertrichosis X-linked (X-linked hypertrichosis)	Interchromosomal insertion mediated by a palindromic sequence Xq24-q27.1				Curly, shorter, dark hair most prominent on the face and upper body Occasional dental anomalies
X-linked reticulate pigmentary disorder, Partington type (Partington syndrome type II, Familial cutaneous amyloidosis, X-linked reticulate pigmentary disorder with systemic manifestations)	POLA1 Xp22.11-p21.3		Rare	Birth	Generalized reticulated brown hyperpigmentation initially developing on the inner thighs, buttocks, or cheeks (between 4 months and 5 years of age) Dental anomalies Hypohidrosis Xerosis Blonde unruly hair with a frontal upsweep

Dyskeratosis congenita[a] (Zinsser-Engman-Cole syndrome)	DKC1 Dyskerin Xq28	Dyskerin interacts with the telomerase enzyme that prevents progressive shortening of the chromosomes with DNA replication	1/ 1,000,000 in Europe	Nail changes begin at early childhood	*Triad* of reticulated hyperpigmentation, nail dystrophy (e.g. pterygium) and leukoplakia
					The lacy reticulated pattern of hyperpigmentation develops during the first decade of life, primarily on the upper chest and upper arms and may be admixed with hypopigmented macules. Additional cutaneous features include telangiectasias, epidermal atrophy, wrinkled skin on the extremities, dorsal hands and genitalia, palmoplantar hyperhidrosis and hyperkeratosis, frictional bullae and acrocyanosis
					Nail involvement begin in early childhood with longitudinal ridging and splitting, followed by pterygia formation and occasionally complete nail loss
					During early adolescence, premalignant leukoplakia occurs: white plaques on the oral mucosa with a predilection for the lateral portions of the tongue. The urethra, anus and vagina may also be involved
					The teeth may be malformed, missing or have aberrant spacing or extensice caries

(continued)

Table 9.1 (continued)

Disorder	Gene Gene product Chromosomal location	Mechanism	Incidence	Onset	Mucocutaneous features
Chronic granulomatos disease (Chronic graulomatous disorder, Bridges-good syndrome, Quie syndrome)	CYBB Cytochrome b 245 β—polypeptide(gp91-phox) Xp21.1	A defect in the subunit of phagocyte NADPH oxidase	1:200,000 (90% are boys. Three quarters have x-linked recessive transmission)	Mean age a diagnosis-3 years. Symptoms may begin in the neonatal period In 65% the onset is by age 1 year	Staphylococcal infections of the skin around the ears and nose, may progress to extensive purulent dermattis with regional lymphadenopathy, perianal abscess, facial periorificial dermatitis, cutaneous abscesses, poorly healing ulcers, purulent inflammatory reactions to minor trauma, cutaneous granulomas (less frequently), seborrheic dermatitis, scalp folliculitis, acute or chronic cutaneous lupus erythematosus-like skin lesions (especially discoid lesions), Sweet's syndrome, ulcers invoving the oral mucosa (resmbling aphthous stomatitis)
IPEX (immune dysregulation, polyendocrinopathy, enteropathy, x-linked syndrome)	FOXP3 Forkhead box P3 Xp11.23	Abnormal development of regulatory T cells		Infancy	A widespread eczematous dermatitis, often complicated by staphylococcal superinfections and sepsis Psoriasiform dermatitis Chelitis, nail dystrophy A variety of autoimmune skin conditions such as alopecia areata, chronic urticaria and bullous pemphigoid

Syndrome	Gene/protein/locus	Function	Incidence	Onset	Clinical features
Wiskott-Aldrich syndrome (Wiskott-Aldrich-Huntley, eczema-thromboctopenia-immunodeficiency syndrome)	WASP WAS protein Xp11.23-p11.22	The WAS protein controls the assembly of actin filaments which are required for micro-vesicle and pro-platelet formation as well as—cell activation and polarization	1:250,000 live male births in European population	Birth	Petechiae and ecchymoses of the skin and oral mucosa (due to thrombocytopenia and platelet dysfunction since birth) Atopic dermatitis develops during the first few months of life, with the face, scalp and flexural areas most severely affected. Patients often have widespread involvement with progressive lichenification Exfoliative dermatitis occasionally develops Excoriated areas frequently have serosanguineous crusts and petechiae Secondary bacterial infections are common, as are eczema herpeticum and molluscum contagiosum Cutaneous small vessesl vasculitiis is the most common associated autoimmune diseas (often with painful edema)
X-linked lymphoproliferative syndrome (Duncan disease)	SH2D1A Signaling lymphocyte activation molecule-associated protein Xq25	The mutated gene encodes an adaptor protein that regulates B-, T- and NK-cell function; particularly important for immune responses to EBV			EBV-related infectious mononuclosis often associated with morbiliform eruptions, purpura and/or jaundice Lymphocytic vasculitis
	XIAP X-linked inhibitor of apoptosis Xq25				

(continued)

Table 9.1 (continued)

Disorder	Gene Gene product Chromosomal location	Mechanism	Incidence	Onset	Mucocutaneous features
X linked agammaglobulinemia (Bruton agammaglobulinemia, Bruton-Gitlin syndrome, congenital hypogammaglobulinemia, X-linked hypogammaglobulinemia)	BTK Bruton tyrosine kinase (pre-B-cell receptor [BCR] signaling Xq22.1	A defect in a key regulator in B-cell development		First few years of life	Recurrent skin infections: furuncles and cellulitis, ecthyma gangrenosum Eczematous dermatitis Papular dermatitis due to lymphihistiocytic infitration Non-infectious granulomas Dermatomyositis-like disorder associated with chronic echoviral meningoencephalitis
Hyper-IgM syndrome	CD40LG CD40 ligand (on T cells) Xq26.3				Pyoderma Extensive warts Oral and anogenital ulcers Non-infectious granulomas Autoimmune coditions such as SLE
Severe combined immunodeficiency (SCID)	IL2RG Common γ chain of the receptors for IL-2,4,7,9,15 and 21 Xq13.1		1:30,000–1:100,000 (three quarters of affected patients are boys, more than 40% of cases have x-linked recessive inheritance)	First few months of life	Widespread seborrheic-like dermatitis or morbiliform eruptions (often reflecting maternofetal GVHD). Eruptions may also resemble lichen planus, acrodermatitis enteropathica, Langerhans cell histiocytosisichthyosiform erythroderma and scleroderma. Cutaneous infections most often due to *C. albicans*, *S.aureus* and *Str. pyogenes*

Disorder	Associated features	Feature in female carriers	Diagnosis	Treatment	MIM number
Steroid sulfatase deficiency (X-linked recessive ichthyosis)	Asymptomatic corneal opacities (10–50%) Cryptorchidism (20-fold increased incidence) Higher risk for developing testicualr cancer and hypogonadism *Rare:* seizures, reactive psychological disorders, attention deficit disorder, developmental delay, pyloric hypertrophy, a congenital defect in the abdominal wall and acute lymphoblastic leukemia	Asymtomatic corneal opacities Prolonged labor with affected child No skin manifestations	Molecular testing: Array CGH, FISH, southern blot, PCR-based analysis. Lipoprotein electrophoresis (increased mobility of β-fraction); plasma cholesterol sulfate increased by chromatography or spectrophotometry; decreased steroid sulfatase activity in leukocytes, fibroblasts, keratinocytes or placental tissue; Non invasive prenatal diagnosis: decreased serum estriol levels and the presence of non-hydrolysed sulfated steroids in material urine	Topical humectants, keratolytics and retinoids	308,100, 300,747
Fabry disease (Anderson-Fabry disease, alpha-galactosidase A deficiency)	Pain and paresthesias of the extremities, renal failure Cardiovascular findings: hypertrophic cardiomyopathy, valvular abnormalities, conduction defects, arryhthmias, progressive atherosclerotic disease of the coronary and cerebral arteries Ophthlmologic findings: corneal and lenicular opacities, retinal vasclar abnormalities Coarse facial features, hearing loss, abdominal pain, diarrhea, vomiting, osteopenia and joint pain	Female heterozygotes also often affected with variable clinical manifestations and later onset Corneal opacities Angiokeratomas (in approximately 30% of heterozygous girls and women)	Demonstration of deficient α-galactosidase A activity (enzyme assay) in plasma or leukocytes; analysis of GLA gene	Enzyme replacemnet therapy effective in arresting the progression of the disorder. Symptomatic treatment includes phenytoin, gabapentin or carbamazepine for alleviation of debilitating limb pain, angiotensin-converting enzyme inhibitors for reducing proteinuria and dialysis or renal transplantation for end stage renal disease	301,500, 300,644

(continued)

Table 9.1 (continued)

Disorder	Associated features	Feature in female carriers	Diagnosis	Treatment	MIM number
Ichthyosis follicularis, atrichia and photophobia (IFAP) syndrome	Vascularizing keratitis, short stature, variable intellectual disability, cerebral atrophy, temporal lobe malformation, hypoplasia of the corpus callosum, seizures, inguinal hernias. Occasional urogenital, renal and vertebral malformations or Hirschprung disease	Linear streaks with follicular keratoses or scaling; patchy hypotrichosis	Clinical		308,205, 300,294
Keratosis follicularis spinulosa decalvans (KFSD)	Keratitis Photopobia Aminoaciduria				308,800, 300,294
Hypohidrotic ectodermal dysplasia (anhidrotic ectodermal dysplasia, Chris-Siemens-Touraine syndrome)	Characteristic facies (saddle nose, full everted lips and frontal bossing) Nasal concretion, asthma Frequent respiratory tract infections Hoarse or raspy voice Gastroesophageal reflux in infants	Variable pheotype: 1. Carriers with no detectable clinical features 2. Limited involvment with finding such as decreased hair density, one or more peg-shaped or missing teeth, and patchy distribution of sweat glands along Blaschko's lines (sometimes with relative hyperpigmentation of te skin that lacks adnexa). 3. Full blown features		Controling ambient temperatures and external methods of cooling Dentures and dental restoration Multidisciplinary care The potential for gene or protein theapy is on the horizon	305,100, 300,451

Hypohidrotic ectodermal dysplasia—immune deficiency	Frontal bossing, periorbtal wrinkling and everted lips Inflammatory colitis Immunodefficiency that results in recurrent infections (pyogeic or opportunistic) Dysgammaglobulinemia (typically elevated IgM and IgA, but decreased IgG) Rarely osteopetrosis and lymphedema	May have mild features of incontinenta pigmenti		Allogeneic hematopoieic stem cell transplantation (although associated with post-transplant complications)	300,291, 300,301, 300,248
Menkes disease (kinky hair disease, trichopoliodystrophy, Menkes steely hair disease)	Failure to thrive, lethargy, hypothermia, hypotonia, seizures, developmental delay, anemia Boney abnormalities Tortuorous elongated arteries Typical facies (pudgy cheeks, a cupid's bow of the upper lip and horizontal eyebrows)	Patches of swirled hypopigmentation or pili torti along Blaschko's lines	Clinical features, low serum levels of copper and ceruloplasmin and microscopic hair shaft findings Prenatal diagnosis possible	Treatment with copper histidine is usually unsuccessful Poor prognosis with life expectancy of 3–5 years	309,400, 300,011
Congenital generalized hypertrichosis X-linked (X-linked hypertrichosis)	Anteverted nostrils Prognathism Deafness	Nevoid hypertrichosis following Blaschko's lines			307,150
X-linked reticulate pigmentary disorder, Partington type (Partington syndrome type II, Familial cutaneous amyloidosis, X-linked reticulate pigmentary disorder with systemic manifestations)	Severe systemic manifestations including low birthweight, neonatal colitis, failure to thrive, seizures, hemiplegia, gastroesophageal reflux, urethral strictures and inguinal hernias Recurrent pneumonias and chronic obstructive pulmonary disease are nearly always present and may lead to premature death Additional features include possible developmental delay, photophobia, corneal clouding and skeletal changes	Hyperpigmented streaks following Blachko's lines		Supportive	301,220, 312,040

(continued)

Table 9.1 (continued)

Disorder	Associated features	Feature in female carriers	Diagnosis	Treatment	MIM number
Dyskeratosis congenita[a] (Zinsser-Engman-Cole syndrome)	Bone marrow failure occurs in 50–90% of patients and is a major cause of mortality. It presents during the second or third decade of life with anemia, thrombodcytopenia or pancytopenia. Malignancies tend to develop during the third or forth decade, most notably squamous cell carcinomas of the mouth, anus, cervix, vagina, esophagous and skin. Also, there is an increased risk for myelodysplasia, acute myelogenous leukemia, Hodgkin disease and gastrointestinal carcinomas. Epiphora resulting from lacrimal duct atresia is common Testicular atrophy Pulmonary fibrosis Liver cirrhosis Developmental delay Immunologic dysfunction leading to opportunistic infections		Short telomeres can be detected in leukocytes by flow fluorescence in situ hybridization	Multdisciplinary care including longitudinal surveillance of all mucosal surfaces to monitor for the development of sqamous cell carcinoma within areas of leukoplakia Avoidance of sun a and cigarettes supportive transfusions of blood products and use of androgens, erythropoetin and granulocyte colony-stimulating factor to treat bone marrow failure Hematopoietic stem call transplantaton has been associated with poor prognosis	305,000, 300,126
Chronic granulomatos disease (chronic graulomatous disorder, Bridges-good syndrome, Quie syndrome)	Lymphadenopathy, hepatosplenomgaly, pneumonia, underweight, short stature, persistent diarrhea and/or abdominal pain, hepatic/perihepatic abscess, pleuritis/empyema, septicemia or meningitis, osteomyelitis, conjuctuvitis and/or chorioretinits, lung abscess, peritonitis	May present with discoid lesions, Jessner's lymphocytic infiltrate, photosensitivity, Raynaud's phenomenon, severe aphthous stomatitis and granulomatous chelitis	Nitroblue tetrazolium (NBT) reduction assay is the screening test Ferricytochrome C reduction and dihydrohodamine 123 assays are more accurate and can be performed to verify the diagnosis Immunoblot analysis Prenatal diagnosis possible	Antibiotics, anti-fungals Periodic evaluation of the lungs, liver and bones Interferon γ Leukocyte tranfusionfo rapidly progressive life threatening infections Systemic corticosteroids for obstructive granulomas Hematopoietic stem cell transplantation Gene therapy	306,400, 300,481

IPEX (immune dysregulation, polyendocrinopathy, enteropathy, x-linked syndrome)	Autoimmune enteropathy causing severe diarrhea. A variety of autoimmune endocrinopathies (early onset type 1 diabetes mellitus, thyroiditis, cytopenias)			304,790, 300,292
Wiskott-Aldrich syndrome (Wiskott-Aldrich-Huntley, eczema-thromboctopenia-immunodeficiency syndrome)	Spontaneous bleeding from the oral cavity, epistaxis, hematemesis, melena and hematuria (due to thrombocytopenia and platelet dysfunction). Recurrent bacterial infections begin during the first 3 months of life and include otitis externa and media, pneumonia, sinusitis, conjuctuvitis, furunculosis, meningitis and septicemia. Encapsulated bacteria such as *Str. pneumoniae, H. influenzae* and *Neisseria meningitidies* are the predominant organisms. With advancing age, there is increased susceptibility to infections with viruses (e.g herpes simplex) and *P. jiroveci*. Autoimmune diseases including autoimmune hemolytic anemia or neutropenia, arthritis, inflammatory bowel disease and cerebral vasculitis. IgE mediated conditions such as urticaria, asthma and food allergies occur with increased frequency. Hepatosplenomegaly and lymphadenopathy are additional features. Lymphomas develop in up to a quarter (20 years and older), especially those with autoimmune disease	Flow cytometry-based assays. Immunoblot analysis. Mutational analysis	Hematopoietic stem cell transplantation is the treatment of choice gene therapy using retrovirally transduced, WASP-reconstituted, autologous CD34+ cells has also been successfully performed. Prophylactic antibiotics and antivirals can decrease the risk for fatal infections. IVIG therapy has a role in preventin infections and may potentially improve the dermatitis. Topical corticosteroids. Splenectomy may reduce bleeding complications. Prenatal diagnosis can be performed by direct mutational analysis and genetic counseling is important for ermale relatives	301,000, 300,392

(continued)

Table 9.1 (continued)

Disorder	Associated features	Feature in female carriers	Diagnosis	Treatment	MIM number
X-linked lymphoproliferative syndrome (Duncan disease)	Severe EBV-related infectious mononucleosis in childhood or adolescence (e.g. fever, pharyngitis, lymphadenopathy and hepatosplenomegaly) +/– hypogammaglobulinemia Fatal EBV-related B-cell lymphoma (70%)				308,240, 300,290 300,635, 300,079
X linked agammaglobulinemia (Bruton agammaglobulinemia, Bruton-Gitlin syndrome, congenital hypogammaglobulinemia, X-linked hypogammaglobulinemia)	Recurrent infections with *Staphylococcus, Streptococcus, Pneumococcus, Haemophilus* and *Pseudomonas* Spp. hepatitis B and enteroviral infections Lymphomas (~5%)			IVIG or subcutaneous immunoglobulins—(should be avoided in patients with profoung IgA deficiency) Antibiotic therapy for infections TNF-α inhibitors for recalcitrant non-infectios granulomas	300,755, 300,300
Hyper-IgM syndrome	Recurrent sinopulmonary and GI infections with pyogenic bacteria and opportunistic organisms (e.g. PCP) Neutropenia Small lymph nodes Autoimmune disease, especially thyroiditis and hemolytic anemia				308,230, 300,386
Severe combined immunodeficiency (SCID)	Recurrent infections, chronic diarrhea, and failure to thrive. Common infections include persistant viral gastroenteritis, penumonias and mucocutaneous candidiasis		Flow cytometric analysis of peripheral blood mononuclear cells with antibodies directed against γc. direct gene analysis. Prenatal diagnosis can be performed by fetal DNA analysis in families with a known genetic defect	Hematopoietic stem cell transplantation during infancy and IVIG replacement therapy for persistent B-cell deficiency. *In-utero* injection of haploidentical CD34+ cells, gene therapy via retroviral-mediated ex vivo gene transfer into CD34+ cells	300,400, 308,380

[a]The most common form is X-linked, as a result 90% of the patients are males

approximately 20% of the patients [16]. Testicular cancer and hypogonadism independent of testicular maldescent have been reported [16–18]. Neurologic symptoms such as seizures, reactive psychological disorders, attention deficit disorder and developmental delay, may occur and thought to represent a manifestation of contiguous gene syndromes [15].

9.2.1.2 Features in Females

Mothers of affected fetuses may present with prolonged labor due to deficiency of steroid sulfatase in the fetal placenta [19]. Low or absent levels of unconjugated estriol in maternal serum may point out the possibility of affected fetus and may be used for prenatal diagnosis [20]. Female carriers do not exhibit any skin manifestations. Asymptomatic corneal opacities present in 25% and are the only reported finding associated with steroid sulfatase deficiency [21].

9.2.2 Fabry Disease

Fabry disease was first described in 1898 [22, 23]. It is a progressive multi-systemic lysosomal storage disorder caused by a deficiency of α-galactosidase A due to mutations in the GLA gene (Xq22.1) [24]. The deficient enzyme leads to accumulation of glycosphingolipids, predominantly globotriaosylceramide, within lysosomes, triggering a cascade of cellular events and resulting in multiorgan system damage. The incidence is reported to be approximately 1 in 80,000 but may represent an underestimation, as newborn screening surveys suggest that the incidence may be much higher [25]. Most clinically apparent affected individuals are males.

9.2.2.1 Clinical Features in Males

The phenotype, as well as the age of onset, of Fabry disease is very variable. The classic form of the disease is seen in affected hemizygous males, where the onset of symptoms usually occurs in early childhood or adolescence [26]. One of the earliest manifestations is angiokeratomas of the skin and mucous membranes. These are individual punctate, dark-red to blue-black macules or slightly elevated papules that may become slightly hyperkeratotic when enlarged. They tend to be clustered between the umbilicus and the knees, but can be found anywhere. The oral mucosa and conjuctiva are commonly involved. Additional early manifestations include acroparesthesias, occurring as episodic crises of agonizing, burning pain in the distal extremities, hypohidrosis and ocular involvement. Characteristic corneal opacities, termed cornea verticillata, are the most common ophthalmologic finding, followed by lenticular opacities and tortuosity of conjuctival and retinal vessels. Characteristic facial features have been described in men with Fabry disease. They include periorbital fullness, prominent ear lobes, bushy eyebrows, a broad forehead and nasal bridge, thick lips, prognathism [27].

As disease progresses, cardiac abnormalities, cerebrovascular disease and progressive renal insufficiency are a major cause of morbidity and mortality. The cardiac and cerebrovasclar disease are present in most males with the classic phenotype by middle age. A variety of cardiac complications may occur including hypertrophic cardiomyopathy, arrhythmias and coronary insufficiency. The cerebrovascualr disease results from multifocal small vessel involvement causing an increased risk of transient ischemic attacks and strokes. Renal disease is characterized by progressive proteinuria and the development of azotemia in the third to fifth decade of life mandating chronic dialysis or renal transplantation. Other abnormalities include gastrointestinal (abdominal pain, diarrhea, vomiting) [28], pulmonary (chronic cough, dyspnea, wheezing) [29], vascular (pitting edema), cochleo-vestibular (hearing loss, tinnitus, dizziness) and psychological manifestations (depression, anxiety) [30].

Atypical variants of Fabry disease include the cardiac variant and the renal variant. They manifest with a later onset, lack the characteristic angiokeratomas and thought to be underdiagnosed [31, 32].

9.2.2.2 Features in Females

The clinical manifestations in heterozygous females ranges from asymptomatic to as severe as the classic affected male. The severity depends on the particular GLA mutation and the random inactivation of the X-chromosome in different cells affecting the degree of enzyme activity [33, 34]. The distinction between recessive and dominant is blurred as many "carriers" are symptomatic. In most cases, the clinical course is milder and heterozygous females have a later onset of clinical abnormalities and better prognosis than affected males [26]. Mild manifestations include the corneal opacities, acroparesthesias, angiokeratomas and hypohidrosis. Interestingly, the skin lesions of women do not show a mosaic pattern. This might suggest a pathogenesis related to cells that are not permanent residents of the skin or are nonepidermal cells. In this case, lyonization leads to intermingling of cells expressing the normal and abnormal genotype and no clinical apparent pattern is seen [35]. Serious manifestations might develop with advancing age and include significant left ventricular hypertrophy, cardiomegaly, myocardial ischemia and infarction, cardiac arrhythmias, transient ischemia attacks, strokes, and end stage renal disease [33, 36].

Biweekly intravenous enzyme replacement therapy is effective in arresting disease progression [37, 38], making early diagnosis of an important value. Enzyme analysis demonstrating marked enzyme deficiency is useful in diagnosis of hemizygous males, while suspected female carriers may need to undergo molecular testing to confirm the diagnosis of Fabry disease.

9.2.3 Hypohidrotic Ectodermal Dysplasia

Hypohidrotic ectodermal Hypohidrotic ectodermal dysplasia is the most common form of ectodermal dysplasia. The majority of the cases are associated with mutations or deletions in the ectodysplasin (EDA) gene inherited on the X-chromosome, but both clinically similar autosomal dominant and autosomal recessive forms exist. Ectodysplasin-A is a component of the TNF-α related signaling pathway involved ectodermal-mesodermal interactions during embryogenesis [39]. It has a critical role in maintaining normal development of ectodermal appendages including hair, teeth, and sweat gland. The prevalence of the disorder has been reported to be between 1:10,000 and 1:100,000 male live births [40]. Males with X-linked hypohidrotic ectodermal dysplasia are hemizygous for EDA gene abnormalities and usually express the full-blown phenotype of hypotrichosis, hypohidrosis, oligodontia, and a predisposition to respiratory infections. Females with the condition are heterozygous and present with a variable phenotype [41].

9.2.3.1 Clinical Features in Males

The three cardinal features that become obvious during childhood are hypotrichosis, hypohidrosis and hypodontia. Affected neonates may present at birth with a collodion-like membrane, marked skin scaling or periorbital hyperpigmentation. The scalp hair is sparse to absent, and when present it is thin, lightly pigmented and slow growing. Due to decreased sweating, heat intolerance develops during infancy and poses a major problem. Teeth fail to erupt at the expected age, may be absent or reduced in number and peg-shaped. Additional cutaneous manifestations include eczema affecting most of the patients, with fragile-appearing skin, facial sebaceous hyperplasia, periorbital hyperpigmentation, smooth skin due to absent eccrine pores. Other signs include characteristic facies (saddle nose, full everted lips, frontal bossing), thick nasal secretions, dry eye symptoms, recurrent respiratory tract infections and raspy voice.

9.2.3.2 Features in Females

The clinical manifestations in female patients are variable due to the random nature of the X-inactivation. Female patients may be asymptomatic, show limited involvement or manifest with the full blown disease (similar to the hemizygous male). Differentiating female carriers with marked skewed X inactivation from unaffected females on one side and from the "full blown" autosomal recessive form on the other side may prove to be difficult. Dental abnormalities, mild hypohidrosis and mild hypotrichosis are commonly described clinical features [42]. An observational study from Italy described the clinical findings in six heterozygous female carriers [43]. Teeth abnormalities were the most constant marker of the disorder, including absence of several germ layers, peg-shaped teeth and delayed eruption. The scalp hair was typically thin but showed a highly variable degree of hypotrichosis. An important finding was a patchy distribution of vellus body hair following the lines of Blaschko. The normal skin was paler, contained vellus hair and looked slightly more elevated. The abnormal skin was slightly depressed, dryer, hyperpigmented and did not contain hair follicles. The starch-iodine test drew the lines of Blaschko, demonstrating the pattern of distribution of functioning eccrine sweat glands. Additional clinical features in female carriers include aplasia or hypoplasia of the mammary glands (breast and nipple), possibly associated with breastfeeding difficulties [44, 45].

9.2.4 Menkes Disease

Menkes disease, also known as Menkes kinky hair disease, is an x-linked recessive form of copper deficiency caused by different mutations in the ATP7A gene [46, 47]. The gene encodes a copper-transporting ATPase and mutations result in defective copper absorption. This leads to the biochemical profile that involves low copper levels in the blood, liver, brain and hair, reduced activity of copper-dependent enzymes and paradoxical accumulation of copper in certain tissues [48]. It is a rare disease with an estimated incidence of 1 in 100,000 [49]. The main clinical features are progressive neurodegeneration, marked connective tissue anomalies and typical sparse abnormal hair [50]. The classic form of the disease manifests in boys, with death occurring by 3 years of age, while females usually manifest with variable clinical findings. A milder allelic variant of Menkes disease is known as occipital horn syndrome, characterized by a less severe neurological phenotype [48].

9.2.4.1 Clinical Features in Males
Affected infants may appear normal in the first 8–12 weeks of life, then gradually develop failure

to thrive, hypotonia, lethargy, hypothermia, seizures and severe developmental delay [49]. Shortly thereafter, hair changes become manifest. The scalp and sometimes eyebrow hair is short, sparse, coarse, twisted (pili torti) and may be lightly pigmented [51]. Other hair abnormalities include transverse fracture of the hair shaft (trichoclasis), longitudinal splitting of the shaft (trichoptilosis), segmental shaft narrowing (monilethrix) and brush-like swellings of the hair shaft (trichorrhexis nodosa) [52, 53].

Distinctive facial features include pudgy cheeks (jowly appearance), a cupid's bow of the upper lip and horizontal eyebrows [48]. Additional clinical features include pectus excavatum, skin laxity (particularly at the nape of the neck, the axilla, and on the trunk) and umbilical or inguinal hernias. Patients may also have diffuse cutaneous pigmentary dilution due to decreased activity of tyrosinase, a copper-dependent enzyme. Vascular tortuosity, bladder diverticula and gastric polyps are common.

9.2.4.2 Features in Females
Menkes disease in females manifests with a variable spectrum of clinical findings. Most obligate female carriers present with patches of swirled hypopigmentation or pili torti along Blaschko's lines [51]. Additional clinical findings in females that are uniformly present include neurodevelopmental disability, hypotonia, and connective tissue findings, while other features, such as seizures, cerebral atrophy, and cerebrovascular tortuosity may be present but are under-reported and under-studied [54]. Heterozygous females may also be asymptomatic, due to favorably skewed X-chromosome inactivation [55] and a classic form was also reported [54].

9.2.5 Management and Treatment

Treatment is mainly symptomatic with gastrostomy tube placement to manage caloric intake, surgery to repair bladder diverticula and antibiotic prophylaxis to prevent bladder infections [49]. Early treatment with parenteral copper (Cu) has shown to improve the neurodevelopmental outcome in a subset of boys with the classic form of the disease [56, 57]. This treatment has never been studied in female patients [54]. Due to its severe phenotype and poor prognosis, genetic counseling is of great value with carrier detection possible through molecular genetic testing of at-risk female relative (following identification of the ATP7A pathogenic variant in the family).

9.3 X-Linked Dominant Genodermatoses

Most X-linked dominant genodermatoses are lethal in male embryos and therefore seen almost exclusively in females. Occasional male patients can be explained by functional mosaicism (Klinefelter syndrome) or genomic mosaicism (de novo half-chromatid or postzygotic mutation). Females typically present with a mosaic pattern of cutaneous lesions, following Blacshko's lines. An affected mother will transmit the disease (whether lethal or nonlethal) to 50% of her children. A list of the known X-linked dominant genodermatoses is presented in Table 9.2 (see Table 9.2); a few of them are discussed in more details ahead.

9.3.1 Conradi-Hunermann-Happle Syndrome

Conradi-Hunermann-Happle syndrome (CHHS), also known as chondrodysplasia punctata type 2, is a rare X-linked dominant disorder of cholesterol biosynthesis affecting mainly the skin, bones and eyes. The disorder is caused by mutations in the EBP gene which encodes emopamil-binding protein (EBP) also called 3β-hydroxysteroid-$\Delta 8$, $\Delta 7$-isomerase [58, 59]. This protein is a widely expressed integral membrane protein, and its deficiency leads to the accumulation of 8-dehydrocholesterol and 8(9)-cholesterol in the skin, plasma and other body tissues. The main clinical features include radiographic epiphyseal stippling, rhizomelic shortness, skin abnormalities, patchy alopecia, cataracts, and midfacial hypoplasia [60]. It pres-

ents almost exclusively in females, where a variable phenotype and skin lesion following Blaschko's lines has been attributed to lyonization [35, 61]. Although assumed to be lethal in male embryos [60], a few cases in male patients have been described. Several due to somatic mutations [62, 63], one due to gonosomal aneuploidy [64] and others who have not had molecular characterization [65–68]. CHILD syndrome (Congenital Hemidysplasia with Ichthyosiform Erythroderma [or Nevus] and Limb Defects), another rare X-linked dominant disorder shares some clinical features with CHHS. Stippled epiphyses during infancy and asymmetric limb shortening represents features of both syndromes, however, the striking lateralization of the skin involvement in CHILD syndrome easily differentiates the two.

9.3.1.1 Clinical Features

The most common manifestation at birth is generalized erythema with thick, adherent feathery scales, often with streaks and whorls of hyperkeratosis following Blaschko's lines (Fig. 9.3a). This usually resolves within the first weeks or months of life and is replaced by linear or patchy follicular atrophoderma with dilated follicular openings. Pigmentary abnormalities (hyper- or hypopigmentation) along Blaschko's lines may coexist. The hair may be sparse, coarse or lusterless with patches of scarring alopecia (Fig. 9.3b). Nail changes include flattening and splitting of the nail plates [60, 69, 70].

Skeletal anomalies normally begin soon after birth and during early childhood as stippling or punctuate calcifications (chondrodysplasia punctata). They usually involve the epiphyses of the long bones, the trachea and vertebrae and can be detected on radiographs during infancy. These changes are age dependent and cannot be seen once bone maturation progresses and normal epiphyseal ossification occurs. Most patients present with an asymmetric rhizomelic shortening of limbs, often involving the femur, humerus and other tubular bones [60]. Moderate to severe kyphoscoliosis is common and can present in infancy or early childhood. Additional skeletal abnormalities include frontal bossing, malar

Table 9.2 X-linked dominant genodermatoses

Disorder	Synonym/s	Gene Gene product Chromosomal location	Mechanism	Incidence	Onset	Mucocutaneous features
CHILD syndrome (congenital Hemidysplasia with ichthyosiform erythroderma [or nevus] and limb defects)	CHILD nevus	NSDHL 3β-hydroxysteroid dehydrogenase enzyme involved in cholesterol biosynthesis Xq28	Deficient sonic hedgehog signaling in cells expressing the mutant NSDHL	Rare	Birth	At birth, unilateral erythema and waxy, yellowish adherent scale Later, verrucous; hyperkeratosis of variable extent, with affinity for skin folds Linear alopecia Claw-like nail dystrophy or onychorrhexis Normal teeth
Conradi-Hunermann-Happle syndrome	X-linked dominant chondroplasia puncata, Chondroplasia punctata type 2 (CDPX2), Conradi-Hunermann syndrom, Happle syndrome	EBP Emopamil binding protein gene Xp11.23	Deficiency of EBP results in accumulation of 8-dehydrocholesterol and 8 (9) cholesterol	Rare	Birth	At birth, generalized ichthyosiform erythroderma with feathery, adherent scale Sreaks and whorls of hperkeratosis along Blachko's lines Later, after infancy, the skin changes evolve into follicular atrophoderma with dilated follicular openings and ice-pick-like scars along Blaschko's lines. The atrophoderma is most pronounced on the forearms and dorsal hands; palms and soles are usually spared Hyper or hypopigmentation Patchy scarring alopecia (swirled, following Blaschko's lines) Sparse, coarse or lusterless hair Onychoschizia and flatening of the nail plate Normal teeth

(continued)

Table 9.2 (continued)

Disorder	Synonym/s	Gene Gene product Chromosomal location	Mechanism	Incidence	Onset	Mucocutaneous features
Incontinentia pigmenti	Bloch-Sulzberger syndrome	NEMO NF-ƙB essential modulator Xq28		Rare	First few months of life	*State 1*: Linear erythema and blisters during the first few months of life *Stage 2*: Vesiculobullous lesions are most common on the limbs and scalp, frequent on the trunk and rare on the face. They resolve within days and often replaced by verrucous linear plaques that favor the extremities and disappear later in infancy *Stage 3*: Streaks and swirls of reticulate grayish-brown hyperpigmentatondevelop next with a predilection for the trunk and intertriginous sites *Stage 4*: From teen years onword, linear hypopigmented bands lacking hair and sweat glands appear on the posterior aspects of the limbs (especially the calves)
Terminal osseous dysplasia with pigmentary defects		FLNA Filamin A Xq28			Birth	Pigmentary skin lesion over the face and scalp
Focal dermal hypoplasia (Goltz syndrome)	Goltz-Gorlin syndrome	PORCN Porcupine homolog Xp11.23	PORCN functions as O-acyltransferase invovled in palmitoylation and secretion of Wnt, a morphogen imporant in ectomesodermal tissue development	Uncommon	Birth	The phenotype varies depending on the proportion and distribution of cells expressing the mutant X chromosome Streaks of vermiculate dermal atrophy and/or telangiectasias are often present from birth Later hypo-, hyperpigmentation and outpouching of fat develop Raspberry-like papillomas appear mostly in the anogenital region, lips, larynx and acral sites Dystrophic nails (longitudinal fissures, hypoplasia) Sparse hair Abnormal teeth (vertical grooving, hypodontia)

Microphthalmia with linear skin defects synrome (MIDAS syndrome)	HCCS Mitochondrial holocytochrome c synthase Xp22			Dermal aplasia
Bazex-Dupre-Christol syndrome	Bazex syndrome Xq24-27		Rare	Follicular atrophoderma—described as multiple ice-pick marks or patulous follicles, found most commonly on the dorsal aspect of the hands, but can also be seen on the feet, lower back, elbows and, rarely, the face Milia Multiple BCCs—in 40% of patietns, primarily on te face HypotrichosisLocalized hypohydrosis (above the neck) Facial hyperpigmentation Hair shaft anomalies and multiple richoepitheliomas
Oral-facial-digital-syndrome typ 1	OFD1 (oral-facial-digital-syndrome 1) [CXORF5] Xp22.1-p22.2	OFD1 encodes a centrosomal protein located at the base of primary (non-motile) cilia, present on most cells and mediate signaling patways such as hedghog and Wnt during embryonic development		Facial milia (primarily during infancy) Patchy alopecia, typically whorled at the vertex

(continued)

Table 9.2 (continued)

Disorder	Associated features	Diagnosis	Treatment	MIM number	Comments
CHILD syndrome (congenital Hemidysplasia with ichthyosiform erythroderma [or nevus] and limb defects)	Ipsilateral skeletal hemidysplasia Congenital or secondary scoliosis Chondropalsia punctata Organ hypoplasia (brain, kidneys, heart and lungs) Mild hearing loss Cleft palate	Clinical Molecular testing	Dermabrasion of the affected skin followed by placement of split-thickness skin grafts Multidisciplinary care depending on the extent of associated organ involvement	308,050, 300,275	Generally lethal in affected male embryos (two affected boys have been reported, one with a post zygotic mutation)
Conradi-Hunermann-Happle syndrome	Asymmetric skeletal abnormalities including frontal bossing, malar hypoplasia, a flat nasal bridge, a short neck, rhizomelic limb shortening and scoliosis Chondroplasia punctata typically involving the trachea and vertebrae (durng infancy) Ocular anomalies such as unilateral cataracts, microphthalmia and microcornea Occasionally: congenital heart defects, sensorineural deafness, CNS malformations and congenital renal anomalies	Clinical Epiphyseal stippling on X-ray during infancy Accumulation of plasma 8(9) cholesterol Molecular testing	Emolients Products containing urea or lactic acid Orthopedic and ophthalmologic care	302,960, 300,205	Generally lethal in male embryos outside the setting of an XXY karyotype or mosaicism due to a postzygotic mutation in the EBP gene
Incontinentia pigmenti	*Surface ectodermal defects:* Missing and conical teeth (60–80% of patients), linear absence of hair and sweat glands, dystrophic nails (ridging, pitting, subungual keratoses), asymmetric breast development or supernumerary nipples. *Eye anomalies (20–40% of patients):* retinal vascular abnormalities, strabismus, cataracts, microphthlmia, optic atrophy *Central nervous system abnormalities (20–30% of patients):* seizures, developmental delay, spastic hemi/di/tetraplegia *Skeletal defecs (uncommon):* skull anomalies, scoliosis *Other organs (uncommon):* pulmonary hypertension		Baseline and longitudinal ophthalmologic and neurologic evaluations and dental assesments	308,300, 300,248	Usually antenatally lethal in boys Occasional occurrences in boys attributed to Klinefelter syndrome or genomic mosaicism
Terminal osseous dysplasia with pigmentary defects	Skeletal dysplasia of the limbs- abnormal and delayed ossification of bones in the hands and feet, leading to brachydactyly, camptodactyly, and clinodactyly, severe limb deformities, and joint contractures Dysmorphic features including hypertelorism, midface hypoplasia, low set ears and multiple frenula Recurrent digital fibroma during infancy			300,244, 300,017	Male-lethal

Disorder	Clinical features	Treatment	OMIM	Comments
Focal dermal hypoplasia (Goltz syndrome)	Bony reduction deformities of the hands are common (particularly ectrodactyly) Osteopathia striata (streaks of decreased bone density) is a common finding in radiographs of the mid portion of the lower extremities Eye abnormalities (often unilateral) include coloboma, aniridia, microphthalmia and anophthalmia Dysmorphic facies (notched nasal alae, pointed chin, large malformed ears) Other features less commonly obsereved include aplasia cutis congenita, myelomeningocele, cleft lip/palate, deafness, urinary tract anomalies and gastrointestinal maldevelopment	Supportive Subspecialist referral based on the associaated abnormalities Pulsed dye laser treatment for the telangiectasias Curettage or photodynamic therapy for exophytic papillomas	305,600, 300,651	Antenatally lethal in males with non-mosiac hemizygous mutations, male patients with genomic or functional mosaicism account for 10% of affected individuals Approximately 95% of cases are sporadic
Microphthalmia with linear skin defects synrome (MIDAS syndrome)	Microphthalmia Sclerocornea Cardiac arrhthymias Agenesis of the corpus callosum Genital anomalies Short stature		309,801, 300,056	Antenatally lethal in males
Bazex-Dupre-Christol syndrome			301,845	Should not be confused with acrokeratosis paraneoplastica, also known as Bazex syndrome, which occurs most commonly in the setting of carcinoma of the upper aerodigestive tract
Oral-facial-digital-syndrome typ 1	Cleft (or pseudocleft) lip/palate Lobulations and hamartomas of the tongue Hypertrophic oral fremula (associated with alveolar clefts) Malformations of the digits Structural brain abnormalities Intelectual disability Polycystic kidneys		311,200, 300,170	

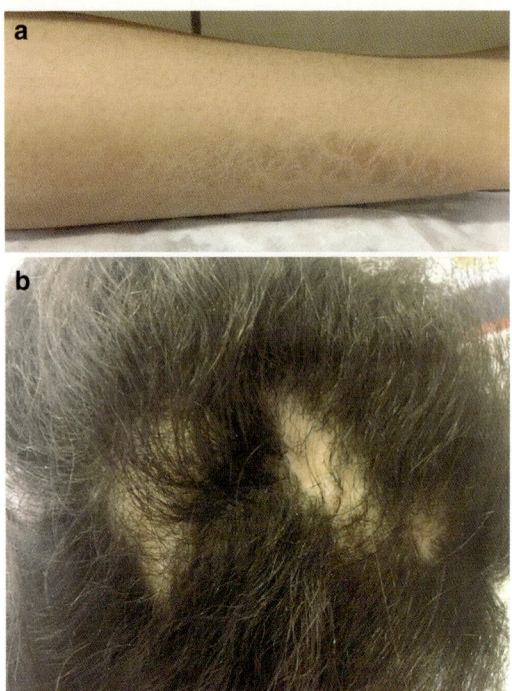

Fig. 9.3 Skin and hair findings in Conradi-Hunermann-Happle syndrome. (**a**) Linear streak of hyperkeratosis over the shin. (**b**) Patches of scarring alopecia

hypoplasia, a flat nasal bridge, a short neck and postaxial polydactyly [60].

Unilateral, asymmetric, and/or sectorial cataracts, which are present at birth or develop early in, are the most common ocular abnormality, less frequently, microphthalmia and/or microcornea may coexist [60, 71, 72].

Other features, less commonly seen, include cardiac or renal malformations, sensorineural deafness, CNS malformations and clubfoot [60, 72]. Intelligence and life expectancy are typically normal.

The classic features of CHH have been reported in male patients (as mentioned above) and the clinical features are well within the marked variability described in affected females.

An allelic X-linked recessive multiple congenital anomaly syndrome has been described in males with a hemizygous EBP pathogenic missense mutation [73, 74]. Patients presented with a collodion-like presentation at birth and evolution to variable ichthyosis phenotype. Neurologic manifestations including moderate to severe developmental delay, CNS malformations (Dandy-Walker malformation, agenesis of the corpus callosum, major gyral abnormalities). Additional features included hydrocephalus, cataracts, cryptorchidism, and cardiovascular, craniofacial and skeletal anomalies.

Treatment of CHHS is symptomatic and individualized. Orthopedic care is important for the management of leg length discrepancy and assessment of kyphoscoliosis. Opthalmologic care for cataract extraction and correction of vision and dermatologic care for the management of skin lesions are additional important therapeutic aspects.

9.3.2 Incontinentia Pigmenti

Among the X-linked dominant disorders with male lethality, incontinentia pigmenti (IP), also known as Bloch-Sulzberger syndrome, is perhaps the best investigated. It is a rare X-linked dominant multi-system disorder involving the skin, teeth, nails, eyes, and central nervous system. The name is derived from the pathologic picture of pigmentary incontinence in the third stage of the disease [75]. IP is caused by mutations in the NEMO (also known as IKBKG) gene at Xq28 [76]. It is caused by a large deletion in most patients. The NEMO gene product is required for the activation of the nuclear factor-kappa B (NF-κB) transcription factor [77]. At the skin level, NF-κB appears to have a dual role in cell growth and apoptosis [78]. X-linked hypohidrotic ectodermal dysplasia and immunodeficiency is another phenotype associated with mutation of the NEMO gene. It is caused primarily by missense mutations that result in impaired, but not absent, NF-κB signaling [79, 80].

The vast majority of IP patients are females with skin lesions presenting in swirling patterns following Blaschko's lines due to cutaneous mosaicism. Although defined as a "male-lethal" disease, there are well-documented male cases [81, 82]. Survival in males is attributed to Kleinfelter syndrome, somatic mosaicism or hypomorphic mutations [83, 84].

9.3.2.1 Clinical Features

The cutaneous manifestations of IP classically evolve through four well characterized stages [85]. The onset, duration and severity of the stages are variable among patients. Some stages may overlap (Fig. 9.4) and some may not appear at all. In all stages, the skin lesions occur along Blaschko's lines. Stage I (vesiculobullous stage I) presents perinatally as an erythematous vesicular rash that is most common on the limbs and scalp. It generally disappears after a few weeks or months when it evolves into hypertrophic wart like linear papules and plaques that favor the distal extremities (verrucous stage II), and disappear later in infancy. The hyperpigmented stage, (hyperpigmented stage III), which is the hallmark of IP is the next to follow. Brown or slate grey macules arise in a swirled pattern along Blaschko's lines with a predilection for the trunk and intertriginous sites (groin, axillae). The pigmentary changes can be linear, swirled, or reticulated but can be quite limited. It usually fades by adolescence but may persist into adulthood. When the pigmentation fades, linear hypopigmentation and alopecia, most noticeable on the posterior aspects of the calves, are to follow (hypopigmented/atrophic stage IV). These changes are mostly permanent and often the only signs of skin involvement in adult patients.

The most common extracutaneous manifestations are dental anomalies affecting more than 80% of IP patients [86]. These include hypodontia, microdontia, delayed dentition and abnormally shaped teeth (conical or peg-shaped). Dystrophic nails (lined, pitted or brittle), linear areas of alopecia and absence of sweat glands may accompany skin stages II and IV, respectively. Breast abnormalities ranging from aplasia to supernumerary nipples are variably present [87]. Ophthalmologic abnormalities are common and variable [88]. Retinal hypervascularization conferring risk of retinal detachment in infancy and childhood is of major concern [89, 90]. Other Ophthalmologic abnormalities include strabismus, cataracts, microphthalmia, optic atrophy, retinal dysfunction, retinal pigmentary abnormalities, uveitis, nystagmus, and blindness [88, 91–93].

Neurologic abnormalities occur in about 30% of patients with IP resulting in convulsive disorders, motor abnormalities (hemiplegia, diplegia, or tetraplegia), developmental delay and intellectual disability [94, 95]. These neurological abnormalities appear to be associated with CNS vasculopathy (cerebral macro- and microangiopathy).

Additional less common clinical features include skeletal and structural anomalies (scoliosis, skull deformities, somatic asymmetry), primary pulmonary hypertension and malignancies [86, 96–98].

As mentioned above, cases of male patients with IP are well-documented. In general, the clinical features are similar to those of female patients but males are more likely than females to have neurologic abnormalities [99].

The management of IP includes topical treatment for the skin lesions and prevention of infections. Baseline and longitudinal ophthalmologic and neurologic evaluations are recommended as well as an early assessment by a pedodontist.

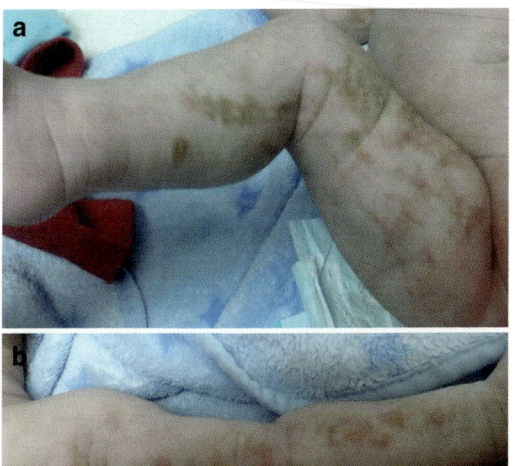

Fig. 9.4 Overlapping Blaschko-linear stages of incontinenta pigmenti. (**a**) Linear and reticulated hyperpigemented streaks over groin and lower limb, occurring simultaneously to linear vesiculobullous lesions over upper limb (**b**) in an infant with incontinenta pigmenti

9.3.3 Focal Dermal Hypoplasia

Focal dermal hypoplasia (FDH), also called Goltz syndrome or Goltz-Gorlin syndrome, is a rare X-linked dominant genodermatosis involving primarily the skin and its appendages, but also characterized by craniofacial and skeletal, as well as ocular, renal and gastrointestinal anomalies [100]. The clinical features are the consequence of developmental abnormalities in mesodermal and ectodermal structures [101, 102]. The disorder is caused by mutations in the PORCN gene, encoding an O-acyltransferase which is crucial for the Wnt signaling pathway [103–105]. Activation of the Wnt pathway is important for normal development [106]. The Wnt signaling stimulates fibroblast proliferation, inhibits adipogenesis and induces osteogenesis. It also has key roles in early limb patterning and tooth formation. The dermatologic features of FDH follow Blaschko's lines due to mosaicism and lyonization [107], also explaining the variability in the disease phenotypes [108]. While the primary cutaneous abnormality is dermal rather than epidermal, the Blaschko-linear pattern reflects embryonic migration pathways of epidermal development. This has led to the postulation that PORCN expression and resultant Wnt signaling originating from the epidermis, regulate development of the underlying dermis [109]. This has been shown in mice with ectoderm-specific deletion of PORCN [110]. Females account for 90% of individuals with FDH. The remaining 10% are males with genomic or functional mosaicism, as non-mosaic male mutations are presumed to be lethal. Approximately 95% of FDH are due to a de novo pathogenic mutation, which likely reflects a decreased likelihood of reproduction by severely affected women and the lethality of PORCN mutations with widespread expression. A preferential inactivation of the mutant X chromosome or a postzygotic mutation might be required for survival of affected female fetuses, as been suggested by some authors [111].

9.3.3.1 Clinical Features

Dermatologic findings are key features in FDH [100, 101, 112, 113]. Streaks of skin atrophy in a Blaschko-linear pattern, which are erythematous at birth, and typically become hypopigmented with time are present in most cases. They may be accompanied by telangiectasias and less commonly hyperpigmentation rather than hypopigmentation. Outpouchings of fat in the dermis, manifesting as soft, yellow-pink cutaneous nodules, are typically seen on the trunk and extremities. Periorificial papillomas with a raspberry-like appearance favor the anogenital region, lips, larynx and acral sites, but may appear anywhere. The nails can be absent (anonychia), small (micronychia), hypoplastic, or dysplastic, often with longitudinal ridging, splitting, or V-nicking. Hair can be sparse, wiry or absent with patches of alopecia. Hair shaft abnormalities on scanning electron microscopy are common. Dental abnormalities including enamel defects, longitudinal grooving, peg teeth or hypodontia are present in most cases [113].

Limb malformations noted at birth, including syndactyly, oligodactyly, and ectrodactyly (split-hand/foot or "lobster-claw"malformation) may impair function. Additionally, reduction defects of the long bones ranging from leg length discrepancies to transverse defects of the distal radius/ulna or tibia/fibula are commonly seen [114]. Osteopathia striata, a striated appearance of the bones evident on plain x-rays is another common feature. Less common skeletal abnormalities include scoliosis, hypoplastic clavicles and ribs, and a deformed thorax [112].

Developmental abnormalities of the eye can include iris and chorioretinal coloboma (most common ocular manifestation), nystagmus, strabismus, cataracts, anophthalmia, microphthalmia, and lacrimal duct abnormalities [115].

The craniofacial features in FDH are highly variable and can include notched or hypoplastic alae nasi, facial asymmetry, a pointed chin, abnormal ear morphology and cleft lip and palate [114, 116].

Other occasional features include aplasia cutis congenita, myelomeningocele, deafness, renal or urinary tract anomalies and gastrointestinal maldevelopment (el and abdominal wall defect) [117].

A recent cohort of 18 patients with FDH provided a phenotypic summary and proposed clinical diagnostic criteria [114]. The authors suggested that the diagnosis should be made in any individual with three or more characteristic skin manifestations in conjunction with at least one characteristic limb malformation. The characteristic skin manifestations include congenital patchy skin aplasia, congenital nodular fat herniation, congenital hyperpigmentation or hypopigmentation in Blaschko-linear distribution, telangiectasia, and congenital ridged dysplastic nails. The characteristic limb malformations are ectrodactyly, transverse limb defects, syndactyly, oligodactyly, or marked long bone reductions.

Because relatively few affected males have been reported, no comprehensive data for a "typical" male phenotype exist. Affected males may have any of the features seen in affected females, but due to the somatic mosaicism for the PORCN pathogenic variant, they are generally more mildly affected than females [103, 104, 118].

The management of FDH depends on the clinical manifestations. The treatment is supportive with appropriate skin care for the pruritic erosive lesions that are also prone to infection, pulsed dye laser may improve the telangiectasias and papillomas can be treated with curettage or photodynamic therapy. Subspecialist referral based on the associated abnormalities is important.

9.4 Other Genodermatoses

Other genodermatoses with gender dependent expression are presented in Table 9.3. Chromosomal abnormalities involving the sex chromosomes are another form of genodermatoses associated with gender differences. Klinefelter syndrome and Turner syndrome belong to this category and will be further discussed.

9.4.1 Klinefelter Syndrome

Klinefelter syndrome, 47,XXY (KS) is the most common chromosomal disorder in males and the most common genetic cause of infertility [119], affecting approximately one in 660 newborn boys [120]. It was first reported in 1942 by Klinefelter et al. who described nine men with enlarged breasts, sparse facial and body hair, small testes and an inability to produce sperm [121]. The genetic background of an extra X chromosome was discovered in 1959 [122]. Despite at least one extra X chromosome, patients with this syndrome are phenotypically males. The classic form of KS, (80–90%) is defined by a 47,XXY karyotype resulting from the aneuploidy of the sex chromosomes. Higher-grade aneuploidies (e.g. 48,XXXY or 48,XXYY), structurally abnormal X chromosome (e.g. 47,iXq,Y) or mosaicisms (e.g. 47,XXY/46,XY) make up the remaining 10–20% of cases [123].

The main features of KS are small testes, hypergonadotropic hypogonadism and cognitive impairment. Additional characteristics include gynecomastia, infertility, tall stature, long lower extremities, eunuchoid body proportions and sparse body hair [120, 124]. The clinical manifestations may be variable thus karyotyping is used to confirm the diagnosis [120].

9.4.1.1 Dermatologic Manifestations

Sparse facial and body hair were included in the original report of KS [121] and are common. They result from the low testosterone levels [125]. Leg ulceration has been reported as a complication or manifestation of KS in many occasions. The prevalence was reported to be 6–13% in one series [126]. The pathogenesis of the ulcer formation in the setting of KS is still unclear but is believed to be complicated and multifactorial. Chronic venous insufficiency, obesity, congenital venous and arterial anomalies, hormonal influences, comorbidities including diabetes mellitus and autoimmune diseases and abnormalities in coagulation and fibrinolytic systems have all been reported [127, 128]. The leg ulcerations are usually hard to treat. Treatment options include local wound care, but successful testosterone replacement therapy has also been reported [128–130].

The treatment and care of patients with KS is multidisciplinary and should ideally involve speech therapists, psychologists, general practitioners, pediatricians, endocrinologists, urologists, and infertility specialists [120].

Table 9.3 Other genodermatoses with gender differences

Group of Diseases	Diagnosis	Mode of inheritance	Synonym/s	Gene	Gene product	Chromosomal location	Molecular defect	Mechanism
Keratodermas	Palmoplantar keratoderma with sex reversal and squamous cell carcinoma	Autosomal recessive		RSPO1	R-spondin 1	1p34.3		The mutated gene encodes a protein that activates β-catenin signaling and has an importat roles in gonadal development
	Hereditary angioedema type III	Autosomal dominant (only females affected)		F12	Factor XII (Hageman factor)	5q33-qter		A heterozygous gain-of-function mutation in the gene encoding FXII
Chromosomal abnormalities	Turner syndrome	Chromosomal aberration: 45, X0						
	Klinefelter syndrome	Chromosomal aberration: 47, XXY						

Group of Diseases	Incidence	Onset	Mucocutaneous features	Associated features	Diagnostic measures	Treatment	MIM number	Comments
Keratodermas	Rare	Infancy	A diffuse NEPPK (non-epidermolytic palmoplantar keratoderma) with onset in infancy and a marked predisposition to the development of squamous cell carcinoma / Variable cutaneous atrophy	XX genotype with either (1) male phenotype (often associated with hypospadias and hypogonadism (2) ambiguous genitalia, sometimes with hermaphrodism / sclerodactyly / Nail dystrophy (hypoplasia, longitudinal ridging, skin growth over the nail plate) / Periodontitis leading to early loss of teeth			610644, 609595	
							610618, 610619	
Chromosomal abnormalities			Congenital lymphedema (usually resolves by age 2 years) / Low posterior hairline / Numerous melanocytic nevi / Small hyperconvex nails / Tendency to form keloids	Short stature, webbed neck, "shield-like" chest with widely spaced nipples / Absence of sexual development / Cardiovascular defects / Renal malformations / Sensorineural hearing loss / Autoimmune hypothyroidism				Mosaicism (45, X0/46, XX or 45 X0/46XY) in ~40% of patients
			Varicose veins / Leg ulcers	Tall stature / Gynecomastea / Small testes, infertility				Mosaicism 46, XY/47, XXY in ~20% of patients; uncommon variants include 48, XXXY and 48, XXY

9.4.2 Turner Syndrome

Turner syndrome is the most common sex chromosome abnormality affecting females and has an incidence of 1 in 2500 live female births [131]. It was first described by Turner et al. in 1938 as a triad of infantilism, webbed neck and elbow deformity (cubitus valgus) [132]. With time, various clinical manifestations were added to the syndrome. The most common are short stature, premature ovarian failure and phenotypic abnormalities including high palate, nail dysplasia, low posterior hairline, wide spaced nipples, webbed neck and low-set or malrotated ears [133]. Additional medical problems associated with TS include cardiovascular defects, renal malformations, skeletal anomalies, hearing loss and autoimmune disorders. The chromosomal basis for TS was described in 1959 [134]. There is genetic heterogeneity with an absence of either the entire second X chromosome, a part of it, a defect in its' structure or mosaicism of 45, X with another cell line [135]. Approximately 50% of TS patients have the classic monosomy X (a 45, X karyotype) [136]. Mosaicism, which arises from postzygotic nondisjunction, may lead to a higher survival rate [137, 138]. The pathophysiologic basis of TS is considered to be a consequence of deficient expression of certain genes on the X chromosome, as not all X-linked genes undergo lyonization [139, 140]. The pseudoautosomal region, which is the distal tip of the short arm of the X chromosome, escapes inactivation and has homologues on the Y chromosome [140]. Several genetic loci have been implicated in TS including the short stature homeobox (SHOX) gene and also genomic imprinting [135]. Some genotype-phenotype correlations have been described [140]. Although the cutaneous findings in Turner syndrome are not the main pathology, they may provide important clinical clues for early detection.

9.4.2.1 Dermatologic Manifestations

Lymphatic abnormalities are a common presenting manifestation of TS and possible sequelae include webbed neck, redundant neck folds and a low posterior hairline and small hypoplastic concave fingernails [135]. Cystic hygroma results from jugular lymphatic obstruction during embryogenesis and may be noted at birth. The congenital lymphedema usually resolves spontaneously by 2 years of age but lymphedema of the legs may recur unilateraly or bilaterally in late childhood or adult life. The lymphedema is usually asymptomatic but, if necessary, may be treated with support stockings or leg elevation. It also may predict other systemic disorders, such as cardiac disease [141, 142].

Patients with TS have an increased number of benign melanocytic nevi of an unknown etiology [143–145]. These nevi are usually small, non-dysplastic, located mostly on the face, back, and extremities and are acquired usually in late childhood. Controversy exists regarding the prevalence of melanoma. A national cohort study from Great Britain suggested that women with TS are possibly at increased risk for melanoma [146]. In other studies, despite the increased number of nevi, the incidence of melanoma seemed to be markedly reduced [144]. Treatment measures such as growth hormone, oral contraceptives or hormone replacement have failed to show a significant influence on nevus count and melanoma risk [135]. Periodic skin examinations and photoprotection are advised.

An increased risk of keloid formation and hypertrophic scarring has been long reported [147], but questioned recently. Reported hair abnormalities include unusual patches of short and long hair, asynchronous scalp hair growth [148], facial hirsutism, scant axillary and pubic hair [149] and alopecia areata [150]. Other dermatologic associations include premature facial skin aging [151], vitiligo [152, 153], psoriasis [150], decreased acne prevalence [135], increased frequency of cafe' au lait macules, neonatal cutis verticis gyrate in the context of congenital lymphedema [154], halo nevi [155, 156], multiple pilomatricomas [157], hemangiomas [158] and pigmentary alterations following Blaschko's lines in mosaic TS [159].

TS is a complex medical condition that requires early medical evaluation, intervention, and long-term follow-up by a multi-disciplinary team.

Conclusion

Gender specific differences are characteristic of genodermatoses in which the pathogenesis involves the sex chromosomes. These include the X-linked genodermatoses (recessive and dominant) and sex chromosome abnormalities. The normal X inactivation (lyonization) which occurs in females and results in functional mosaicism, is a major determinant of gender specific variability in genodermatoses. Elucidation of the pathomechanisms responsible for this gender specific variability and better understanding of the role of genes located on the sex chromosomes in determining the cutaneous phenotype, may provide insights into gender differences in dermatology in general.

References

1. Feramisco JD, Sadreyev RI, Murray ML, Grishin NV, Tsao H. Phenotypic and genotypic analyses of genetic skin disease through the online mendelian inheritance in man (OMIM) database. J Invest Dermatol. 2009;129(11):2628–36.
2. Lemke JR, Kernland-Lang K, Hörtnagel K, Itin P. Monogenic human skin disorders. Dermatology. 2014;229(2):55–64.
3. Fine J-D, Eady RA, Bauer EA, Bauer JW, Bruckner-Tuderman L, Heagerty A, et al. The classification of inherited epidermolysis bullosa (EB): report of the third international consensus meeting on diagnosis and classification of EB. J Am Acad Dermatol. 2008;58(6):931–50.
4. Oji V, Tadini G, Akiyama M, Bardon CB, Bodemer C, Bourrat E, et al. Revised nomenclature and classification of inherited ichthyoses: results of the first Ichthyosis consensus conference in Soreze 2009. J Am Acad Dermatol. 2010;63(4):607–41.
5. Lyon MF. X-chromosome inactivation: a repeat hypothesis. Cytogenet Genome Res. 1998; 80(1-4):133–7.
6. Sun BK, Tsao H. X-chromosome inactivation and skin disease. J Invest Dermatol. 2008;128(12): 2753–9.
7. Wells R, Kerr C. Genetic classification of ichthyosis. Arch Dermatol. 1965;92(1):1–6.
8. Elias P, Williams M, Maloney M, Bonifas J, Brown B, Grayson S, et al. Stratum corneum lipids in disorders of cornification. Steroid sulfatase and cholesterol sulfate in normal desquamation and the pathogenesis of recessive X-linked ichthyosis. J Clin Invest. 1984;74(4):1414.
9. Williams ML. Epidermal lipids and scaling diseases of the skin. Semin Dermatol. 1992;11:169.
10. Bonifas JM, Morley BJ, Oakey RE, Kan YW, Epstein EH. Cloning of a cDNA for steroid sulfatase: frequent occurrence of gene deletions in patients with recessive X chromosome-linked ichthyosis. Proc Natl Acad Sci U S A. 1987;84(24):9248–51.
11. Reed M, Purohit A, Woo L, Newman SP, Potter BV. Steroid sulfatase: molecular biology, regulation, and inhibition. Endocr Rev. 2005;26(2):171–202.
12. Siegel DH, Sybert VP. Mosaicism in genetic skin disorders. Pediatr Dermatol. 2006;23(1):87–92.
13. Mevorah B, Frenk E, Müller C, Ropers H. X-linked recessive ichthyosis in three sisters: evidence for homozygosity. Br J Dermatol. 1981;105(6):711–7.
14. Hazan C, Orlow SJ, Schaffer JV. X-linked recessive ichthyosis. Dermatol Online J. 2005;11(4):12.
15. Fernandes NF, Janniger CK, Schwartz RA. X-linked ichthyosis: an oculocutaneous genodermatosis. J Am Acad Dermatol. 2010;62(3):480–5.
16. Traupe H, Happle R. Clinical spectrum of steroid sulfatase deficiency: X-linked recessive ichthyosis, birth complications and cryptorchidism. Eur J Pediatr. 1983;140(1):19–21.
17. Lykkesfeldt G, Lykkesfeldt A, Hoyer H, Skakkebaek N. Steroid sulphatase deficiency associated with testis cancer. Lancet. 1983;322(8365):1456.
18. Lynch HT, Ozer F, CW MN, Johnson JE, Jampolsky NA. Secondary male hypogonadism and congenital ichthyosis: association of two rare genetic diseases. Am J Hum Genet. 1960;12(4 Pt 1):440.
19. Bradshaw K, Carr B. Placental sulfatase deficiency: maternal and fetal expression of steroid sulfatase deficiency and X-linked ichthyosis. Obstet Gynecol Surv. 1986;41(7):401–13.
20. Liaugaudienė O, Benušienė E, Domarkienė I, Ambrozaitytė L, Kučinskas V. X-linked ichthyosis: differential diagnosis of low maternal oestriol level. J Obstetric Gynecol. 2014;34(8):737–9.
21. Costagliola C, Fabbrocini G, Illiano G, Scibelli G, Delfino M. Ocular findings in X-linked ichthyosis: a survey on 38 cases. Ophthalmologica. 1991;202(3):152–5.
22. Fabry J. Ein Beitrag zur Kenntniss der Purpura haemorrhagica nodularis (Purpura papulosa haemorrhagica Hebrae). Arch Dermatol Res. 1898;43(1):187–200.
23. Anderson W. A case of "Angeio-Keratoma." Br J Dermatol. 1898;10(4):113–7.
24. Calhoun DH, Bishop DF, Bernstein HS, Quinn M, Hantzopoulos P, Desnick RJ. Fabry disease: isolation of a cDNA clone encoding human alpha-galactosidase A. Proc Natl Acad Sci U S A. 1985;82(21):7364–8.
25. Inoue T, Hattori K, Ihara K, Ishii A, Nakamura K, Hirose S. Newborn screening for Fabry disease in Japan: prevalence and genotypes of Fabry disease in a pilot study. J Hum Genet. 2013;58(8):548–52.
26. Schiffmann R, Ries M. Fabry disease: a disorder of childhood onset. Pediatr Neurol. 2016;64:10–20.

27. Ries M, Moore DF, Robinson CJ, Tifft CJ, Rosenbaum KN, Brady RO, et al. Quantitative dysmorphology assessment in Fabry disease. Genet Med. 2006;8(2):96–101.

28. Hoffmann B, Schwarz M, Mehta A, Keshav S, Investigators FOSE. Gastrointestinal symptoms in 342 patients with Fabry disease: prevalence and response to enzyme replacement therapy. Clin Gastroenterol Hepatol. 2007;5(12):1447–53.

29. Magage S, Lubanda J-C, Susa Z, Bultas J, Karetova D, Dobrovolný R, et al. Natural history of the respiratory involvement in Anderson–Fabry disease. J Inherit Metab Dis. 2007;30(5):790–9.

30. Cole A, Lee P, Hughes D, Deegan P, Waldek S, Lachmann R. Depression in adults with Fabry disease: a common and under-diagnosed problem. J Inherit Metab Dis. 2007;30(6):943–51.

31. Sachdev B, Takenaka T, Teraguchi H, Tei C, Lee P, McKenna W, et al. Prevalence of Anderson-Fabry disease in male patients with late onset hypertrophic cardiomyopathy. Circulation. 2002;105(12):1407–11.

32. Nakao S, Kodama C, Takenaka T, Tanaka A, Yasumoto Y, Yoshida A, et al. Fabry disease: detection of undiagnosed hemodialysis patients and identification of a "renal variant" phenotype1. Kidney Int. 2003;64(3):801–7.

33. Deegan P, Baehner A, Romero MA, Hughes D, Kampmann C, Beck M. Natural history of Fabry disease in females in the Fabry outcome survey. J Med Genet. 2006;43(4):347–52.

34. Wang RY, Lelis A, Mirocha J, Wilcox WR. Heterozygous Fabry women are not just carriers, but have a significant burden of disease and impaired quality of life. Genet Med. 2007;9(1):34–45.

35. Happle R. X-chromosome inactivation: role in skin disease expression. Acta Paediatr. 2006;95(S451):16–23.

36. Wilcox WR, Oliveira JP, Hopkin RJ, Ortiz A, Banikazemi M, Feldt-Rasmussen U, et al. Females with Fabry disease frequently have major organ involvement: lessons from the Fabry registry. Mol Genet Metab. 2008;93(2):112–28.

37. Eng CM, Guffon N, Wilcox WR, Germain DP, Lee P, Waldek S, et al. Safety and efficacy of recombinant human α-galactosidase A replacement therapy in Fabry's disease. N Engl J Med. 2001;345(1):9–16.

38. Wilcox WR, Banikazemi M, Guffon N, Waldek S, Lee P, Linthorst GE, et al. Long-term safety and efficacy of enzyme replacement therapy for Fabry disease. Am J Hum Genet. 2004;75(1):65–74.

39. Trzeciak WH, Koczorowski R. Molecular basis of hypohidrotic ectodermal dysplasia: an update. J Appl Genet. 2016;57(1):51–61.

40. Deshmukh S, Prashanth S. Ectodermal dysplasia: a genetic review. Int J Clin Pediatr Dent. 2012;5(3):197–202.

41. Fete M, Hermann J, Behrens J, Huttner KM. X-linked hypohidrotic ectodermal dysplasia (XLHED): clinical and diagnostic insights from an international patient registry. Am J Med Genet A. 2014;164(10):2437–42.

42. Freire-Maia N, Pinheiro M. Carrier detection in Christ-Siemens-Touraine syndrome (X-linked hypohidrotic ectodermal dysplasia). Am J Hum Genet. 1982;34(4):672.

43. Cambiaghi S, Restano L, Pääkkönen K, Caputo R, Kere J. Clinical findings in mosaic carriers of hypohidrotic ectodermal dysplasia. Arch Dermatol. 2000;136(2):217–24.

44. Clarke A, Phillips D, Brown R, Harper PS. Clinical aspects of X-linked hypohidrotic ectodermal dysplasia. Arch Dis Child. 1987;62(10):989–96.

45. Visinoni AF, Lisboa-Costa T, Pagnan NA, Chautard-Freire-Maia EA. Ectodermal dysplasias: clinical and molecular review. Am J Med Genet A. 2009;149(9):1980–2002.

46. Kaler SG. Metabolic and molecular bases of Menkes disease and occipital horn syndrome. Pediatr Dev Pathol. 1998;1(1):85–98.

47. Vulpe C, Levinson B, Whitney S, Packman S, Gitschier J. Isolation of a candidate gene for Menkes disease and evidence that it encodes a copper-transporting ATPase. Nat Genet. 1993;3(1):7–13.

48. Kaler SG. Inborn errors of copper metabolism. Handb Clin Neurol. 2013;113:1745.

49. Kaler SG. ATP7A-related copper transport disorders. 2010.

50. Nadal D, Baerlocher K. Menkes' disease: long-term treatment with copper and D-penicillamine. Eur J Pediatr. 1988;147(6):621–5.

51. Moore CM, Howell RR. Ectodermal manifestations in Menkes disease. Clin Genet. 1985;28(6):532–40.

52. Taylor C, Green S. Menkes' syndrome (Trichopoliodystrophy): use of scanning electron-microscope in diagnosis and carrier identification. Dev Med Child Neurol. 1981;23(3):361–8.

53. Craiu D, Kaler S, Craiu M. Role of optic microscopy for early diagnosis of Menkes. Romanian J Morphol Embryol. 2014;55(3):953–6.

54. Smpokou P, Samanta M, Berry GT, Hecht L, Engle EC, Lichter-Konecki U. Menkes disease in affected females: the clinical disease spectrum. Am J Med Genet A. 2015;167(2):417–20.

55. Desai V, Donsante A, Swoboda KJ, Martensen M, Thompson J, Kaler S. Favorably skewed X-inactivation accounts for neurological sparing in female carriers of Menkes disease. Clin Genet. 2011;79(2):176–82.

56. Kaler SG, Holmes CS, Goldstein DS, Tang J, Godwin SC, Donsante A, et al. Neonatal diagnosis and treatment of Menkes disease. N Engl J Med. 2008;358(6):605–14.

57. Kaler SG, Liew CJ, Donsante A, Hicks JD, Sato S, Greenfield JC. Molecular correlates of epilepsy in early diagnosed and treated Menkes disease. J Inherit Metab Dis. 2010;33(5):583–9.

58. Derry JM, Gormally E, Means GD, Zhao W, Meindl A, Kelley RI, et al. Mutations in a Δ8-Δ7 sterol isomerase in the tattered mouse and X-linked

dominant chondrodysplasia punctata. Nat Genet. 1999;22(3):286–90.

59. Braverman N, Lin P, Moebius FF, Obie C, Moser A, Glossmann H, et al. Mutations in the gene encoding 3β-hydroxysteroid-Δ 8, Δ7-isomerase cause X-linked dominant Conradi-Hünermann syndrome. Nat Genet. 1999;22(3):291–4.

60. Happle R. X-linked dominant chondrodysplasia punctata. Hum Genet. 1979;53(1):65–73.

61. Happle R, Frosch P. Manifestation of the lines of Blaschko in women heterozygous for X-linked hypohidrotic ectodermal dysplasia. Clin Genet. 1985;27(5):468–71.

62. Aughton DJ, Kelley RI, Metzenberg A, Pureza V, Pauli RM. X-linked dominant chondrodysplasia punctata (CDPX2) caused by single gene mosaicism in a male. Am J Med Genet A. 2003;116(3):255–60.

63. Tan C, Haverfield E, Dempsey M, Kratz L, Descartes M, Powell B. X-linked dominant chondrodysplasia punctata and EBP mutations in males. Poster session. American College of Medical Genetics Annual Clinical Genetics Meeting, Albuquerque, NM; 2010.

64. Sutphen R, Amar MJ, Kousseff BG, Toomey KE. XXY male with X-linked dominant chondrodysplasia punctata (Happle syndrome). Am J Med Genet. 1995;57(3):489–92.

65. Crovato F, Rebora A. Acute skin manifestations of Conradi-Huenermann syndrome in a male adult. Arch Dermatol. 1985;121(8):1064–5.

66. De Raeve L, Song M, De Dobbeleer G, Spehl M, Regemorter V. Lethal course of X-linked dominant chondrodysplasia punctata in a male newborn. Dermatology. 1989;178(3):167–70.

67. Tronnier M, Froster-Iskenius U, Schmeller W, Happle R, Wolff H. X-chromosome dominant chondrodysplasia punctata (Happle) in a boy. Hautarzt. 1992;43(4):221–5.

68. Omobono E, Goetsch W. Chondrodysplasia punctata (the Conradi-Hunermann syndrome). A clinical case report and review of the literature. Minerva Pediatr. 1993;45(3):117–21.

69. Dempsey MA, Tan C, Herman GE. Chondrodysplasia punctata 2, X-linked. In: Pagon RA, Adam MP, Ardinger HH, Wallace SE, Amemiya A, Bean LJH, Bird TD, Ledbetter N, Mefford HC, Smith RJH, Stephens K, editors. GeneReviews. Seattle: University of Washington; 2011.

70. Cañueto J, Girós M, Ciria S, Pi-Castán G, Artigas M, García-Dorado J, et al. Clinical, molecular and biochemical characterization of nine Spanish families with Conradi–Hünermann–Happle syndrome: new insights into X-linked dominant chondrodysplasia punctata with a comprehensive review of the literature. Br J Dermatol. 2012;166(4):830–8.

71. Happle R. Cataracts as a marker of genetic heterogeneity in chondrodysplasia punctata. Clin Genet. 1981;19(1):64–6.

72. Herman GE, Kelley RI, Pureza V, Smith D, Kopacz K, Pitt J, et al. Characterization of mutations in 22 females with X-linked dominant chondrodysplasia punctata (Happle syndrome). Genet Med. 2002;4(6):434–8.

73. Milunsky JM, Maher TA, Metzenberg AB. Molecular, biochemical, and phenotypic analysis of a hemizygous male with a severe atypical phenotype for X-linked dominant Conradi-Hunermann-Happle syndrome and a mutation in EBP. Am J Med Genet A. 2003;116(3):249–54.

74. Furtado LV, Bayrak-Toydemir P, Hulinsky B, Damjanovich K, Carey JC, Rope AF. A novel X-linked multiple congenital anomaly syndrome associated with an EBP mutation. Am J Med Genet A. 2010;152(11):2838–44.

75. Haber H. The Bloch-Sulzberger syndrome (Incontinentia Pigmenti). Br J Dermatol. 1952;64(4):129–40.

76. Fusco F, Bardaro T, Fimiani G, Mercadante V, Miano MG, Falco G, et al. Molecular analysis of the genetic defect in a large cohort of IP patients and identification of novel NEMO mutations interfering with NF-κB activation. Hum Mol Genet. 2004;13(16):1763–73.

77. Smahi A, Courtois G, Vabres P, Yamaoka S, Heuertz S, Munnich A, et al. Genomic rearrangement in NEMO impairs NF-κB activation and is a cause of incontinentia pigmenti. Nature. 2000;405(6785):466–72.

78. Kaufman CK, Fuchs E. It's got you covered Nf-κb in the epidermis. J Cell Biol. 2000;149(5):999–1004.

79. Zonana J, Elder ME, Schneider LC, Orlow SJ, Moss C, Golabi M, et al. A novel X-linked disorder of immune deficiency and hypohidrotic ectodermal dysplasia is allelic to incontinentia pigmenti and due to mutations in IKK-gamma (NEMO). Am J Hum Genet. 2000;67(6):1555–62.

80. Fusco F, Pescatore A, Bal E, Ghoul A, Paciolla M, Lioi MB, et al. Alterations of the IKBKG locus and diseases: an update and a report of 13 novel mutations. Hum Mutat. 2008;29(5):595–604.

81. Scheuerle AE. Male cases of incontinentia pigmenti: case report and review. Am J Med Genet. 1998;77(3):201–18.

82. Fusco F, Fimiani G, Tadini G, Ursini MV. Clinical diagnosis of incontinentia pigmenti in a cohort of male patients. J Am Acad Dermatol. 2007;56(2):264–7.

83. International IP Consortium. Survival of male patients with incontinentia pigmenti carrying a lethal mutation can be explained by somatic mosaicism or Klinefelter syndrome. Am J Hum Genet. 2001;69(6):1210–7.

84. Pacheco TR, Levy M, Collyer JC, de Parra NP, Parra CA, Garay M, et al. Incontinentia pigmenti in male patients. J Am Acad Dermatol. 2006;55(2):251–5.

85. Hadj-Rabia S, Froidevaux D, Bodak N, Hamel-Teillac D, Smahi A, Touil Y, et al. Clinical study of 40 cases of incontinentia pigmenti. Arch Dermatol. 2003;139(9):1163–70.

86. Landy S, Donnai D. Incontinentia pigmenti (Bloch-Sulzberger syndrome). J Med Genet. 1993;30(1):53.

87. Badgwell A, Iglesias A, Emmerich S, Willner J. The natural history of incontinentia pigmenti as reported

by 198 affected individuals. Abstract 38. Nashville, TN: American College of Medical Genetics Annual Meeting; 2007.

88. Swinney CC, Han DP, Karth PA. Incontinentia pigmenti: a comprehensive review and update. Ophthalmic Surg Lasers Imaging Retina. 2015;46(6):650–7.

89. Watzke RC, Stevens TS, Carney RG. Retinal vascular changes of incontinentia pigmenti. Arch Ophthalmol. 1976;94(5):743–6.

90. Francois J. Incontinentia pigmenti (Bloch-Sulzberger syndrome) and retinal changes. Br J Ophthalmol. 1984;68(1):19–25.

91. Goldberg MF, Custis PH. Retinal and other manifestations of incontinentia pigmenti (Bloch-Sulzberger syndrome). Ophthalmology. 1993;100(11):1645–54.

92. Rosenfeld SI, Smith ME. Ocular findings in incontinentia pigmenti. Ophthalmology. 1985;92(4):543–6.

93. Holmström G, Thoren K. Ocular manifestations of incontinentia pigmenti. Acta Ophthalmol Scand. 2000;78(3):348–53.

94. Meuwissen ME, Mancini GM. Neurological findings in incontinentia pigmenti; a review. Eur J Med Genet. 2012;55(5):323–31.

95. Minić S, Trpinac D, Obradović M. Incontinentia pigmenti diagnostic criteria update. Clin Genet. 2014;85(6):536–42.

96. Hayes IM, Varigos G, Upjohn EJ, Orchard DC, Penny DJ, Savarirayan R. Unilateral acheiria and fatal primary pulmonary hypertension in a girl with incontinentia pigmenti. Am J Med Genet A. 2005;135(3):302–3.

97. Brown C. Incontinentia pigmenti: the development of pseudoglioma. Br J Ophthalmol. 1988;72(6):452–5.

98. Roberts WM, Jenkins JJ, Moorhead EL, Douglass EC. Incontinentia pigmenti, a chromosomal instability syndrome, is associated with childhood malignancy. Cancer. 1988;62(11):2370–2.

99. Scheuerle AE, Ursini MV. Incontinentia pigmenti. In: Pagon RA, Adam MP, Ardinger HH, Wallace SE, Amemiya A, LJH B, Bird TD, Ledbetter N, Mefford HC, RJH S, Stephens K, editors. GeneReviews. Seattle: University of Washington; 2015.

100. Bree AF, Grange DK, Hicks MJ, Goltz RW. Dermatologic findings of focal dermal hypoplasia (Goltz syndrome). Am J Med Genet C Semin Med Genet. 2016;172C:44.

101. Goltz RW, Peterson WC, Gorlin RJ, Ravits HG. Focal dermal hypoplasia. Arch Dermatol. 1962;86(6):708–17.

102. Holden JD, Akers WA. Goltz's syndrome: focal dermal hypoplasia: a combined mesoectodermal dysplasia. Am J Dis Child. 1967;114(3):292–300.

103. Grzeschik K-H, Bornholdt D, Oeffner F, König A, del Carmen Boente M, Enders H, et al. Deficiency of PORCN, a regulator of Wnt signaling, is associated with focal dermal hypoplasia. Nat Genet. 2007;39(7):833–5.

104. Wang X, Sutton VR, Peraza-Llanes JO, Yu Z, Rosetta R, Kou Y-C, et al. Mutations in X-linked PORCN, a putative regulator of Wnt signaling, cause focal dermal hypoplasia. Nat Genet. 2007;39(7):836–8.

105. Proffitt KD, Virshup DM. Precise regulation of porcupine activity is required for physiological Wnt signaling. J Biol Chem. 2012;287(41):34167–78.

106. Clevers H, Nusse R. Wnt/β-catenin signaling and disease. Cell. 2012;149(6):1192–205.

107. Molho-Pessach V, Schaffer JV. Blaschko lines and other patterns of cutaneous mosaicism. Clin Dermatol. 2011;29(2):205–25.

108. Wechsler MA, Papa CM, Haberman F, Marion RW. Variable expression in focal dermal hypoplasia: an example of differential X-chromosome inactivation. Am J Dis Child. 1988;142(3):297–300.

109. Paller AS. Wnt signaling in focal dermal hypoplasia. Nat Genet. 2007;39(7):820–1.

110. Barrott JJ, Cash GM, Smith AP, Barrow JR, Murtaugh LC. Deletion of mouse Porcn blocks Wnt ligand secretion and reveals an ectodermal etiology of human focal dermal hypoplasia/Goltz syndrome. Proc Natl Acad Sci U S A. 2011;108(31):12752–7.

111. Bornholdt D, Oeffner F, König A, Happle R, Alanay Y, Ascherman J, et al. PORCN mutations in focal dermal hypoplasia: coping with lethality. Hum Mutat. 2009;30(5):E618–E28.

112. Sutton VR, Van den Veyver IB. Focal dermal hypoplasia. In: Pagon RA, Adam MP, Ardinger HH, Wallace SE, Amemiya A, Bean LJH, Bird TD, Ledbetter N, Mefford HC, Smith RJH, Stephens K, editors. GeneReviews. Seattle: University of Washington; 2013.

113. Fete TJ, Fete M. International research symposium on Goltz syndrome. Am J Med Genet C Semin Med Genet. 2016;172C:3.

114. Bostwick B, Fang P, Patel A, Sutton VR. Phenotypic and molecular characterization of focal dermal hypoplasia in 18 individuals. Am J Med Genet C Semin Med Genet. 2016;172C:9.

115. Gisseman JD, Herce HH. Ophthalmologic manifestations of focal dermal hypoplasia (Goltz syndrome): a case series of 18 patients. Am J Med Genet C Semin Med Genet. 2016;172C:59.

116. Nagalo K, Laberge J, Nguyen V, Laberge-Caouette L, Turgeon J. Focal dermal hypoplasia (Goltz syndrome) in the neonate: report of a case presenting with cleft lip and palate. Arch Pediatr. 2012;19(2):160–2.

117. Smigiel R, Jakubiak A, Lombardi MP, Jaworski W, Slezak R, Patkowski D, et al. Co-occurrence of severe Goltz-Gorlin syndrome and pentalogy of Cantrell - case report and review of the literature. Am J Med Genet A. 2011;155A(5):1102–5.

118. Lombardi MP, Bulk S, Celli J, Lampe A, Gabbett MT, Ousager LB, et al. Mutation update for the PORCN gene. Hum Mutat. 2011;32(7):723–8.

119. Van Assche E, Bonduelle M, Tournaye H, Joris H, Verheyen G, Devroey P, et al. Cytogenetics of infertile men. Hum Reprod. 1996;11(Suppl 4):1–26.

120. Groth KA, Skakkebæk A, Høst C, Gravholt CH, Bojesen A. Klinefelter syndrome—a clinical update. J Clin Endocrinol Metab. 2012;98(1):20–30.

121. Klinefelter HF Jr, Reifenstein EC Jr, Albright F Jr. Syndrome characterized by gynecomastia, aspermatogenesis without A-Leydigism, and increased excretion of follicle-stimulating hormone 1. J Clin Endocrinol Metab. 1942;2(11):615–27.

122. Jacobs PA. A case of human intersexuality having a possible XXY sexdetermining mechanism. Nature. 1959;183:302–3.

123. Bonomi M, Rochira V, Pasquali D, Balercia G, Jannini E, Ferlin A. Klinefelter syndrome (KS): genetics, clinical phenotype and hypogonadism. J Endocrinol Investig. 2017;40:123–34.

124. Aksglaede L, Link K, Giwercman A, Jørgensen N, Skakkebaek NE, Juul A. 47, XXY Klinefelter syndrome: clinical characteristics and age-specific recommendations for medical management. Am J Med Genet C Semin Med Genet. 2013;163C:55.

125. Bojesen A, Gravholt CH. Klinefelter syndrome in clinical practice. Nat Clin Pract Urol. 2007;4(4):192–204.

126. Campbell W, Newton M, Price W. Hypostatic leg ulceration and Klinefelter's syndrome. J Intelect Disabil Res. 1980;24(2):115–7.

127. Zollner TM, Veraart J, Wolter M, Hesse S, Villemur B, Wenke A, et al. Leg ulcers in Klinefelter's syndrome–further evidence for an involvement of plasminogen activator inhibitor-1. Br J Dermatol. 1997;136(3):341–4.

128. Shanmugam VK, Tsagaris KC, Attinger CE. Leg ulcers associated with Klinefelter's syndrome: a case report and review of the literature. Int Wound J. 2012;9(1):104–7.

129. De Morentin HM, Dodiuk-Gad RP, Brenner S. Klinefelter's syndrome presenting with leg ulcers. Skinmed. 2004;3(5):274–8.

130. Villemur B, Truche H, Pernod G, De Angelis M, Beani J, Halimi S, et al. Leg ulcer and Klinefelter syndrome. J Mal Vasc. 1994;20(3):215–8.

131. Stochholm K, Juul S, Juel K, Naeraa RW, Højbjerg Gravholt C. Prevalence, incidence, diagnostic delay, and mortality in Turner syndrome. J Clin Endocrinol Metab. 2006;91(10):3897–902.

132. Turner HH. A syndrome of infantilism, congenital webbed neck, and cubitus valgus 1. Endocrinologist. 1938;23(5):566–74.

133. Bondy CA. Care of girls and women with Turner syndrome: a guideline of the Turner Syndrome Study Group. J Clin Endocrinol Metab. 2007;92(1):10–25.

134. Ford CE, Jones KW, Polani PE, De Almeida J, Briggs JH. A sex-chromosome anomaly in a case of gonadal dysgenesis (Turner's syndrome). Lancet. 1959;273(7075):711–3.

135. Lowenstein EJ, Kim KH, Glick SA. Turner's syndrome in dermatology. J Am Acad Dermatol. 2004;50(5):767–76.

136. Robinson W, Binkert F, Bernasconi F, Lorda-Sanchez I, Werder E, Schinzel A. Molecular studies of chromosomal mosaicism: relative frequency of chromosome gain or loss and possible role of cell selection. Am J Hum Genet. 1995;56(2):444.

137. Fernández-García R, García-Doval S, Costoya S, Pasaro E. Analysis of sex chromosome aneuploidy in 41 patients with Turner syndrome: a study of 'hidden' mosaicism. Clin Genet. 2000;58(3):201–8.

138. Hassold T, Pettay D, Robinson A, Uchida I. Molecular studies of parental origin and mosaicism in 45, X conceptuses. Hum Genet. 1992;89(6):647–52.

139. Rao E, Weiss B, Fukami M, Rump A, Niesler B, Mertz A, et al. Pseudoautosomal deletions encompassing a novel homeobox gene cause growth failure in idiopathic short stature and Turner syndrome. Nat Genet. 1997;16(1):54–63.

140. Ferguson-Smith MA. Karyotype-phenotype correlations in gonadal dysgenesis and their bearing on the pathogenesis of malformations. J Med Genet. 1965;2(2):142.

141. Berdahl LD, Wenstrom KD, Hanson JW. Web neck anomaly and its association with congenital heart disease. Am J Med Genet A. 1995;56(3):304–7.

142. Brady AF, Patton MA. Web-neck anomaly and its association with congenital heart disease. Am J Med Genet. 1996;64(4):605.

143. Becker B, Jospe N, Goldsmith LA. Melanocytic nevi in Turner syndrome. Pediatr Dermatol. 1994;11(2):120–4.

144. Gibbs P, Brady BM, Gonzalez R, Robinson WA. Nevi and melanoma: lessons from Turner's syndrome. Dermatology. 2001;202(1):1–3.

145. Zvulunov A, Wyatt D, Laud P, Esterly N. Influence of genetic and environmental factors on melanocytic naevi: a lesson from Turner's syndrome. Br J Dermatol. 1998;138(6):993–7.

146. Schoemaker MJ, Swerdlow AJ, Higgins CD, Wright AF, Jacobs PA. Cancer incidence in women with Turner syndrome in Great Britain: a national cohort study. Lancet Oncol. 2008;9(3):239–46.

147. Lemli L, Smith DW. The XO syndrome: a study of the differentiated phenotype in 25 patients. J Pediatr. 1963;63(4):577–88.

148. Smith DW, Hanson JW. Asynchronous growth of scalp hair in XO Turner syndrome. J Pediatr. 1975;87(4):659–60.

149. Kannan TP, Azman BZ, Ahmad Tarmizi AB, Suhaida MA, Siti Mariam I, Ravindran A, et al. Turner syndrome diagnosed in northeastern Malaysia. Singap Med J. 2008;49(5):400–4.

150. Rosina P, Segalla G, Magnanini M, Chieregato C, Barba A. Turner's syndrome associated with psoriasis and alopecia areata. J Eur Acad Dermatol Venereol. 2003;17(1):50–2.

151. Polani P. Turner's syndrome and allied conditions: clinical features and chromosome abnormalities. Br Med Bull. 1961;17(3):200–5.

152. Larizza D, Calcaterra V, Martinetti M. Autoimmune stigmata in Turner syndrome: when lacks an X chromosome. J Autoimmun. 2009;33(1):25–30.

153. Gravholt CH. Epidemiological, endocrine and metabolic features in Turner syndrome. Eur J Endocrinol. 2004;151(6):657–87.

154. Larralde M, Gardner SS, Torrado MV, Fernhoff PM, Muñoz AES, Spraker MK, et al. Lymphedema as a postulated cause of cutis verticis gyrata in Turner syndrome. Pediatr Dermatol. 1998;15(1):18–22.
155. Bello-Quintero CE, Gonzalez ME, Alvarez-Connelly E. Halo nevi in Turner syndrome. Pediatr Dermatol. 2010;27(4):368–9.
156. Brazzelli V, Larizza D, Martinetti M, Martinoli S, Calcaterra V, De Silvestri A, et al. Halo nevus, rather than vitiligo, is a typical dermatologic finding of Turner's syndrome: clinical, genetic, and immunogenetic study in 72 patients. J Am Acad Dermatol. 2004;51(3):354–8.
157. Handler MZ, Derrick KM, Lutz RE, Morrell DS, Davenport ML, Armstrong AW. Prevalence of pilomatricoma in Turner syndrome: findings from a multicenter study. JAMA Dermatol. 2013;149(5):559–64.
158. Paller AS, Esterly NB, Charrow J, Cahan FM. Pedal hemangiomas in Turner syndrome. J Pediatr. 1983;103(1):87–8.
159. Nehal KS, PeBenito R, Orlow SJ. Analysis of 54 cases of hypopigmentation and hyperpigmentation along the lines of Blaschko. Arch Dermatol. 1996;132(10):1167–70.

Specific Dermatoses of Pregnancy

10

Arieh Ingber

10.1 Introduction

This is a group of dermatological conditions which appear only, or almost only, in pregnancy. There is confusion about which diseases to include in this group and much confusion regarding the names of these diseases. In this chapter we will review, up to date, diseases which are unique to pregnancy and will discuss the nomenclature.

We will review the following diseases:

Pruritic Urticarial Papules and Plaques of Pregnancy (PUPPP)
Pemphigoid Gestationis (PG)
Impetigo Herpetiformis (IH)
Prurigo of Pregnancy (Besnier)
Pruritic Folliculitis of Pregnancy
Linear IgM Dermatosis of Pregnancy

10.2 Nomenclature and Specificity

The nomenclature of these pregnancy-specific eruptions has been revised several times, generating confusion. Several diseases like atopic eruption of pregnancy, which is not specific to

pregnancy, and intrahepatic cholestasis of pregnancy, which is not a dermatosis, were included in this group of diseases generating more confusion by further clouding the specificity [1].

The term polymorphic eruption of pregnancy [2], a basket of diseases, which are basically different and not related, caused more uncertainty. The debate if IH is a pregnancy variant of pustular psoriasis or a disease sui generis caused confusion. Diseases like prurigo of pregnancy (Besnier) and pruritic folliculitis of pregnancy were thrown into the basket of polymorphic eruption of pregnancy unjustifiably, caused more embarrassment.

In describing the various diseases we will emphasize the uniqueness of each of them with the intention to try to overcome the uncertainty and to cast light on their specificity.

10.3 Pruritic Urticarial Papules and Plaques of Pregnancy (PUPPP)

This disease appears only in pregnancy.

10.3.1 Epidemiology

The most common specific dermatosis of pregnancy (occurs in about 1 in every 160–200 pregnancies). It's more common among Caucasians.

A. Ingber
Department of Dermatology, Hadassah University Hospital, Hebrew University, Jerusalem, Israel

© Springer International Publishing AG, part of Springer Nature 2018
E. Tur, H. I. Maibach (eds.), *Gender and Dermatology*,
https://doi.org/10.1007/978-3-319-72156-9_10

In 80% of the cases it present in primigravid women. It was reported to happen more often in multiple gestation pregnancies, in pregnancy with twins and in maternal over weight. This is not my experience. Over the years I have seen dozens of cases of PUPPP. Most of them were pregnant with one fetus, most of them had proper weight and I didn't see higher incidence of PUPPP in multiple gestation pregnancies. Usually occurs in the third trimester of pregnancy, from week 35 and on. One study [3] revealed a male-to-female infant ratio of 2:1. In my experience the incidence of boys or girls birth is equal. Rarely, it occurs at postpartum period within 2 weeks after delivery. Rarely returns in subsequent pregnancies, unless they are multiple gestations, and then it is generally less severe than the first episode [4–7].

10.3.2 Pathogenesis

The pathogenesis of PUPPP is not known. Conventional theory is that the distension of the abdominal skin during pregnancy causes an alteration of the epidermal skin, and generation of a new antigen. PUPPP is a reaction to this antigen. This theory is supported by studies revealed that PUPPP is more common in multiple gestation, in pregnancies with twins or in maternal overweight [8]. Since in PUPPP there is no known antibody formation against any skin structure this theory is doubted.

In a study fetal DNA was found in the skin of mothers with PUPPP, suggesting that chimerism may be the basic pathogenesis of this dermatosis [9].

Recently it was postulated that mast cells (MCs) has a role in the pathogenesis of PUPPP. During pregnancy, the maternal organism is under the influence of many endocrine as well as immunological changes as an adaptation to the implanted and developing fetus. Mast cells are known for their susceptibility to hormones. While physiological numbers of MCs were shown to positively influence pregnancy outcome, at least in mouse models, uncontrolled augmentations in quantity, and/or activation can lead to pregnancy complications. It is tempting to

speculate that MCs are involved in the onset of PUPPP although no studies are existing showing a direct link between MCs and this disease. There are several lines of evidence that clearly suggest a role for MCs. First, as in urticaria, antihistamines are the first line option in the treatment of PUPPP and are effective in most patients. Second, even though PUPPP and urticaria are different diseases there are several similarities in terms of the clinical symptoms including pruritic erythema and urticarial lesions. Third, autologous whole blood injections have been reported as an effective treatment option in PUPPP [10, 11].

10.3.3 Clinical Presentation

The rash usually appears in the third trimester. In 90% of the cases, the disease starts in the abdomen, buttocks and thighs, and then spreads to the upper limbs and trunk. It never appears on the face, neck, and hands and feet (in the typical form of the disease). Significantly it appears in the abdominal skin and inside and around the distance striae. An important clue to the diagnosis of this disease is, as a rule, the sparing of the navel.

In the vast majority of cases the rash is urticarial and edematous. As a rule the rash is very itchy.

Rarely the rash is polymorphic, with the presence of blisters and target-like lesions [4, 12, 13]. Dyshidrotic rash on the hands and feet was reported but never was seen by me. Purpura is rarely seen [14].

10.3.4 Laboratory Tests

All laboratory tests are normal except eosinophilia in some cases. Direct and indirect immunofluorescence tests are negative [4].

10.3.5 Histopathology

Skin biopsy is rarely necessary. The histology of PUPPP is not specific. Two patterns has been described a superficial (early) and deep (late). In the early superficial pattern the findings are epidermal

(Edema of the papillary dermis, focal parakeratosis, exocytosis of eosinophils, hyperkeratosis) and perivascular (Lymphohistiocytic infiltration). In the late deeper pattern the infiltrate is interstitial scatted with eosinophils. The papillary dermis is edematous occasionally with blister formation [15].

10.3.6 Treatment

In mild cases antihistamines (Those drugs which are allowed in pregnancy) and weak to moderate potent steroid creams are recommended.

In severe cases oral prednisone at a dose of 0.5–1 mg/kg/d is usually needed [16]. In my experience most of cases the itch is distressing and oral prednisone is necessary to control the itch, usually, at least, till delivery. In some cases this treatment is necessary even after delivery. Phototherapy by narrowband UVB was reported to be effective in some cases [14].

Recently, Autologous Whole Blood (AWB) injection was reported to be effective in three cases of PUPPP unresponsive to therapy [11]. AWB often used for treatment of urticaria before the introduction of antihistamines and was also thought to have beneficial effects in treatment of viral diseases, circulatory disorders and atopic dermatitis. The exact mechanism of AWB injection remains to be established; however, it is still popular in central Europe, mostly in private clinics. Venous blood of 10 mL was drawn from the patient, followed by intramuscular injection of 5 mL of the blood on each side of her buttock. All patients showed good responses to intramuscular injection of AWB, tolerated the treatment, and there were no adverse effects to the patients or their babies.

It is tempting to suggest treating PUPPP with Omalizumab (Xolair). Omalizumab is category B in pregnancy- only recommended for use during pregnancy when benefit outweighs risk.

10.3.7 Prognosis

The prognosis of PUPPP is usually excellent. No fetal or maternal complications have been reported. In the most of cases PUPPP is dramatically improving within hours after delivery. In some cases the disease can last longer even several weeks postpartum. The disease usually does not recur in subsequent pregnancies [4, 17].

10.4   Pemphigoid Gestationis (PG)

For many years the disease has been named: Herpes Gestationis. This name caused much confusion among non- dermatologists physicians who mistakenly thought it is an infectious disease caused by herpes virus. In the past it happened to me several times when after I made the diagnosis of Herpes Gestationis, the general practitioner or the gynecologist checked for the presence of antibodies to HSV and got angry at me when the results were negative. They accused me for causing false fear to the pregnant woman…Replacing the name to PG by Holmes and Black in 1982 [2] was absolutely justified.

10.4.1 Epidemiology

PG is a rare disease and specific to pregnancy. The incidence of PG is unknown and is different in different parts of the world. According to various studies, the incidence is 1:7000–50,000 births. It is the least common of the specific dermatoses of pregnancy. The disease is more common in the white race [18, 19]. Interestingly, in my experience, most Israeli PG patients are Sephardic women (women of North- African origin).

In my experience in the vast majority of cases: boys are born! There is a higher frequency of HLA-DR3 and HLA-DR4 in patients with the disease. All these facts suggest an ethnic genetic background of the disease [20].

10.4.2 Pathogenesis

PG is an autoimmune, usually blistering, disease. Most patients develop antibodies against 2 hemidesmosomal proteins, BP180 (BPAG2, collagen XVII) and less frequently BP230. These circulating antibodies belong to immunoglobulin G1 subclass (occasionally and/or to G3). Immunoglobulin G1 is binding to the extracellular NC16A domain of BP180 and/or BP230 antigen at the basal layer inducing the formation of PG lesions. These antibodies have a very strong complement activation ability, and at the end of the road inducing C3 deposition at basement membrane zone along the upper part of lamina lucida [21].

Recently it was demonstrated that There is a strong association between MHC class II molecules and PG, indicates a pivotal role of MHC class II in the pathogenesis of the disease. MHC class II molecules are aberrantly expressed on amniochorionic stromal cells and on the trophoblast. As a consequence, BP180, which is expressed in the amniotic epithelium of the placenta and the umbilical cord, is presented to maternal MHC class II in the presence of paternal MHC class II and is recognized as a foreign antigen, resulting in the formation of IgG autoantibodies, predominantly of the IgG_1 and IgG_3 subclasses, directed to BP180 [22].

For years PG was considered as a bullous pephigoid variant of pregnancy. A recent study suggested different pathogenesis between PG and Bullos Pemphigoid [23].

10.4.3 Clinical Presentation

Usually begins in the second trimester of pregnancy at week 21 of gestation. The eruption presents as periumbilical erythematous urticarial lesions that later spreads to limbs, abdomen and chest and develop into tense vesicles or blisters. Pruritus is severe in most cases. Palms and soles involvement may occur. Rarely the rash may appear on face and neck. At early stage of the disease, the differential diagnosis from PUPPP may be difficult. Involvement of the umbilicus is an important clue to diagnosis of PG. The lesions are arranged in a grouped pattern (resembling dermatitis herpetiformis) around the umbilicus. Occasionally, distance striae is involved. Rarely vesicles and blisters are not developed. Mucosal lesions are very rare. In most of cases an exacer-

bation of the diseases can be seen close to delivery and immediately after [24, 25].

10.4.4 Laboratory Tests

Most hematologic studies are within normal limits. Eosinophilia is not uncommon and may correlate with disease severity. Laboratory values that may be elevated include immunoglobulin levels, erythrocyte sedimentation rates, acute phase reactant levels, and antithyroid antibodies [26].

10.4.5 Histopathology

Subepidermal blister formation with eosinophilc infiltrate. Perivascular Inflammatory reaction at the dermoepidermal Junction is present. Edema in the dermis is often prominent [27].

10.4.6 Direct and Indirect Immunofluorescence

In most of PG Patients direct immunofluorescence (DIF) results exhibit a linear band of C3 deposition with or without immunoglobulin G (present in 20–25% of patients) along the basement membrane. Indirect immunofluorescence may detect circulating antibodies for basement membrane zone (HG factor) [21]. Recognition of the bullous pemphigoid antigen (BP180) by ELISA was reported and was used to determine the severity of the disease [28]. HLA-DR3/DR4 is present in half of patients with PG, as compared with 3% of the general population [20].

10.4.7 Treatment

In my experience most PG patients suffering from frustrating disease with widespread vesicles and severe itch. Usually systemic treatment with prednisone 0.5 mg/kg/d is mandatory. This treatment may be limited by age of pregnancy. In early pregnancy it may be contraindicated.

As always, the physician must consider the risks and benefits for the mother and fetus. Many anecdotal treatments were reported to control the disease: Dapsone, methotrexate, ciclosporine and intravenous immunoglobulin [29–31]. Recently azathioprine combined with intravenous immunoglobulin was found to be effective in a 37 years old pregnant woman who failed on prednisone treatment [32].

10.4.8 Prognosis

The disease regresses a few weeks or months after delivery. A common opinion is that on subsequent pregnancies the disease will appear earlier and will be more severe. There is no evidence that this is the rule. Some studies revealed higher rate of premature deliveries and small to term babies. As a result they recommended follow up of those women in high risk pregnancy units [33, 34]. In my experience all the PG that I have seen, had no miscarriages and delivered healthy children. Infants born to mothers with PG, 5–10% reported to have transient rash which resolved after few weeks [34]. I have never seen the appearance of the disease in neonates. The existence of a second autoimmune disease in PG patients, Hashimoto thyroiditis, Grave's disease and others was reported [35].

10.5 Impetigo Herpetiformis

10.5.1 Nomenclature

This rare disease of pregnancy, is in a long debate if it is a disease sui generis or a variant of generalize pustular psoriasis of Von Zumbusch. The term "impetigo" usually means a bacterial contagious disease and this disease is not bacterial and not contagious. The term "impetigo" was given due to the pustules which are the main features of this illness. On the other hand the name generalized pustular psoriasis of pregnancy is fixing the attitude that this disease is pustular psoriasis. It is still controversial if the disease is specific to pregnancy or general pustular psoriasis exacer-bated by pregnancy [36, 37]. As long as the debate continues, it makes sense to keep the historical name.

10.5.2 Epidemiology

A very rare disease, less than 200 cases were reported in the literature [38]. Surprisingly it was reported in non pregnant women and even in men. It is clear that in these patients the diseases is classical pustular psoriasis of Von Zumbusch, while in pregnant women it may be a different illness specific to pregnancy [39].

10.5.3 Pathogenesis

The cause of this disease is unknown. Since hypoparathyroidism was reported in some Impetigo herpetiformis patients, some authors related this illness to hypoparathyroidism. The increase consumption of calcium at the last trimester of the pregnancy causes hypocalcemia in patient with latent hypoparathyroidism. It has been shown that hypocalcemia may induce general pustular psoriasis [39–41].

Recently new data was published on the pathogenesis of Impetigo herpetiformis following a study on different genetic profiles of psoriasis vulgaris and general pustular psoriasis. The majority of general pustular psoriasis that is not accompanied by psoriasis vulgaris is caused by homozygous or compound heterozygous mutations of *IL36RN*, which encodes IL-36 receptor antagonist (IL-36RN, a part of the IL-36 signaling system that is thought to be present in epithelial barriers and to take part in local inflammatory response). Only a small number of cases with general pustular psoriasis preceding or accompanied by psoriasis vulgaris, were found to have *IL36RN* mutations. These findings further supports the idea that general pustular psoriasis with psoriasis vulgaris differs genetically from general pustular psoriasis alone. Till now there have been no reports of impetigo herpetiformis with *IL36RN* mutations. A recent publication reported on two cases of impetigo herpetiformis with homozygous and heterozygous *IL36RN* mutations. These findings support the view that impetigo herpetiformis is not related to psoriasis vulgarris but may be related to general pustular psoriasis [42, 43].

10.5.4 Clinical Presentation

Impetigo herpetiformis is a dramatic disease occasionally with systemic symptoms. It may present in any stage of pregnancy, but usually appears in the last trimester of pregnancy. Most patients do not have a personal or familial history of psoriasis and do not subsequently develop chronic plaque psoriasis. We have seen a case of Impetigo herpetiformis in a young pregnant patient, with no history of psoriasis who years later developed widespread plaque psoriasis [37].

The onset is acute occasionally with a prodrome of high fever, chills and malaise. Other symptoms may happen but are not common. The rash is present on lower abdomen, navel, inframammary folds, armpits and the neck. The primary lesions are red papules and patches and numerous pin size sterile pustules. Slight scales often present on the patches. The lesions are arranged in a peculiar pattern: rings and serpentine distribution. Sometimes the pustules create "lakes" of pus [44].

10.5.5 Laboratory Tests

Leukocytosis, neutrophilia and relative lymphopenia, are the common findings in the acute stage. Hypocalcemia and hyperphosphathemia due to hypoparathyroidism is relatively common. In some cases hypoalbuminemia, high levels of urea and high uric acid was reported. immunofluorescence tests, direct and indirect, are negative [39, 40].

10.5.6 Histopathology

Subcorneal neutrophilic pustules and neutrophilic influx into the upper epidermis (forming Kogoj microabscesses) are the common findings along with parakeratosis. Chronic perivsacular infiltrate in the upper dermis [45].

10.5.7 Treatment

Impetigo herpetiformis is a severe illness. Careful treatment and follow up is required. Calcium and albumin serum levels must be followed. Systemic prednisone 0.5–1.0 mg/kg/d is the treatment of choice. Antibiotics treatment usually is necessary to prevent secondary infection. Ciclosporine, narrowband UVB and methotrexate (at late pregnancy), were reported as potential therapies [46–48]. Recently in a case which omplicated with intrauterine growth restriction successfully treated with granulocyte and monocyte apheresis [49].

10.5.8 Prognosis

Before the era of steroids and antibiotics, the prognosis of this disease was very poor with high maternal mortality. Nowadays the maternal prognosis is good but the fetal prognosis may be occasionally still poor. Stillbirths may happen. The fetal prognosis is in correlation to the disease severity. Proper control of the maternal illness is mandatory. Cesarean section should be done if possible in case of disease exacerbation [38, 39, 50].

10.6   Prurigo of Pregnancy (Besnier)

This disease was introduced by Ernest Besnier a French dermatologist in 1904 [51]. Many authors consider Prurigo of Pregnancy (Besnier) as a variant of atopic dermatitis of pregnancy and it's cataloged to the basket of polymorphic eruption of pregnancy [25]. In my opinion and in my experience, Prurigo of Pregnancy (Besnier) is a disease sui generis and specific to pregnancy.

10.6.1 Epidemiology

The incidence is 1:300–400 pregnancies [52]. In my experience it is much more common but overlooked or misdiagnosed. It's more common among Caucasians. In Israel in my experience it's mainly in Sephardic women (women of North-African origin). The disease develops beyond the twentieth week of pregnancy but may appear in any time of pregnancy [52, 53].

10.6.2 Pathogenesis

The cause of prurigo of pregnancy (Besnier) and the severe itch is not known. It was postulated that prurigo of pregnancy (Besnier) is on the spectrum of intrahepatic cholestasis of pregnancy with primary lesion, which are absent in intrahepatic cholestasis of pregnancy [2].

10.6.3 Clinical Presentation

The rash appears predominantly on the extensor parts of the limbs and dorsal aspects of the hand and feet. Rarely the papules can also occur on the abdomen and trunk. Prurigo defines as papules with erosions on the top. Occasionally nodules can be seen resembling prurigo nodularis but they are much smaller and in lighter color than prurigo nodularis. The skin around the papules is normal. The lesions do not merge and do not form plaques. Typically they arranged in longitudinal pattern. The lesions are extremely itchy resulting in excoriated lesions, sometimes associated with secondary infection [19, 53, 54].

10.6.4 Differential Diagnosis of Prurigo of Pregnancy (Besnier) and Atopic Dermatitis

The following data indicate that prurigo of pregnancy (Besnier) is not atopic dermatitis:

1. In my experience the incidence of personal or familial atopic background in prurigo of pregnancy (Besnier) patients, is not higher than in the general population (In contrary to some reports in the literature).

2. The predominant primary lesion (prurigo or occasionally nodules) is unique and usually does not seen in atopic dermatitis also not in the papular type atopic dermatitis.
3. The distribution of prurigo of pregnancy (Besnier) is predominantly on the extensor aspects of the limbs and not on other skin areas.
4. The lesions do not merge into plaques.
5. The arrangement of the lesions is unique in longitudinal lines, not following Blaschko lines and not following the pattern of Koebners phenomenon.
6. The background skin around the lesions isn't dry.
7. The prognosis is excellent, complete recovery after delivery.

10.6.5 Laboratory Tests

The laboratory tests are within the normal limits. Direct and indirect immunofluorescence tests are negative.

10.6.6 Histopathology

Chronic superficial perivascular inflammatory cell infiltrate with eosinophils, histiocytes and neutrofhils [14].

10.6.7 Treatment

Moderate to potent steroid creams and antihistamines are the common treatment. In my experience the best treatment is phototherapy by narrowband UVB [53].

10.6.8 Prognosis

The prognosis is excellent with no effect on the pregnancy and the newborn. The disease resolves after delivery and usually is do not returning in subsequent pregnancies [14] (Personal communication).

10.7 Pruritic Folliculitis of Pregnancy

A unique disease of pregnancy, unfortunately it's not familiar to dermatologists. The disease is much more common than diagnosed. Usually is diagnosed as atopic dermatitis, acne, bacterial folliculitis or pruritic papular and urticarial papules and plaques of pregnancy [54] (Personal communication).

10.7.1 Epidemiology

In UK it was estimated to happen in one of 3000 pregnancies [55]. In my experience it's less common in Israel.

10.7.2 Pathogenesis

It's commonly thought that the cause of the disease is hormonal changes in pregnancy [56]. The exact mechanism of the disease is unknown. In one study high levels of serum androgens was detected but this finding was not confirmed by others [3, 57]. Some authors noted similarities between this disease and PUPPP. Indeed folliculitis may be found in some cases of PUPPP, but it is easy to differentiate between these two diseases which in many ways are not alike.

10.7.3 Clinical Presentation

The disease begins in the second to the third trimesters of pregnancy in healthy women with no personal or familial atopic dermatitis background. The disease is usually widespread, mainly on the back and abdomen. Occasionally it appears also on the limbs. The primary lesions are follicular red papules and sterile pustules. The rash is monomorphic resembling papulopustular acne or steroid acne [53, 58]. Contrary to the disease name the disease is usually not itching [59] (Personal communication).

10.7.4 Laboratory Tests

The laboratory tests are within the normal limits. Direct and indirect immunofluorescence tests are negative [12].

10.7.5 Histopathology

The pathological findings are usually not specific. Perifollicular neutrophilic infiltrate is common [60].

10.7.6 Treatment

Steroid creams and antihistamines are not effective and usually not needed. Anti-acne topical medication was reported to have some benefit [53, 58].

10.7.7 Prognosis

The prognosis is excellent with no effect on the pregnancy and the newborn. The disease resolves usually in 1 month after delivery and do not returning in subsequent pregnancies [61] (Personal communication). In one study of 14 patients small for date babies were born [3].

10.8 Linear IgM Dermatosis of Pregnancy

A very rare dermatosis, was reported in two pregnant women in Israel. Both of them reported from the department of dermatology, Rabin Medical Center, Campus Beilinson, one case by us [62] and the other case by another group (Unpublished data). Although this is a rare disease, I decided to introduce it. I assume that if dermatologists will be more aware of the existence of the diseases, it will be more diagnosed. I'm sure that the disease is more common but overlooked.

10.8.1 Pathogenesis

Some authors considered the diseases as a variant of prurigo of pregnancy or PUPPP [14], but it's more resembling pruritic folliculitis of pregnancy. The presence of IgM at the basal membrane zone may suggest an autoimmune background. In one of the patients the disease appeared 1 week after beginning of nifedipine treatment for premature contractions. Three days after cessation of the drug much improvement was noticed. The patient decided to take again nifedipine and the rash exacerbated quickly. They concluded that this disease may be drug related (Unpublished data). IgM was detected in the serum of healthy persons by indirect immunofluorescence technique. It was also reported in association with many dermatological conditions like: Urticaria, Grover's disease, Vasculitis and more [63, 64]. IgM deposits at the basement membrane zone by direct immunofluorescence test is rare in other dermatological conditions, indicating the uniqueness of these patients.

10.8.2 Clinical Presentation

In both cases the disease appeared at late pregnancy on week 37 and 30. The primary lesions were red follicular papules and sterile pustules on the abdomen and limbs. The rash was intensely pruritic.

10.8.3 Laboratory Tests

Laboratory tests were within the normal limits. Direct immunofluorescence test revealed linear IgM deposits at the basement membrane zone in both patients. Indirect immunofluorescence was negative in both cases. In one patient after the resolution of the rash the direct immunofluorescence test turned negative.

10.8.4 Histopathology

In biopsies folliculitis was observed.

10.8.5 Treatment

Treatment was palliative. The disease didn't respond to topical non steroidal creams and oral antihistamines.

10.8.6 Prognosis

The prognosis was excellent the rash resolved in a few weeks. The disease had no effect on mother and newborn.

References

1. Danesh M, Pomeranz MK, McMeniman E, Murase JE. Dermatoses of pregnancy: nomenclature, misnomers, and myths. Clin Dermatol. 2016;34:314–9.
2. Holmes RC, Black MM. The specific dermatoses of pregnancy: a reappraisal with special emphasis on a proposed simplified clinical classification. Clin Exp Dermatol. 1982;7:65–73.
3. Vaughan Jones SA, Hern S, Nelson-Piercy C, Seed PT, Black MM. A prospective study of 200 women with dermatoses of pregnancy correlating clinical findings with hormonal and immunopathological profiles. Br J Dermatol. 1999;141:71–81.
4. Lawley TJ, Hertz KC, Wade TR, Ackerman AB, Katz SI. Pruritic urticarial papules and plaques of pregnancy. JAMA. 1979;241:1696–9.
5. Dehdashti AL, Wikas SM. Pruritic urticarial papules and plaques of pregnancy occurring postpartum. Cutis. 2015;95:344–7.
6. Ghazeeri G, Kibbi AG, Abbas O. Pruritic urticarial papules and plaques of pregnancy: epidemiological, clinical, and histopathological study of 18 cases from Lebanon. Int J Dermatol. 2012;51:1047–53.
7. Thurston A, Grau RH. An update on the dermatoses of pregnancy. J Okla State Med Assoc. 2008;101:7–11.
8. Rudolph CM, Al-Fares S, Vaughan-Jones SA, Müllegger RR, Kerl H, Black MM. Polymorphic eruption of pregnancy: clinicopathology and potential trigger factors in 181 patients. Br J Dermatol. 2006;154:54–60.
9. Aractingi S, Berkane N, Bertheau P, Le Goué C, Dausset J, Uzan S, Carosella ED. Fetal DNA in

skin of polymorphic eruptions of pregnancy. Lancet. 1998;352:1898–901.

10. Woidacki K, Zenclussen AC, Siebenhaar F. Mast cell-mediated and associated disorders in pregnancy: a risky game with an uncertain outcome? Front Immunol. 2014;5:231.

11. Jeon IK, On HR, Oh SH, Hann SK. Three cases of pruritic urticarial papules and plaques of pregnancy (PUPPP) treated with intramuscular injection of autologous whole blood. J Eur Acad Dermatol Venereol. 2015;29:797–800.

12. Brandão P, Sousa-Faria B, Marinho C, Vieira-Enes P, Melo A, Mota L. Polymorphic eruption of pregnancy: review of literature. J Obstet Gynaecol. 2017;37:137–40.

13. Taylor D, Pappo E, Aronson IK. Polymorphic eruption of pregnancy. Clin Dermatol. 2016;34:383–91.

14. Kraumpouzos G, Cohen LM. Dermatoses of pregnancy. J Am Acad Dermatol. 2003;45:1–19.

15. Callen JP, Hanno R. Pruritic urticarial papules and plaques of pregnanacy. A clinicopathologic study. J Am Acad Dermatol. 1981;5:401–5.

16. Callen JP. Pregnancy's effects on the skin. Common and uncommon changes. Postgrad Med. 1984;75:138–45.

17. Shornik JK. Dermatoses of pregnancy. Semin Cutan Med Surg. 1988;17:172–81.

18. Schmidt E, Zillikens D. Pemphigoid diseases. Lancet. 2013;381:320–32.

19. Kroumpouzos G, Zillikens D. Pemphigoid gestationis. In: Kroumpouzos G, editor. Text atlas of obstetric dermatology. Philadelphia: Lippincott Williams & Wilkins; 2013. p. 180–93.

20. Shornick JK, Stastny P, Gilliam JN. High frequency of histocompatibility antigens HLA-DR3 and DR4 in herpes gestations. J Clin Invest. 1981;68:553–5.

21. Chimanovitch I, Schmidt E, Messer G, et al. IGG1 and IGG3 are the major immunoglobulin subclasses targeting epitopes within the NC16A domain of BP180 in pemphigoid gestationis. J Invest Dermatol. 1999;113:140–2.

22. Sadik CD, Lima AL, Zillikens D. Pemphigoid gestationis: toward a better understanding of the etiopathogenesis. Clin Dermatol. 2016;34(3):378–82.

23. Tani N, Kimura Y, Koga H, Kawakami T, Ohata C, Ishii N, Hashimoto T. Clinical and immunological profiles of 25 patients with pemphigoid gestationis. Br J Dermatol. 2015;172:120–9.

24. Jenkins RE, Hern S, Black MM. Clinical features and management of 87 patients with pemphigoid gestationis. Clin Exp Dermatol. 1999;24:255–9.

25. Ambros-Rudolph CM, Mullegger RR, Vaughan-Jones SA, et al. The specific dermatoses of pregnancy revisited and reclassified: results of a retrospective two-center study on 505 pregnant patients. J Am Acad Dermatol. 2006;54:395–404.

26. Lawley TJ, Stingl G, Katz SI. Fetal and maternal risk factors in herpes gestationis. Arch Dermatol. 1978;114:552–5.

27. Hertz KC, Katz SI, Maize J, et al. Herpes gestationis: a clinicopathologic study. Arch Dermatol. 1976;112:1543–8.

28. Barnadas MA, Rubiales MV, Gonzalez MJ, et al. Enzyme-linked immunosorbent assay (ELISA) and indirect immunofluorescence testing in a bullous pemphigoid and pemphigoid gestationis. Int J Dermatol. 2008;47:1245–9.

29. Rodrigues Cdos S, Filipe P, Solana Mdel M, et al. Persistent herpes gestationis treated with high-dose intravenous immunoglobulin. Acta Derm Venereol. 2007;87:184–6.

30. Kreuter A, Harati A, Breuckmann F, et al. Intravenous immune globulin in the treatment of persistent pemphigoid gestationis. J Am Acad Dermatol. 2004;51:1027–8.

31. Hern S, Harman K, Bhogal BS, et al. A severe persistent case of pemphigoid gestationis treated with intravenous immunoglobulins and cyclosporin. Clin Exp Dermatol. 1998;23:185–8.

32. Gan DC, Welsh B, Webster M. Successful treatment of a severe persistent case of pemphigoid gestationis with antepartum and postpartum intravenous immunoglobulin followed by azathioprine. Australas J Dermatol. 2012;53:66–9.

33. Shornick JK, Black MM. Fetal risks in herpes gestationis. J Am Acad Dermatol. 1992;26:63–8.

34. Al-Mutairi N, Sharma AK, Zaki A, et al. Maternal and neonatal pemphigoid gestationis. Clin Exp Dermatol. 2004;29:202–4.

35. Shornick JK, Black MM. Secondary autoimmune diseases in herpes gestationis (pemphigoid gestationis). J Am Acad Dermatol. 1992;26:563–6.

36. Chang SE, Kim HH, Choi JH, Sung KJ, Moon KC, Koh JK. Impetigo herpetiformis followed by generalized pustular psoriasis: more evidence of same disease entity? Int J Dermatol. 2003;42(9):754–5.

37. Lotem M, Katzenelson V, Rotem A, Hod M, Sandbank M. Impetigo herpetiformis: a variant of pustular psoriasis or a separate entity? J Am Acad Dermatol. 1989;20:338–41.

38. Winton GB, Lewis CW. Dermatoses of pregnanacy. J Am Acad Dermatol. 1982;6:977–98.

39. Hellreich P. The skin changes of pregnancy. Cutis. 1974;13:82–6.

40. Sasseville D, Wilkinson RD, Schnader JY. Dermatoses of pregnancy. Int J Dermatol. 1981;20:223–41.

41. Baker H, Ryan TJ. Generalized pustular psoriasis. A clinical and epidemiological study of 104 cases. Br J Dermatol. 1968;80:771–93.

42. Sugiura K, Nakasuka A, Kono H, Kono M, Akiyama M. Impetigo herpetiformis with IL36RN mutations in a Chinese patient: a founder haplotype of c.115+6T>C in East Asia. J Dermatol Sci. 2015;79:319–20.

43. Sugiura K, Oiso N, Iinuma S, Matsuda H, Minami-Hori M, Ishida-Yamamoto A, Kawada A, Iizuka H, Akiyama M. IL36RN mutations underlie impetigo herpetiformis. J Invest Dermatol. 2014;134:2472–4.

44. Soutou B, Aractingi S. Skin disease in pregnancy. Best Pract Res Clin Obstet Gynaecol. 2015;29:732–40.
45. Eudy SF, Baker GF. Dermatopathology for the obstetrician. Clin Obstet Gynecol. 1990;33:728–37.
46. Bozdag K, Ozturk S, Ermete M. A case of recurrent impetigo herpetiformis treated with systemic corticosteroids and narrowband UVB. Cutan Ocul Toxicol. 2012;31:67–9.
47. Shaw CJ, Wu P, Sriemevan A. First trimester impetigo herpetiformis in multiparous female successfully treated with oral cyclosporine. BMJ Case Rep. 2011;12:bcr0220113915.
48. Luewan S, Sirichotiyakul S, Tongsong T. Recurrent impetigo herpetiformis successfully treated with methotrexate: a case report. J Obstet Gynaecol Res. 2011;37:661–3.
49. Saito-Sasaki N, Izu K, Sawada Y, Hino R, Nakano R, Shimajiri S, Nishimura I, Nakamura H, Sugiura K, Nakamura M. Impetigo herpetiformis complicated with intrauterine growth restriction treated successfully with granulocyte and monocyte apheresis. Acta Derm Venereol. 2017;97:410–1.
50. Hayashi RH. Bullous dermatoses and prurigo of pregnancy. Clin Obstet Gynecol. 1990;33:746–53.
51. Barker B. Ernest Besnier 1831-1909. Arch Dermatol Syphilol. 1929;20:95–9.
52. Nurse DS. Prurigo of pregnancy. Australas J Dermatol. 1968;9:258–67.
53. Cohen LM. Dermatoses of pregnancy. West J Med. 1998;169:223–4.
54. Black MM. Prurigo of pregnancy, papular dermatitis of pregnancy, and pruritic folliculitis of pregnancy. Semin Dermatol. 1997;8:23–5.
55. Roger D, Vaillant L, Fignon A, et al. Specific pruritic diseases of pregnancy. A prospective study of 3192 pregnant women. Arch Dermatol. 1994;130:744–9.
56. Black MM, Stephens C. The specific dermatoses of pregnancy, the British perspective. Adv Dermatol. 1989;7:105–27.
57. Wilkinson SM, Buckler H, Wilkinson N. Androgen levels in pruritic folliculitis of pregnancy. Clin Exp Dermatol. 1995;20:234–6.
58. Dacus JV. Pruritus in pregnancy. Clin Obstet Gynecol. 1990;33:738–45.
59. Tunzi M, Gray GR. Common skin conditions during pregnancy. Am Fam Physician. 2007;75:211–8.
60. Al-Fares SI, Jones SV, Black MM. The specific dermatoses of pregnancy: a re-appraisal. J Eur Acad Dermatol Venereol. 2001;15:197–206.
61. Zoberman E, Farmer ER. Pruritic folliculitis of pregnancy. Arch Dermatol. 1981;117:20–2.
62. Alcalay J, Ingber A, Hazaz B, et al. Linear IgM dermatosis of pregnancy. J Am Acad Dermatol. 1988;18:412–5.
63. Helm TN, Valenzuela R. Continuous dermoepidermal junction IgM detected by immunofluorescence: a report of nine cases. J Am Acad Dermatol. 1992;26:203–6.
64. Dahdah MI, Kibbi AG. Less well-defined dermatoses of pregnancy. Clin Dermatol. 2006;24:118–21.

Nipples: A Sensitive Topic

11

Eve Finkelstein, Deena Yael Meerkin, and Gina Weissman

11.1 Anatomy and Physiology of the Nipple

The nipple is a cylindrical or conical eminence that projects from just below the centre of the anterior surface of the breast. In female mammals it is the portal through which milk from the breast is delivered to the mouth of the suckling infant.

Although they are very different in size, the nipples of women and men are qualitatively identical [1, 2]. In male mammals, nipples are considered vestigial structures. Their level on the thorax varies but nipples commonly lie at the level of the fourth intercostal space. The areola is the disc of skin which circles the base of the nipple.

The skin covering the nipple and areola is modified. It has a convoluted surface and contains many sweat and sebaceous gland which open directly onto the skin's surface. The oily secretion of the sebaceous glands is a lubricant that protects the nursing nipple. Other areolar glands are intermediate in structure between mammary and sweat glands. They enlarge in pregnancy and lactation as subcutaneous tubercles (Montgomery glands).

Melanocytes are numerous in the skin of the nipple and areola causing the nipple and areola to be darker in colour than the remainder of the breast. In the nulliparous they are pink, light brown or dark, depending on the general melanization of the body. It is noted that the deep colour of the areola is helpful in guiding the baby to its nutritional source, and perhaps even encourage the infant to grasp more of the areola and nipple.

The nervous innervation of the nipple is supplied from the anterior and lateral cutaneous branches of the third to fifth intercostal nerves, which lie along the ducts to the nipple [3]. They form an extensive plexus within the nipple and its sensory fibres terminate close to the epithelium as free endings, Meissner corpuscles and merkel disc endings. These are essential in signaling suckling to the central nervous system. The autonomic motor nerve supply of the breast is derived from the sympathetic fibers of the intercostal nerves, which supply the smooth musculature of the areola and the nipple. The autonomic supply is also derived from sympathetic fibers of the accompanying arteries, which innervate the smooth musculature of the inner glandular blood vessel walls to produce constriction. All cutaneous nerves run radially to the glandular body toward the nipple. The nerve supply to the inner gland is sparse and contains only sympathetic

E. Finkelstein (✉)
Department of Dermatology, Hadassah Medical
Centre, Hebrew University, Jerusalem, Israel
e-mail: evefjaw@gmail.com

D. Y. Meerkin
Lactation Consultant, NICU Shaarei Zedek Medical
Centre, Jerusalem, Israel

G. Weissman
The Israeli Association of Certified Lactation
Consultants, Beerotayim, Israel

© Springer International Publishing AG, part of Springer Nature 2018
E. Tur, H. I. Maibach (eds.), *Gender and Dermatology*,
https://doi.org/10.1007/978-3-319-72156-9_11

nerves accompanying blood vessels [2]. Secretory activities of the gland are largely controlled by ovarian and hypophyseal hormones rather than by efferent nerve fibres. The areola has less sensory endings than the nipple [4].

A large proportion of the mammary glandular tissue is located at a 30 mm (1.18 in.) radius from the base of the nipple [5]. Approximately 5–10 main ducts and 10–15 others branch and extend from the nipple in a complex and intertwined pattern. These lactiferous ducts transport milk from the lobules they drain to the nipple tip. Ducts are superficial and are easily compressed and may obstruct the milk flow [6]. There are 23–27 milk collecting ducts on average. Each of the tubuloalveolar glands composing the breast opens onto the nipple by a separate opening, however the number of collecting ducts is greater than the number of nipple duct openings [7]. Lobules extend from these ducts; they are composed of branching ductules that terminate in alveolar clusters. The alveolus is the milk-secreting unit of the breast that is lined with alveolar milk-secreting epithelial cells surrounded by supporting structures, a rich vascular supply, and myoepithelial cells [8]. Under the influence of oxytocin the myoepithelial cells contract causing ejection of milk into the ductules. Tactile, thermal, or sexual stimulation of the nipple causes contraction of the muscular fibroelastic system in the nipple and areola with subsequent decrease in surface area of the areola producing nipple erection, and emptying the swollen ducts during breastfeeding. Local venostasis and hyperaemia occur to enhance the process of erection of the nipple. The nipple becomes smaller, firmer, and more prominent [9]. Touch receptors in the nipple detect sucking by the infant. These touch receptors are afferents that are parts of the third, fourth, and fifth intercostal nerves. Impulses from the touch receptors are relayed to the spinal cord and further on to projections in the median eminence of the hypothalamus, where prolactin and oxytocin are released [10]. Between feedings smooth muscles present in the distal ducts prevent leakage of milk. Sympathetic mammary stimulation causes contraction of the small myoepithelial cells of the areola and the nipple.

Locally released norepinephrine induces stimulation of the myoepithelial adrenergic receptors, causing muscular relaxation.

11.2 The Nipple as an Erogenous Zone

Physiologically the nipple is considered an erogenous zone as stimulation of the nipple activates not only the thoracic region on the homuncular map of the brain but also stimulates the genital region of the medial paracentral lobule. There is congruence between the activation produced by the stimulation of the nipple and the activation produced by stimulation of the cervix, vagina and clitoris. This suggests a neurological basis for the perception of nipples of being erotogenic [11].

Oxytocin causes the uterus to contract and the nipples to become erect. This occurs during breastfeeding as well as during orgasms and labor. Some women experience some form of sexual gratification during suckling and in a study by Masters and Johnson, 3 out of 24 women experienced orgasm on occasion during breastfeeding [2, 12].

This phenomenon may be underreported due to embarrassment and guilt regarding these feelings. A mother may experience an erogenous reaction to breastfeeding with an older child who may roll the nipple while feeding. Feelings of guilt or embarrassment in this situation may lead to early weaning. These feelings seem to be more prevalent among lower social groups. Physicians must be aware of the possibility for these feelings and be prepared to explain and discuss this phenomenon openly. The majority of women who enjoy breastfeeding have no feelings or responses to the stimulation of the breast that could be interpreted as sexual arousal [13].

Some women may have increased interest in sexual relations while breastfeeding, while others may experience lack of libido for 6 months or more. It is unclear whether the lack of interest stems from the satisfaction of the mother's needs for intimacy through nursing, general exhaustion, or fear of pregnancy [12]. Sexual stimuli may trigger the milk ejection reflex during orgasm or sex and may have a negative effect on some men. Feeding the infant or expressing some milk beforehand may be helpful in reducing this phenomenon.

In addition to its function in nurturing infants, in females, nipples are sexualized, objectified and censored while the display of male nipples is totally acceptable [14]. Photographs of nursing women are deemed unacceptable even when in the photograph the infant's body covers the breast entirely, and women breastfeeding their infants in public have caused uproars in many countries. Bottle feeding is perceived as sterile, while breast milk is considered a bodily fluid that must be contained [15]. When young men were interviewed regarding perceptions of their partners breastfeeding, themes concerning sexuality embarrassment and social conduct were identified. The authors of that study concluded that perceptions of breastfeeding as sexual activity, and the emphasis by the media of breasts as a sexual objects, present additional obstacles to breastfeeding [2, 16].

11.3 Nipple Pathology

11.3.1 Rudimentary or Absent Nipples

Absent breasts and nipples have been described as an isolated defect with Dominant inheritance [17]. Rudimentary nipples have been described as part of many congenital syndromes [18–21].

11.3.2 Supernumerary Nipples (Polythelia)

Mammalian nipples and breasts develop in the embryo in the mammary ridge (also called mammary fold or milk line) which is a bandlike thickening of the ectoderm extending from just below the axilla to the inguinal region. In humans, milk lines appear in the fourth to sixth week of embryonic development. Since the milk lines appear before human sexual differentiation, males also have nipples. Mammary glands develop during the seventh week of embryonic development through cell migration from the epidermis [22]. They first appear as elevated ridges along the milk lines and then separate into individual buds in specific regions lateral of the dorsal midline. The location of the buds varies according to the species and they are located in the thoracic region in primates, the inguinal area in ungulates and along the entire length of the trunk in rodents and pigs [23]. In humans during puberty about 11 alveolar buds form in clusters around each terminal duct creating a lobule. The areola enlarges and darkens, and the breast increase to the adult size [8]. While the glandular elements of the breast are developing near the fourth rib there is regression of the rest of the thickened ectodermal ridge. In the case where complete regression does not occur supernumerary nipples or breasts may be formed. During pregnancy, progesterone, prolactin, human placental lactogen, growth hormone, and insulin-like growth factor cause the completion of breast growth and maturation [8].

Atavism is the reappearance of an ancestral characteristic in an organism after several generations of absence. The appearance of atavistic structures reminds us that the genetic information used in the production of such structures has not been lost during evolution but remains quiescent in the genome.

Supernumerary (or accessory) nipples are atavistic structures that usually form on the milk line, though 10% are known as ectopic supernumerary nipples and can even develop at sites that are distant from the milk line such as on the face [24] and on the foot [25]. Supernumerary nipples can appear complete with breast tissue and ducts and are then known as polymastia or they can appear with only part of the breast tissues.

Supernumerary Nipples are relatively common, with an incidence of 2–5.6% and with a higher incidence in males. They are more common on the left side [26]. They are usually inconsequential and most people think that they are simply raised nevi. Sometimes patients present to their doctor distressed when they undergo changes during puberty, pregnancy or after childbirth. They can become swollen and tender with the hormonal changes and during pregnancy they can become hyperpigmented. Milk leakage during breast feeding can be so bothersome that excision is requested. Classification by Kajava in 1915 is still used today [27].

1. Complete supernumerary nipple—Nipple and areola and glandular breast tissue
2. Supernumerary Nipple—Nipple and glandular tissue (no areola)
3. Supernumerary Nipple—Areola and glandular tissue (no nipple)
4. Aberrant Glandular tissue only
5. Supernumerary Nipple—Nipple and areola and pseudomamma (fat tissue that replaces the glandular tissue)
6. Supernumerary Nipple—Nipple only (the most common supernumerary nipple)
7. Supernumerary Nipple—Areola only (polythelia areolaris)
8. Patch of Hair only

Excision of breast tissue is recommended if the patient is carrier of the BRCA gene or other hereditary forms of breast cancer, and if not, screening of the breast tissue is recommended at the rate that is appropriate for that woman's age. Supernumerary Nipples can been found associated with many rare genodermatoses [28, 29] and a wide range of other congenital abnormalities [30]. Supernumerary nipples are associated with kidney and urinary tract malformations, adult dominant polycystic kidney disease, unilateral renal agenesis, cystic renal dysplasia, familial renal cysts and congenital stenosis of the pyeloureteral joint [31] and a significantly higher frequency of polythelia has been recorded in urogenital cancer patients [32].

Familial polythelia has been noted with either an autosomal dominant or X linked dominant pattern. There is some controversy as to whether the familial cases are associated with kidney and urinary tract malformations to a greater degree than sporadic cases. It has been suggested that due to the possible increased incidence of malignancy of the urogenital tract it is reasonable to consider familial polythelia as genodermatosis with malignant potential and that appropriate follow-up is recommended [33] (Fig. 11.1).

11.4 Flat and Inverted Nipples Are Mentioned Below in the Section on Breastfeeding

11.4.1 Hyperkeratosis of the Nipple

Hyperkeratosis of the nipple is a rare condition. The original classification by Levy-Franckel in 1934, simplified by Perez-Izquierdo et al. in 1990, is based on etiology. They classify hyperkeratosis of nipple as idiopathic and nevoid or secondary.

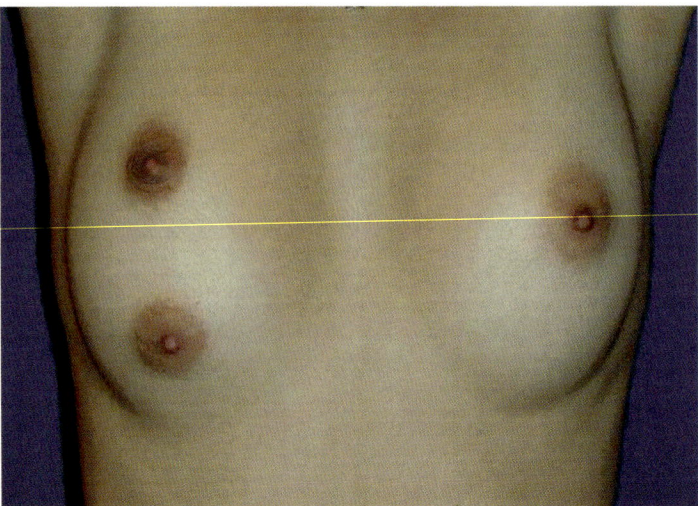

Fig. 11.1 Supernummerary nipple. Photo credit: Dr Yoav Barnea

11.4.2 Nevoid Hyperkeratosis of the Nipple (Unilateral or Bilateral)

Nevoid hyperkeratosis of the nipple is a rare, idiopathic disorder where the nipple and/or areola becomes thickened and hyperpigmented and sometimes verrucous. The lesions are usually bilateral, however there are some reported cases where this condition is unilateral, and there are cases which are unilateral that become bilateral after pregnancy. 80% of cases of primary hyperkeratosis occur in females most commonly between the ages of 10 and 40 [34].

Lesions are usually asymptomatic, though there are cases where breastfeeding is not possible. Patients sometimes request treatment due to cosmetic concerns. Cosmetically satisfactory results have been reported with cryotherapy [35], excision with full thickness thin grafts from the excessive (sic) labia minora [36], and temporary response has been reported with the topical application of retinoid acid [37] or calcipotriol [38]. Early Nevoid Hyperkeratosis has been recorded as having mimicked pigmented Basal Cell Carcinoma [39] (Fig. 11.2).

11.4.2.1 Secondary Hyperkeratosis of the Nipple

Secondary hyperkeratosis of the Nipple can be associated with many conditions including acanthosis nigricans, Epidermal naevi, Organoid

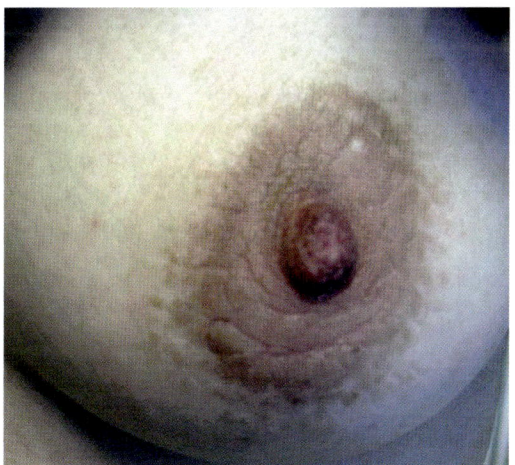

Fig. 11.2 Nevoid hyperkeratosis of nipple. Photo credit: Dr Ricardo Ruiz Villaverde

naevi, Leiomyomas, Verrucae, acquired or erythrodermic ichthyosis, Dariers disease, Cutaneous T cell lymphoma, Chronic mucocutaneous candidiasis, and pregnant females. It can be drug related and found in patients receiving Estrogen therapy for androgen insensitivity syndrome and males receiving hormonal therapy for prostate cancer [40].

11.4.2.2 Acanthosis Nigricans

Acanthosis Nigricans, while listed as a type of secondary hyperkeratosis deserves a separate note. Acanthosis Nigricans is a symmetric eruption characterized by hyperpigmented velvety thickening that can occur on any part of the body but which usually affects the axillae, nape and sides of neck, the groin, antecubital and popliteal surfaces and umbilical area. In its common form it is associated with insulin resistance and compensatory increased insulin secretion which activates insulin like growth factor-1 receptors and mediate epidermal cell proliferation [41].

There are 8 types of Acanthosis Nigricans: (1) Benign acanthosis nigricans (2) obesity associated acanthosis nigricans (3) Syndromic acanthosis nigricans (4) malignant acanthosis nigricans (5) Acral acanthosis nigricans (6) Unilateral acanthosis nigricans (7) medication induced acanthosis nigricans and (8) medication induced acanthosis nigricans where 2 types are present.

Cases of Acanthosis Nigricans of the nipple in the literature are mainly of the benign type, though cases related to obesity and insulin resistance, medication, or related to malignancy are reported. When related to malignancy it tends to be the most florid and is usually associated with other symptoms such as weight loss and other paraneoplastic signs [42]. Treatment involves treating the underlying malignancy. Gastric cancer is the most commonly found association in over 50% of cases.

11.5 Seborrheic Keratosis

Seborrheic keratoses and achrochordons (skin tags) may erupt in association with pregnancy, and tend to be located on the chest back and abdomen. They are diagnosed histologically by hyperkeratosis, epidermal acanthosis and papillomatosis. The appearance of seborrheic keratosis on the nipples during pregnancy is common and is a not an infrequent source of referral of anxious pregnant women who note new lesions on their nipples. The appearance could be explained by the increase in epidermal growth factor during pregnancy [43].

While no difference was observed in the expression of immunoreactive growth hormone receptors in keritinocytes from normal epidermis and keratinocytes in seborrheic keratoses, in a study of patients with dysplastic nevus syndrome, it was shown that sex steroids may effect growth factor metabolism in patients with benign epidermal hyperproliferative lesions [44].

Usually reassurance is the only treatment necessary but large lesions may interfere with the baby's latch on to the nipple and in that case should be treated with an ablative treatment such as liquid nitrogen. The treatment should be done early enough in pregnancy to leave time for the nipple to heal well before the birth.

A case of eruptive seborrheic keratoses of the breast was reported to be associated with ipsilateral intraductal carcinoma [45]. The sudden appearance of multiple seborrheic keratoses associated with malignancy is known as the Sign of Leser Trelat. Although the cause of this rare paraneoplastic sign is not known it is assumed to be due to a growth factor that is produced by the neoplasm, as it is associated with Acanthosis Nigricans in up to 35% of cases and with pruritus in 50% of cases [46] (Fig. 11.3).

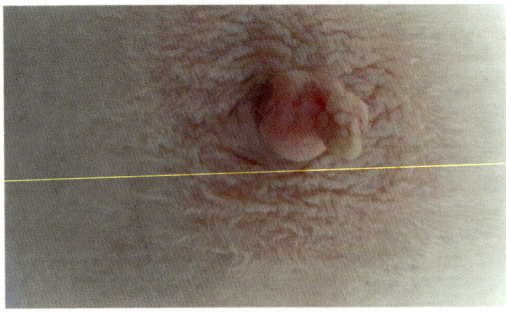

Fig. 11.3 Keratosis of the nipple photo. This woman successfully nursed 2 children without removing the keratosis

11.6 Mammary Duct Ectasia

Mammary Duct Ectasia is a term introduced by Haagensen [47] to describe a benign condition characterized by dilatation of the subareolar duct system that drain via the nipple. After menopause the subareolar ducts may dilate or shorten and aging causes involution of breast tissue, i.e. the composition of the breast becomes less glandular and more fatty. As a result of these age related changes by age 70, 40% of women have substantial duct dilatation or duct ectasia. There may be an association with cigarette smoking. Some women with excessive dilatation and shortening present with nipple discharge, nipple retraction or a palpable mass that may be hard or doughy. The discharge is usually cheesy, and the nipple retraction is classically slit like. In most cases no treatment is necessary. Antibiotics are sometimes necessary to treat infection and some women complain of pain that can be treated by over the counter analgesics. Surgery is indicated if the discharge is troublesome or the patient wishes the nipple to be everted [48].

11.7 Adnexal Polyp of Neonatal Skin

The adenexal polyp of neonatal skin is an elastic, firm and polypoid tumour, about 1 mm in diameter. It is skin coloured or pink. It usually occurring on the areola of a neonate, a few millimeters medial to the nipple. Occasionally they are found elsewhere on the body. It becomes dry and brown and falls off spontaneously within a few days of birth. Histologically it contains hair follicles, eccrine glands and vestigial sebaceous glands. A Japanese study reported a 4% incidence in newborns [49].

11.8 Erosive Adenomatosis of the Nipple

Syn: Benign Papillomatosis of the Nipple; Florid Papillomatosis of the Nipple Ducts; Papillary Adenoma of the Nipple; Subareolar Duct Papillomatosis.

Erosive adenomatosis of the nipple is a complex benign tumour of the lactiferous ducts of the breast that has a variety of histologic appearances. Although it can appear at any age, its peak incidence is after the fifth decade so it often confused with Paget's disease clinically, and histologically it can be confused with syringoadenoma papilliferum, hidroadenoma papilliferum or low grade adenocarcinoma. It occasionally occurs in males [50].

Unilateral serous, bloody, or serosanguinous discharge with crusting is most frequently present. Bilateral cases have been reported which would make it very difficult to differentiate from eczema. Symptoms include tenderness and pruritus. A palpable nodule is found in a third of cases. Swelling or induration and erythema have been seen less frequently. The symptoms may be worse in the premenstrual phase.

The lesion is characterized histologically by ductal proliferation that invades the surrounding stroma. A major distinguishing characteristic is the presence of a double layer of cells composed of an inner cuboidal epithelial layer and outer myoepithelial contractile cell layer. Carcinoma, by contrast does not produce this double layer of cells. Papillary projections have been frequently reported. The tubules are filled with keratin flakes, and an eosinophilic material, secreted by the columnar cells. Erosions and ulcerations were reported in about half the cases [51].

Simple excision of the nipple is considered treatment of choice. Recurrences are common and are assumed to be due to incomplete resection. Moh's micrographic surgery [52] and two 45 second treatments with Cryosurgery (reaching a temperature of −40 °C) [53] have been successfully used to treat this benign condition.

11.9 Paget's Disease

Pagets disease is a chronic eczematous scaling and crusting of the nipple (and more rarely) the areola due to invasion on the epidermis by malignant cells of in situ (DCIS) or invasive ductal adenocarcinoma. Paget's disease occurs almost exclusively in women and is often mistaken for dermatitis. It is most commonly diagnosed between 50 and 60 years of age. It is also called Mammary Paget disease to distinguish it from Extramammary Paget's disease which is an intraepithelial adenocarcinoma that occurs in the groin, genitalia or perineum. Metastatic disease is often present at the time of diagnosis. Paget's disease occurs in 1–3% of all primary breast carcinomas.

The malignancy starts as an intraductal carcinoma that distend and spread through the ducts. A number of ducts are usually involved, but it is considered an in-situ carcinoma. Only at a later stage does it become a truly invasive breast carcinoma.

Pagets's disease may present as a change in sensation at the nipple area and itching and burning is a common presenting symptom. About half of the presenting cases have a palpable underlying mass [54].

Since the lesions of Paget's disease are almost invariable unilateral and only very exceptionally bilateral [55] the dictum "Beware of Unilateral Nipple dermatitis" should be taught to every medical professional to ensure early diagnosis (Figs. 11.4 and 11.5).

11.10 Nipple Piercing

Body piercing has become more popular over the last few decades, and is often performed before the age of 18 [56]. It is reported that up to 75% of

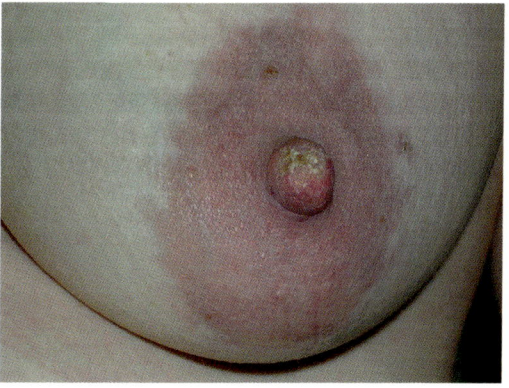

Fig. 11.4 Paget's disease with early eczematous changes to the nipple. Photo credit: Dr Oded Olsha

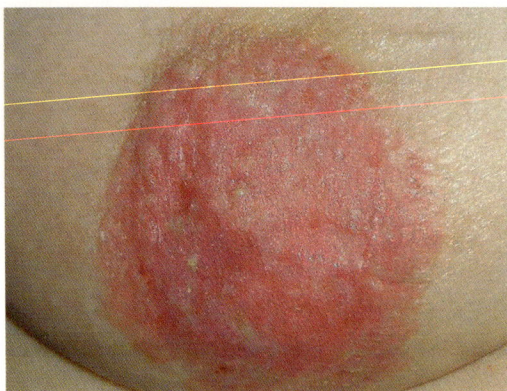

Fig. 11.5 Pagets disease with destruction of the nipple and involvement of the areola. Photo credit: Dr Oded Olsha

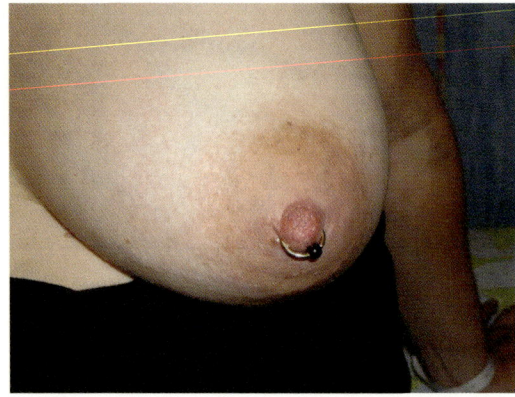

Fig. 11.6 Pierced nipple. This woman successfully nursed her infant with this nipple ring in place. Photo credit: Dr. Gina Weissman, IBCLC

adolescents who had tattoos or body piercings did not seek permission from their parents [57] and almost one third had done so outside of a dedicated studio. Body piercing (other than piercing of the soft lobe of the ear) has been shown to be a marker of risk taking behaviour in adolescents -including eating disorders, drug use, sexual activity and, violence and suicide [58]. 9% were drunk or high on drugs at the time of the piercing. While women greatly outnumber men in multiple ear, belly button and nose piercings, men outnumber women 6 to one with respect to nipple piercings [56].

Nipple piercing may cause contact dermatitis to jewellery, with incidence increasing with the number of body piercings. There is also an increased the risk of infection with Hepatitis A, B and C as well as HIV although as noted previously, those who pierce have increased risk taking behaviour and the infection may not have been acquired through the act of body piercing [59]. Infective endocarditis has also been described after nipple piercing [60]. A striptease dancer who wore tassel ornaments suspended from her breasts developed Mammary duct ectasia [61].

Although most women who have pierced their nipples go on to successfully breastfeed their infants there are cases where infants have had attachment problems on the side with the piercing and where the piercing have led to the blockage of ducts and the formation of septa that can interfere with milk supply. Decreased milk supply secondary to reduction in blood flow to the pierced breast has been described [62] (Fig. 11.6).

11.11 Nipple Changes in Pregnancy

During pregnancy, the nipples become more prominent due to the increased levels of oestrogen, progesterone and placental lactogen. There is an increased blood supply to the nipple which may cause women to complain of tingling and stinging or even of bleeding from the nipples.

Darkening of the nipple and areola occurs in nearly all women and is even considered to be a sign of early pregnancy. The exact pathogenesis is unclear but may be due to an increase in the Melanocyte stimulating hormone and serum estrogen and progesterone levels [91]. It is thought that the darker colour makes it easier for the baby to target and latch on to the nipple.

Beginning as early as 6 weeks into the pregnancy sebaceous glands associated with the lactiferous ducts of the areolae of the breasts hypertrophy, appearing as small elevated brown papules called Montgomery's glands or tubercles [63]. These sebaceous glands, which can be as few as 4 or as many as 28, secrete oils to make the areola more supple and have a distinctive smell so that the baby recognizes its mother [64].

11.12 Skin Disease Involving the Nipple: Special Considerations

Psoriasis, Atopic dermatitis, Pemphigus, and Darier's disease can all occur on the nipples. Trauma to the nipple from breastfeeding or expressing milk can cause koebnerization of psoriasis and increase transepidermal water loss and therefore worsen eczema. Infection, through bacterial superantigen activity can worsen eczema, psoriasis and Sezary syndrome [65, 66] and is thought to play a part in the activity of Dariers disease [67] (Fig. 11.7).

Skin disease that affects the nipples is usually treated no differently than if the disease was located on any other part of the body. Systemic therapies need to be reviewed to assess what percentage of the drug is secreted in the breast milk and whether there will be risk to the newborn infant from ingesting the drug. Drugs that are more likely to transfer into human milk are those that attain high concentrations in the plasma, are low in molecular weight, are low in protein binding, and pass into the brain easily [68]. In many cases the amount of medication that finds its way into the breast milk is small. For example, one study showed 0.14% of an original prednisolone dose in 1 litre of breast milk in mothers given a radioactive dose [69]. In all cases of systemic therapies there are pregnancy categories to guide the medical practitioner.

There is less information regarding topical therapies. All topical therapies are absorbed to some degree, but the amounts are usually small and therefore the amount subsequently secreted in the breast milk is usually negligible. The concern of absorption of the topical medication is more an issue when the medication is applied directly to the nipple. To avoid the baby ingesting significant amounts of the active ingredients, creams should be applied immediately after breastfeeding so that by the time the baby next feeds at the nipple a few hours will have passed and the amount of medication absorbed by the infant is negligible. Having said that, most topical creams have no pregnancy categories assigned and so reassuring worried mothers that the therapies prescribed are totally safe can be challenging.

The mainstay of treatment of skin in pregnant and nursing women is topical moisturizers and topical steroids, and as mentioned there is usually only minimal absorption, but treating severe skin disease covering large area of the body is especially problematic. Super potent topical steroids used on large area of skin are absorbed systemically. A study has found significant association between first trimester use of topical steroids and orofacial cleft, and another study found significant association between maternal use of very potent topical corticosteroids and low birth weight [70] (Fig. 11.8).

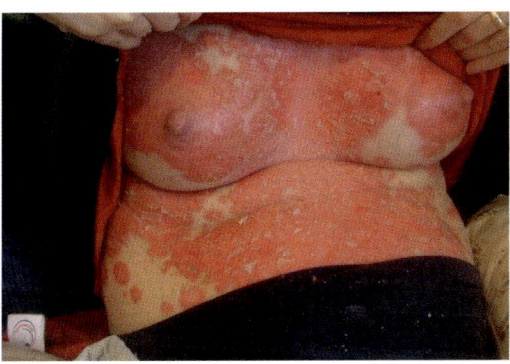

Fig. 11.7 Psoriasis involving the nipple and areola. This woman successfully nursed her baby despite the extensive skin disease. Photo credit: Liat Bendarsky, IBCLC, HalavM breastfeeding clinic

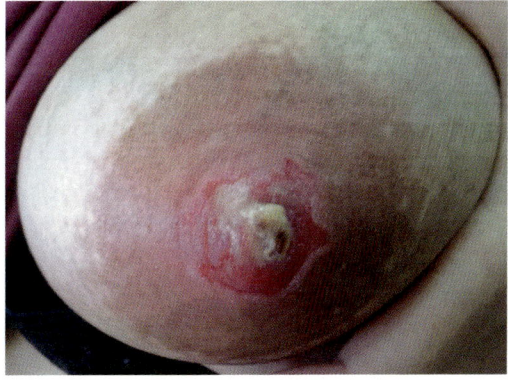

Fig. 11.8 Pyoderma gangrenosum of the nipple in a patient with ulcerative colitis. This woman continued to pump from that side despite the destruction of the nipple. The nipple eventually healed with high potency steroid under occlusion and she was able to breast feed normally

11.12.1 Psoriasis

55% of women with psoriasis note an improvement in their symptoms during pregnancy, and 65% experience worsening of their Psoriasis after the child is born. While studies have connected the improvement during pregnancy to raised estriol and estradiol levels [71] there are other factors at play that effect the immune system as well. In pregnancy there is a shift from TH1 immunity (associated with cellular immunity) to TH2 immunity (associated with certain aspects of humoral immunity). This promotes fetal survival by decreasing TH1 responses involved in the rejection of the fetus as an allograft [72]. This would explain, in part the improvement of psoriasis in pregnancy.

The worsening of psoriasis in the post-partum period can be explained by the up regulation of inflammatory responses. There are increased levels of pro inflammatory cytokines such as Interleukin 6 and Interleukin 1 after delivery [73]. These cytokines are upregulated even more in breast feeding mothers compared to mothers who were bottle feeding their infants [74]. These cytokines are important in the pathogenesis of psoriasis.

In studies unrelated to pregnancy, sleep deprivation and disruption of the sleep cycle has also shown to be a factor which increases the secretion of proinflammatory cytokines that exacerbate Psoriasis [75]. This obviously plays a part in the exacerbation of psoriasis in the postpartum period.

Treatment of Psoriasis in the pregnant and breastfeeding mother can be especially problematic because some of the treatments are extremely toxic to the developing fetus and infant. First line treatment with moisturisers and low to mid-potency topical steroids is recommended. Second line treatment with Narrowband UVB or Broadband UVB is considered safe in both pregnant and breastfeeding women, though folic acid supplementation is recommended due to the photo degradation of folic acid associated with light therapy [76].

The oral agents most commonly used in the treatment of Psoriasis, Methotrexate and Acitretin, cannot be used in pregnancy. Methotrexate is a mutagen and abortifactant and should be stopped 12 weeks before conception and since 8% is secreted in the breast milk should be avoided in breastfeeding mothers. Acetretin is a teratogen that affects organogenesis in weeks 2–9 and may affect neurodevelopment in the 3rd trimester. Acetretin should be stopped 2 years before conception [77] but since only 1% is excreted in the milk, it is unlikely to be toxic to the breast fed infant.

The newer biologic agents that are TNF alpha agents (etaneracept adalimumab, infliximab) are considered category B in the first 2 trimesters in pregnant but can be used in breastfeeding women. There are, however concerns. In pregnant women, maternal antibodies are actively transported across the chorionic villi by the neonatal Fc receptor (FcRn) in the last trimester. Infliximab and adalimumab are both of the IgG1 subclass and this may result in higher levels in the infants at birth than their mothers [78]. These FcRn receptors then actively bind and recycle the antibodies and increase their half life by protecting them from catabolism [79]. Although the half-life of infliximab is 8–9.5 days in adults in infants there are detectable levels for 2–7 months after the infant is born [80]. Studies where the infliximab was stopped at 21 weeks gestation had no detectable levels in the newborn but those who stopped at 26 weeks still had high levels [81]. There is a recorded fatal case of disseminated BCG infection after immunization in a baby born to a mother who was treated by infliximab throughout her pregnancy [82]. It is therefore recommended to stop treatment with TNF alpha agents half way through the pregnancy, and in cases where it is not possible to stop the medication it is recommended to avoid live vaccines in the first 6 months of life. Inactive vaccines can be administered on schedule. If treatment with a biologic agent is necessary the use of Certolizumab could be considered as it does not have an Fc portion and does not cross the placenta in significant amounts.

Breastfeeding for mothers using anti TNF alpha agents is considered safe as the transfer to the infant during breast feeding is negligible and the infant's gastric digestion would destroy and drug present. The Biologic agents that block IL17 and IL12/23 (Secukinumab and ustikinimab) are category B and are considered relatively safe for both pregnant and breast-feeding women because of generalization of the data on anti TNF alpha agents, even though there is extremely limited data and no human studies. They are also large protein molecules and therefore the amount in milk is low and absorption is unlikely because of its destruction in the GI tract of the newborn [83]. However, it seems prudent to wait until there are human studies before prescribing these agents to breastfeeding women.

Cyclosporine has been used extensively in pregnant transplant patients and can be used in pregnancy, but it is associated with an increased risk of prematurity and low birth weight [84]. As only low levels are found in breast milk, Cyclosporin is considered compatible with breastfeeding [76].

At the time of writing there are no human studies proving the safety of Phosphodiesterase 4 inhibitor Apremilast in pregnancy or nursing and animal studies show an increase in incidence of abortion. There is no data regarding safety in lactation in humans but in mice it appears in high levels in breast milk [76].

Coal tar is a mainstay in the treatment of psoriasis but has no pregnancy category, and despite there being limited data it is commonly used in the second and third trimester of pregnancy for up to 3–4 weeks at a time. There is no category for breastfeeding so it would seem unwise to prescribe it to the nipples of a breast feeding woman.

Calcipotriol is Category C for pregnancy and systemic use is associated with skeletal abnormalities, however it is considered safe in breastfeeding.

Anthralin is catagory B for pregnancy and there is no human data for pregnancy and breastfeeding, but due to its irritant properties it is not suitable for use on nipples.

11.12.2 Eczema of the Nipples

Eczema is a broad term which describes the clinical presentation of an itchy, erythematous eruption caused by inflammation of the skin. The eczematous plaques may be studded with vesi-cles or covered by crust. When the area is repeatedly scratched the skin may become lichenified. The causes of eczema of the nipples can be divided into 3 categories. Endogenous, atopic dermatitis; Allergic contact dermatitis, and irritant contact dermatitis.

11.12.2.1 Atopic Dermatitis

Atopic disease, including atopic dermatitis (eczema), allergy and asthma affects approximately 20% of the population in the developed world. The predisposition is highly heritable and has been associated with variants in the gene encoding filaggrin which is a protein that facilitate the terminal differentiation of the epidermis and formation of the skin barrier [85]. The disrupted skin barrier allows transepidermal water loss which leads to inflammation. The disrupted barrier also provides an environment which favors the growth of Staph aureus which, through the effect of superantigens worsens the inflammation.

Atopic dermatitis on the nipples may worsen considerably during breast feeding due to further disruption of the epidermal barrier by the babies mouth and by superinfection by candida which is found amongst the flora of the mouth of 48% of healthy infants [86] and Streptococci and Staphylococci which are also present in the oral flora of half of all newborns [87] (Fig. 11.9).

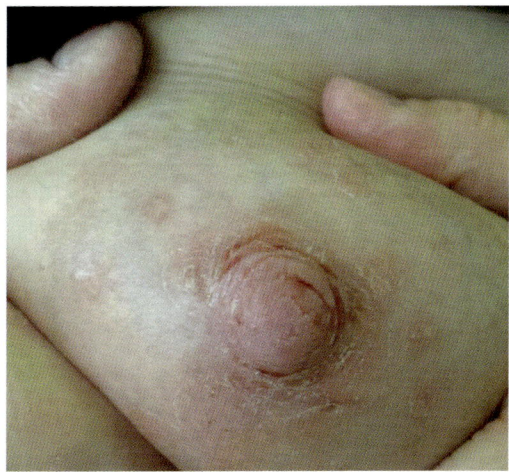

Fig. 11.9 Atopic dermatitis if the nipple and breast. Note the dermatitis is present on the mothers hands and the yellow crust that is typical of infection with Staphlococcus

11.12.2.2 Irritant Dermatitis

Irritation of the nipple, which results in dermatitis, can occur from a number of causes. Saliva is alkaline and can irritate the nipple and areola. Washing with soap removes the natural oils that act as a natural barrier. Surfactants and emulsifying agents found in shampoos and body lotions, such as Sodium Lauryl Sulfate and cocamidopropyl betaine [88] can irritate nipples and therefore breastfeeding women should be counseled that no soap is necessary for cleansing the nipple and areola. Dry cold air, as is found at high altitudes in the winter, may result in dry irritable skin.

Nipples are protuberant and therefore more likely to be irritated my mechanical pressure and shearing forces. Synthetic and lacy materials can irritate the nipples. The seams of ill-fitting bras can also cause irritation. This can cause unilateral dermatitis in women that have asymmetric breasts where there is friction only on the side of the larger breast [89].

Sports Injury: Recreational Irritant Dermatitis

Long distance runners of either sex can suffer from "Jogger's nipples" which is irritation and erosions of the nipples due to friction of the nipples on the shirt. The condition is more marked in female joggers who don't wear a bra whilst jogging. Wearing a properly fitted sports bra will decrease the friction. In males, covering the nipples with petroleum jelly and wearing a shirt that is smooth and soft is helpful. Covering the nipples with tape is preventative [90].

Bicyclists can suffer from cold injury of the nipples after they have been sweating in cold weather and their shirt is wet from perspiration. Evaporation and wind chill lower the temperature of the nipples. The nipples are sore and sensitive to temperature change and pressure, and the pain can continue for several days after the ride is over. Treatment consists of passage of time and the avoidance of subsequent thermal injury. Prevention focuses on the use of windbreaking materials over the chest. Specialized cycling shirts are available on the market that are windbreaking [91] as well as shirts made from "quick dry" self-wicking polyester, which draws off the moisture from the skin quickly by capillary action.

Surf Board riders may suffer irritant dermatitis from the friction, shearing forces, and pressure with the surfboard. The macerating effect of moisture increases the susceptibility. Salabrasion which results from friction and the abrasive action of salt causes abrasion at the points of contact. Wind causes chilling of superficial tissues and deposition of salts on the skin from the evaporation of sweat or salt water. Sand particles may also cause abrasion. Females are less susceptible to this form of dermatitis because their swimsuits add an extra layer of protection. Surfers may also suffer from allergic contact dermatitis to the surfboard wax as well as plasticizers used in the production of the board itself. Neoprene wetsuits may afford protection from irritant contact dermatitis but may cause allergic contact dermatitis due to Thiurea [92, 93] (Fig. 11.10).

11.12.2.3 Allergic Contact Dermatitis

Allergic contact dermatitis is caused by a type 4 or delayed hypersensitivity reaction which occurs 48–72 h after exposure to an allergen. Patients with an impaired barrier function of their skin caused by atopic or irritant dermatitis are more prone to developing allergic contact dermatitis. Allergic contact dermatitis starts locally where the skin comes into contact with the offending agent, but severe or prolonged contact with the allergen can lead to "generalization" of the rash i.e. appearance of an allergic reaction at a site that had no direct contact with the substance.

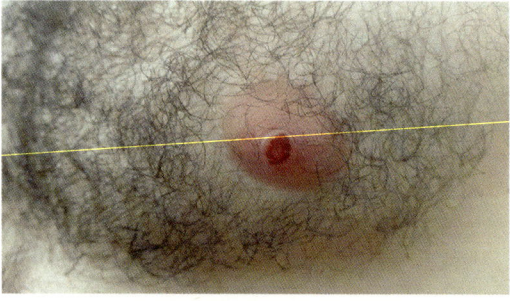

Fig. 11.10 Surfer's nipple. This surfer suffered injury to his nipple despite wearing a rash vest to protect himself from the friction of the surfboard. Abrasion from the salt and sand probably plays a role

There are many possible causes of allergic contact dermatitis of the nipples, and sometimes it is difficult to diagnose through solely taking a history from the patient, and patch testing must be performed. Patch testing is performed by applying standardized allergen to the skin for 48 h as well as the patient's own products.

Allergic contact dermatitis has been recorded to occur from many products that are applied to the skin of the breast and nipples.

Baby wipes, body washes and creams may contain methylisothiazoinone, preservatives and fragrances [94]. Nipple creams may contain lanolin [95], chamomile [94], or beeswax [96]. Treatment creams containing neomycin, mupirocin and cortisones may illicit allergic reactions as may preservative in the creams such as chlorochresol. Clothes washing detergents may contain fragrances, benzalkonium chloride or chloroxylenol which is an antiseptic. The use of nipple pads with an adhesive strip may result in allergic contact dermatitis to the adhesives. In a patient previously sensitized to paraphenylenediamine, contact allergy to the permanent colorants used for tattooing the nipple after breast reconstruction is recorded [97].

When allergic contact dermatitis occurs to topical medicaments it is often misdiagnosed for some time. A common scenario is that the nursing mother has sore nipples, so she applies a topical treatment. When the discomfort intensifies due to the development of contact dermatitis she blames the breastfeeding and therefore applies more of the ointment. Often, it only after the allergic contact dermatitis generalizes that the patient presents to a Dermatologist and a history is taken and the diagnosis made.

Treatment of nipple dermatitis consists of restoring the barrier function of the skin with topical moisturizer and treating the inflammation with a mild steroid ointment. All soaps, including mild ones, should be avoided. If any creams remain on the nipple they can be wiped off with cotton wool and water when the baby needs to feed. The superantigen activity of the bacteria and yeast can be quietened by applying antibacterial and anti-yeast medication that also contains a mild steroid. All purpose nipple cream (often called Dr Newman's nipple cream after the Canadian physician who championed it's use) containing 2% mupirocin 0.1% betamethasone and 2% miconazole is often used.

11.13 The Importance of Breast Feeding to the Mother and the Infant

Breast milk is the gold standard of nutrition for the newborn [98, 99]. The WHO as well as many international health organizations recommend exclusive breastfeeding for the first 6 months of the infants life and thereafter continued breastfeeding with gradual introduction of complimentary food until 2 years of age, or as long as both mother and infant are interested [100].

Breast milk contains unique oligosaccharides that promote a healthy gut bacteria, including proliferating Bifidobacterium longum biovar infantis as well as antimicrobial agents such as lactoferrin and secretory IgA. Some recent meta-analyses indicate that breastfeeding provides protection against child infections including gastroenteritis, respiratory illness, otitis media and urinary tract infections as well as malocclusion of the teeth. It probably increases intelligence, and probably reduces the incidence of obesity and diabetes [101].

For the breastfeeding mother, breastfeeding provides protection against type 2 diabetes and improves birth spacing. By inducing ovarian quiescence and decreasing estrogen secretion breastfeeding protects against breast, ovarian and endometrial cancer [102, 103]. Breastfeeding decreases the risk of postpartum depression and also helps the mother return to her pre-pregnancy weight [104].

Since breasts that are full of milk are uncomfortable, and this discomfort is relieved by nursing, nursing ensures that mother and baby remain in close proximity and creates a symbiotic relationship between the mother and her newborn. This closeness encourages the bonding that will ensure the emotional and physical well being of the baby.

11.14 Nipple Pain Associated with Breast Feeding

Twenty-four hours post partum, the nipple and areola sensitivity is significantly heightened but decreases in the next few days. After this initial period nipple pain is a sign of pathology of the breast or of the breastfeeding process. Studies of breastfeeding mothers have documented nipple pain as one of the most common reasons reported for consultation with incidence ranging from 36–79% [105, 106]. Nipple pain is the second most common reason given for subsequent cessation of exclusive breastfeeding surpassed only by a mother's perception of insufficient milk supply [105].

Nipple pain causes pain during breastfeeding which may affect mothers not only in the immediate postpartum period but even up to 8 weeks post-partum and beyond [107]. Nipple pain can negatively affect the mother's function, mood and sleep, leading to breastfeeding cessation with serious consequences to the health of both mother and nursing infant [108]. Postpartum, the woman's body undergoes major hormonal changes and this coupled with sleep deprivation and the fact that the new mother must learn to divide her time amongst more dependents means that her pain threshold and ability to cope with this pain are decreased. Childbirth has been shown to have detrimental effect on the physical and mental health of women in an Australian self-reported study, with 94% of women complaining of health problems in the 6 months after birth. As well as tiredness, women reported backache, perineal pain, sexual problems, hemorrhoids, mastitis and depression [109]. 49% of women in this study would have liked more help or advice. Nipple pain is one of the problems that nursing women face after birth that the medical/nursing profession can assist with, and it is important that we do so.

Lactation consultants are professionals who are trained to diagnose problems with the mother-baby dyad and to offer the guidance and the crucial emotional support that women need when dealing with diseases and pain of the nipples. They are, however, unable to prescribe the medi-

cations that are often necessary for the treatment of these conditions. It is therefore crucial that Dermatologists be aware of these problems, so that they can partner with lactation consultants in the treatment of women with sore nipples [71, 104, 110].

In many countries with socialized health care, there is reimbursement for patients who seek the advice of doctors but no reimbursement for patients who seek the guidance of Lactation consultants/instructors. Therefore, patients who cannot afford to see lactation consultants will present to the Dermatologist with nipple pain and pathology. Dermatologists must be aware of their abilities and limitations in helping these patients.

Breastfeeding is no longer viewed as a lifestyle choice but rather as an important health practice contributing to the health and wellbeing of the mother and infant, as well as the global economy [111]. Therefore early diagnosis and effective treatment are essential to assure continuation of a positive breastfeeding relationship between the mother-infant dyad.

11.14.1 Etiology of Nipple Pain

Although nipple pain is common, it can be prevented and treated. It is important to distinguish between physiological sensitivity and pain. In a state of tenderness during breastfeeding, the nipple will appear normal and round at the end of the feeding, and sensitivity should pass within 2–3 days after birth, without the development of clinical signs of injury. The source of the sensitivity is probably hormonal or due to the negative pressure exerted on the milk ducts before they are filled with milk [13]. If pain persists more than two days and is accompanied by worsening, or if there are signs of injury to the breast, the etiology of the pain must be discerned and prompt treatment given. Nipple trauma and subsequent pain may result from a combination of causes. If we are to prevent early weaning, systematic diagnosis of the cause of pain in order to decide on the appropriate management is of utmost importance. This requires careful history taking and examination of both mother and infant, as well as observation of a breastfeed. Pain is understood to be a multidimensional phenomenon and treatment may require a holistic and multidisciplinary approach. Causes of nipple pain are multifactorial and interdependent and will be discussed in the following sections [112].

11.14.1.1 Attributes of the Mother

Nipple Shape

In order for a baby to nurse effectively the baby must be able to grasp the nipple and areola and stretch the nipple forward and up against the roof of the mouth. The nipple, with much of the areola and underlying breast tissue is drawn out into a teat by the suction created by the baby's mouth. This teat is about three times as long as the nipple at rest and extends back as far as the junction between the hard and soft palates [113]. Current studies have demonstrated that the tongue functions using both peristaltic action to move the milk, as well as tongue depression to generate vacuum, which allows milk to enter the infants mouth [114]. The nipple must be sufficiently elastic to allow this process. If the mother's nipple is flat or inverted this process may be impaired and the nipple will be compressed causing pain and potential injury.

Flat and Inverted Nipples

About a third of mothers have flat nipples, that is nipples that do not protrude, but during pregnancy the skin becomes more elastic and by the time of birth only about 10% have flat or inverted by the time the baby is born. Mostly, flat nipples are not tethered and will not cause problems for the nursing mother. In order to test whether there is true tethering pregnant women are encouraged to perform the "pinch test". The thumb and index finger are held at the base of the areolar and pressure is applied about 2 cm behind the nipple. Usually the nipple will protrude, but if it does not, or if it further retracts, then the nipple is truly inverted (Fig. 11.11).

Inverted nipples are common and affect 3% of women. In 87% of cases it is unilateral and in 13% of cases it is bilateral [115]. The appearance may cause cosmetic concern and can interfere

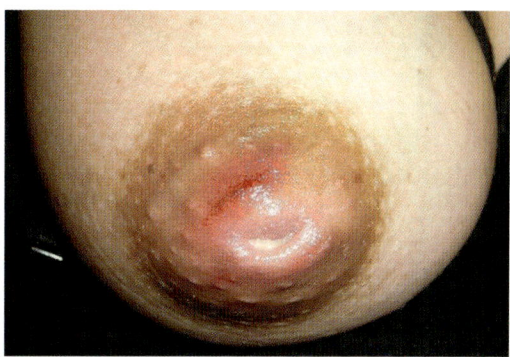

Fig. 11.11 Inverted nipple with erosion. Photo credit: Dr. Gina Weissman, IBCLC

with breast feeding as inverted nipples are caused by short lactiferous ducts and adhesions that tether the nipple and prevent it from projecting.

In some cases, readjusting the infant's position at the breast using the "football position" may be sufficient to enable the infant to attach correctly to the mother's breast and breast feeding can continue painlessly. With this method, the infant is positioned on the side of the mother with the infant's legs under her arm. The infant is turned sideways or sitting partially upright facing the breast. The mother's hand and wrist support the infant's back and shoulders. If this is not successful combining the "football position" with the "teacup method" of holding the breast may be beneficial. The "teacup method" on its own with classic positioning of the infant can also be employed. The mother uses her thumb and index finger, to grasp the areola and some of the breast tissue near the nipple in an attempt to pull out the nipple and place it as deep as possible into the infants mouth. The baby latches while the procedure is being performed and can suckle while the mother continues to hold the nipple. If these simple methods are not successful several other interventions may be helpful (Figs. 11.12 and 11.13).

Sometimes the baby, through vigorous nursing can help to slowly draw the nipple out, and using a breast pump may also help to draw out the nipple and lengthen the adhesions. Nipple shields, flexible silicone nipple with holes in the end that fits over the nipple during feeding can help the newborn attach on that side and when

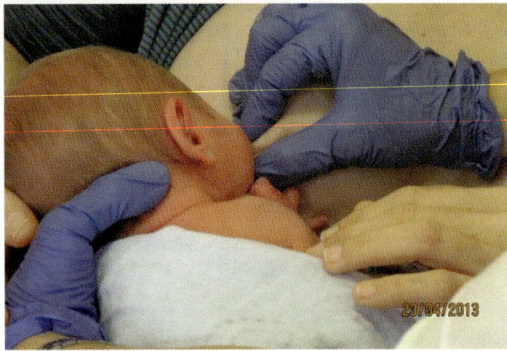

Fig. 11.12 Breast feeding while holding the nipple in the tea cup method. Photo credit: Dr. Gina Weissman, IBCLC

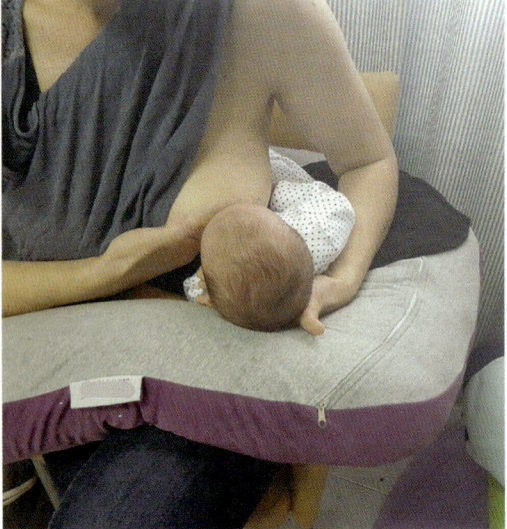

Fig. 11.13 Football hold. Photo credit: Dr. Gina Weissman, IBCLC

successfully nursing his suction can help to evert and pull out the nipple.

A device can be simply fashioned to help to lengthen and evert the nipple. One can take a 10 or 20 cc syringe, cut off the end with the tip, remove the plunger and reinsert it into the other end of the cylinder. Then the mother can apply negative pressure to the nipple to evert it. This is a cheap method and universally available. There are also commercial devices available. The degree of suction is controlled by the women herself. Ideally it should be used before the patient becomes pregnant but can also be used when the patient is pregnant or before nursing sessions. Most women experience soreness during this process.

Most babies succeed in latching on to their mother's breast, despite the anatomical variations (Fig. 11.14).

In the case of flat or inverted nipples it is of great importance not to expose the baby to pacifiers and bottles. The stiff everted nipple of the artificial teat creates more intense stimulation in the baby's mouth and requires less effort to suck, and therefore the baby is less likely to develop the technique that it requires to produce milk from its mother's flat/inverted nipple.

Nipple shields are thin, flexible silicone nipples with holes in the end that fits over the nipple during feeding can help the newborn attach on that side. When the newborn successfully nurses, his suction can help to evert and pull out the nipple. Nipple shields come in different sizes and it is important to ensure that the right size is chosen to suit the diameter of the mother's nipple and the size of baby's mouth.

Nipple shields can be helpful during nursing to assist the baby to latch onto flat or engorged nipples and can be useful when nipples are inverted. They have traditionally been used to provide a barrier to further trauma from the infant's mouth whilst nursing when nipples are sensitive or have erosions. Although there are no studies proving the effectiveness of nipple shields for the management of nipple pain, there are cases where the mother's report that they are invaluable. They should never be recommended until the patient has been assessed by a lactation consultant who will assess and correct the problematic latch which is usually the source of the problem in the case of nipple pain, and who will instruct the patient in methods of remedying flat or inverted nipples through other means.

Nipple shields may decrease the flow of milk and increase the risk of plugged ducts and mastitis. All mothers using then need to be instructed how to wean their baby off nipple shields and back onto the breast as soon as possible. This should be done under the supervision of a lactation clinician (Fig. 11.15).

Vasospasm of the Nipple

Vasospasm of the nipple causes extreme, debilitating stabbing or throbbing pain associated with blanching of the nipple. The patient may

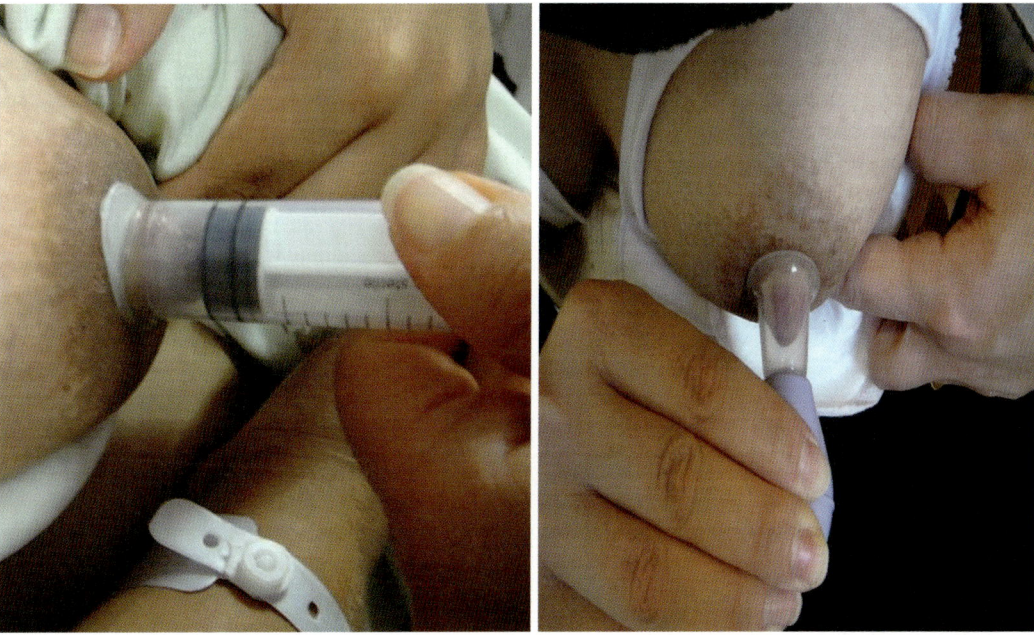

Fig. 11.14 A home made device to evert nipples along side a proprietary device. Photo credit: Dr. Gina Weissman, IBCLC

actually double over in pain and clutch at her breast. The pain can occur a short time after nursing or in between feedings. The vasospasm might be secondary to trauma to the nipple or a primary phenomenon known as Raynaud's of the Nipple.

Vasospasm should not be confused with blanching due to compression of the nipple. Blanching due to compression is noticed immediately after the nipple is removed from the baby's mouth and though the pain may occur when the blood supply returns to the nipple, it is short lived. It is most commonly caused by the baby having a shallow latch and can be rectified by teaching the mother to position the baby properly at the beginning of nursing. It can also be caused by improper sucking or tongue—tie.

Vasospasm of the arterioles of the nipple causing intermittent ischaemia, and subsequent reflex vasodilatation may occur after nursing or between feedings. The nipple turns white with ischaemia, and then blue due to cyanosis and then red as there is reperfusion.

It is classified as primary Raynaud's phenomenon when it is idiopathic and secondary when it is related to an underlying cause. Although there are very few studies, this phenomenon has been

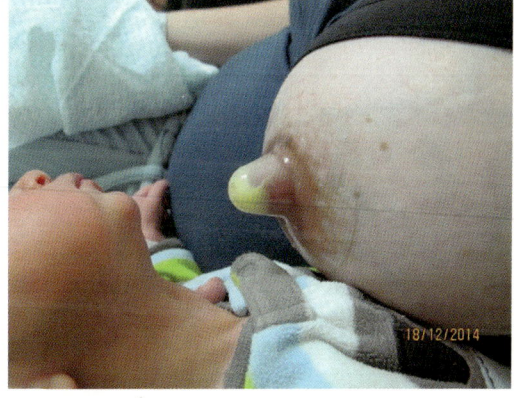

Fig. 11.15 A nipple shield in use. Photo credit: Dr. Gina Weissman, IBCLC

reported to occur relatively frequently and was recorded in 23% of women with post-partum nipple pain. Of the women that experienced vasospasm, 14% reported that the pain lasted for more than 5 minutes at a time [106]. It may be bilateral and may accompany Raynaud's phenomenon of the fingers and toes. Cold may trigger the vasospasm, or make it worse. It can occur during pregnancy and may recur with subsequent pregnancies/breastfeeding.

Women of childbearing age are at increased risk of developing Raynaud phenomenon because

Estrogen and stress are associated with an exaggerated vasomotor response [116, 117].

Medical conditions that have been associated with secondary Raynaud's phenomenon include fibromyalgia, rheumatologic diseases such as systemic lupus erythematosus or rheumatoid arthritis and endocrine problems such as carcinoid or hypothyroidism.

Previous breast surgery has also been associated with vasospasm, as has the use of the mixed alpha/beta adrenergic antagonist, Labetalol, an antihypertensive agent [118], betablockers, ergotamine, and over the counter cold medications that contain pseudoephidrine. It may be secondary to a thrush infection and may persist for some weeks after the thrush infection has been successfully treated. In a study of 22 women with primary Raynaud's phenomenon 91% reported cold sensitivity with a history of colour change of acral surfaces [116, 117].

Treatment involves preventative measures such as keeping the whole body warm and avoiding vasoconstrictive substances such as nicotine and caffeine or the medications causing vasoconstriction. When the vasospasm occurs, warming the nipple gives relief (this author recommends tipping hot water into a ceramic mug then tipping the water out and using the warm mug to warm the area). Wheat bags warmed in the microwave are also helpful but the 2 minutes that it takes to warm them in the microwave is a very long time when a woman is experiencing this type of pain.

The calcium channel blocker, Nifedipine sustained release formulation, can give relief at a dose of 30–60 mg a day. If the patient experiences side effects such as dizziness and tachycardia, 10 mg of the short acting Nifedipine can be given up to 3 times a day. This therapy is safe for the baby (as only 5% of the maternal dose is transferred to the breast milk), tolerance is high and most women using this therapy found it to be effective [119].

11.14.1.2 Attributes of the Infant

Variations in infant oral anatomy such as very small mouths relative to the mother's breast size ("mother—infant mismatch"), receding chin, high palate or restricted tongue movements may cause the baby difficulty attaching to the breast. Poor attachment to the breast can lead to compression of the nipple causing pain and subsequent skin breakdown.

Receding Chin/Jaw and High Palate

If an infant's jaw is receding this may cause difficulty with attachment to the breast as the nipple may not stay in place during suckling. A lactation consultant can help the mother to find a breastfeeding position that is effective and does not cause pain. Sometimes gentle support to the infant at the angle of the jaw with the mother's index finger may be helpful. The mother may need to support the breast with her hand during the feeding time. Positions that bring the chin very close to the breast may be beneficial [6, 8].

Receding chin and high palate also require referral to a lactation consultant for adjustment of infant's position at the breast.

Ankyloglossia

As explained above the function of the tongue is of great importance during breastfeeding. The tongue plays a critical role in milk removal and clearance of the milk bolus from the oral cavity [120]. Ankyloglossia, also referred to as tongue tie, is a congenital anomaly of the tongue characterized by a short and sometimes anteriorly inserted frenulum that does not allow the baby to extend the tongue. It occurs in 5% of neonates with a male-to-female ratio of 2.6:1. Breastfeeding difficulties were experienced in 25% of mothers with of infants with ankyloglossia compared with 3% of control mothers [121].

In babies with ankyloglossia, the compression of the breast occurs from the gum pad instead of the tongue, because the tongue is unable to extend anteriorly. As well as the direct trauma on the nipple, there will be poor placement of the tongue around the nipple which results in further trauma.

The limitation of movement of the tongue also prevents the normal wave motion that should move the bolus of milk to the back of the palate to be swallowed. This makes it difficult for the baby to nurse successfully and will lead to decreased milk supply. This then leads to a hungry irritable baby with failure to thrive.

This coupled with the fact that the feedings will take longer may result in further nipple trauma. In short, the consequences of ankyloglossia may be an exhausted, frustrated and suffering mother and an irritable underweight baby, and early cessation of breastfeeding.

When breastfeeding difficulties are encountered and a short or tight sublingual frenulum is noted, the appearance and function of the tongue may be quantified using a scoring system such as the Hazelbaker Assesment Tool For Lingual Frenum Fuction [122] (Fig. 11.16).

Conservative management of tongue-tie may be sufficient, requiring no intervention beyond breastfeeding assistance, parental education, and reassurance [19].

In the event that conservative breastfeeding management isn't effective, Frenotomy, or simple incision or "snipping," of a tongue-tie is a common procedure performed for ankyloglossia. The procedure of tongue-tie release should be performed by a physician, dentist, Ear Nose and Throat surgeon or oral surgeon experienced with the procedure. Release of the tongue-tie appears to be a minor procedure, but it may be ineffective in solving the immediate clinical problem and may cause complications such as infant pain and distress, postoperative bleeding, infection, or injury to Wharton's duct [19]. Complications are rare, however as with any surgical procedure, experience is important [123–126]. Frenotomy may lead to an immedi-ate decrease in pain experienced by the nursing mother and to increased weight gain in the baby [127]. However, pain relief and improved breastfeeding are not always immediate after the procedure and anticipatory guidance and follow up with a Lactation consultant are important.

Lip Tie

Lip-tie is another abnormality that may affect the infant's ability to correctly attach to the breast, by stopping the required flanging of lips. Lip tie is the attachment of the upper lip to the maxillary gingival tissue. Historically this tissue has been described as the superior labial frenulum, median labial frenulum or maxillary labial frenulum, depending on the frenulum attachment point [128] (Fig. 11.17).

The classification, however describes the anatomy, but does not determine the severity. Infants with low frenulums might not have any problems nursing and may not give their mothers painful nipples. The degree of restriction is determined by feeling the lip and trying to elevate it, mimicking the flanging motion needed of the lip on the breast to achieve a good seal. If there is blanching at the gum then this may be an indication that the frenulum should be cut to free the lip. This would only be indicated in the event that there was no ankyloglossia, and that there is still breastfeeding pain despite the fact that the mother has been assessed by

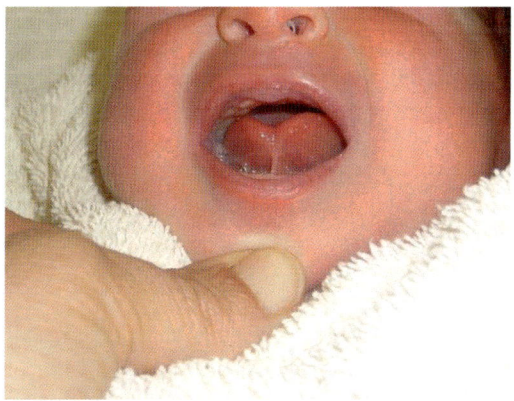

Fig. 11.16 A tongue tied infant. Photo credit: Dr. Gina Weissman, IBCLC

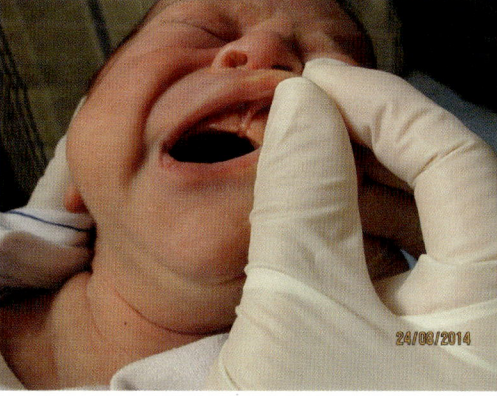

Fig. 11.17 Infant with lip tie and blanching of the gum. Photo credit: Dr. Gina Weissman, IBCLC

professional lactation clinician to rule out other causes of pain.

It is thought that low frenulums are also associated with early dental decay (because of food being caught in the pockets formed on either side of the frenulum) and a gap developing between the 2 front teeth (diastema) because of the tension caused. However, there is not enough scientific data to support cutting the frenulum for these two reasons.

Pain Associated with High Intraoral Vacuum

In some cases despite correct positioning of the child at the breast and despite the fact that the child's mouth and tongue are normal, the nursing mother experiences persistent nipple pain. An Australian study measured the intraoral vacuums of nursing infants, using a small milk filled tube taped alongside the nipple and connected to a pressure transducer. In was found that in infants in the group where the mothers were experiencing pain applied significantly higher baseline and pause vacuums. Despite similar sucking times, the mean milk intake was significantly lower for infants of mothers with nipple pain [129]. These babies are referred to as "barracuda feeders" and the child often spontaneously decreases the vacuum pressure at about 6 weeks of age bringing about relief to the breastfeeding mother.

11.14.1.3 The Interaction Between the Mother and the Infant

Attachment

The correct positioning of the babies mouth on the nipple is of utmost importance so that the latch/attachment is correct.

Incorrect positioning of the infant at the breast and poor attachment to the breast are the most common cause for painful nipples during the initial postpartum period. When a mother presents with nipple pain, in addition to checking the mother's breast anatomy and the infant's mouth, it is necessary to observe the positioning of the infant during breastfeeding and attachment to the breast. Repositioning of the infant must be accompanied by provision of an optimal environment for wound healing.

When the infant latches properly to the breast the nipple and the surrounding areola and underlying breast tissue is drawn deeply into the mouth. The infant's tongue, lips and cheeks then form a seal.

Suboptimal positioning can lead to a shallow latch and therefore to abnormal compression of the nipple between the tongue and the palate resulting in abrasions to the nipple. If attachment is incorrect infants may try to facilitate milk intake by compensatory movements that increase negative pressure such as chewing and biting to hold the nipple in place, thereby causing further damage to the nipple. The airtight seal that is formed between the baby's tongue and the breast can cause damage if the infant's mouth is removed actively from the nipple without breaking the seal. By gently inserting a finger into the corner of the baby's mouth at the end of nursing, the seal is broken and trauma to the nipple can be avoided.

Suboptimal contact of the baby's mouth and the nipple can occur when the nipple is very large or inverted, or when the breast is engorged with milk so the baby cannot position himself correctly because of the firmness of the areola and the flattening of the nipple.

For optimal contact the mother needs to insert the breast into the infant's mouth only when the mouth is open wide and the lips are everted. Changing the position of the infant so that its chin points in different directions can be helpful to ensure even emptying of the breast. Attachment problems should be suspected if there is evidence of fissures of the nipple or trauma on the face of the nipple or if the mother reports a misshappen nipple when the infant detaches from the breast [130] (Figs. 11.18 and 11.19).

Mother–Infant "Mismatch"

Mothers' nipples and infants mouths come in all shapes and sizes. One of the causes of attachment difficulties may be mismatch between infant and mother anatomy. The infant may have a small mouth while the mother has a wide nipple.

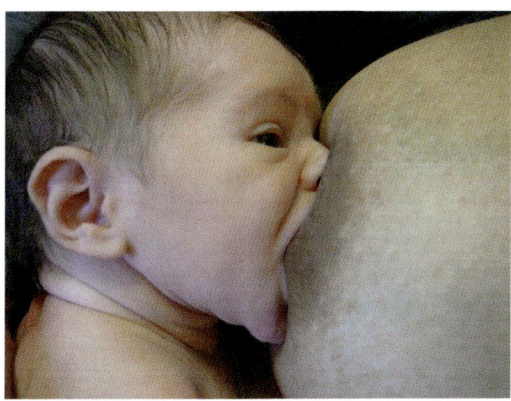

Fig. 11.18 Correct attachment to the breast with mouth wide open. Photo credit: Dr. Gina Weissman, IBCLC

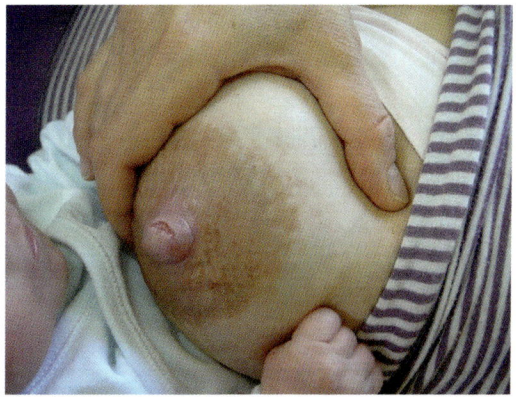

Fig. 11.19 Incorrect attachment of the infant to the breast results in nipple damage Photo credit: Dr. Gina Weissman, IBCLC

Incorrect attachment to the breast will lead to nipple damage. In addition to treatment of the nipple damage prompt referral to a lactation consultant is recommended in order to treat the source of the damage. Attempts at improving positioning and attachment may be beneficial. Sometimes a silicone nipple used temporarily may be of help. In some situations the remedy is tincture of time. With the passage of time the infant's mouth will grow and he will be able to cope with the dimensions of the mother's nipple. In the meantime, in order to protect the milk supply the mother will be required to express her milk at least 8 times daily.

11.14.1.4 Infections

Bacterial
Cracked nipples due to nursing, like any fissure on the skin, are prone to secondary bacterial and yeast infections. Recent evidence suggests pathogenic bacteria activate nociceptors directly, triggering an inflammatory response [131]. The risk is increased in moist areas and just as secondarily infected tinea pedis can lead to cellulitis, cracked and fissured nipples can lead to mastitis. The risk is greatly increased when the breast is not emptied totally after each feed, so the mother massaging the breast in a radial fashion during nursing or changing the babies position during nursing can help to prevent this. While the symptoms of mastitis can be subtle with few local symptoms

and with just a feeling lack of wellbeing, or dull aching breast pain during or after feeding, the classical symptoms include erythema and painful induration of the breast, fever over 38 degree C and malaise. Chills and rigors may also be present. In order to prevent Mastitis it is important to treat nipple damage early and to refer to a Lactation consultant for assessment of the infant's attachment to the breast and function during breastfeeding.

Human milk contains many commensal bacteria. Commensal Staphylococci are found in 64% and oral Streptococci are found in 30% of healthy, lactating women with *Staph epidermidis*, *strep salivaius* and *strep mitis* being the most common isolates. Some of these bacteria as well as others such as enterococci and Lactic acid bacteria are actually inhibitory of *Staph Aureus* [132].

Studies of the milk of women with mastitis show that the same bacteria are present but that the *Staphlococcus epidermidis* occurred in higher numbers. *Staph epidermidis* has been regarded as a commensal in the past, however its role in causing infection has increased due to its ability of the bacteria to form biofilms that protect them from attacks by the immune system and antibiotic treatment [133]. Some researchers have concluded that Mastitis could be a dysbiotic process that leads to an outgrowth of certain bacterial groups such as *Staphylococci*. It is proposed that *S. epidermidis* requires a predisposed host in order to change from a commensal to a pathogen, and could possibly explain why only 3–30% of lactating women suffer from Staph infection of the breast and nipple when it is the predominant bacterial species found in breast milk [134].

Initial treatment is conservative with the application of warm compresses, making sure all areas of the breast are properly emptied during nursing, rest and the administration of non-steroidal anti-inflammatory drugs. If there has been no improvement after 24 h the administration of antibiotics is recommended [135]. Cephalosporin, or Amoxicillin with or without Clavulanic acid are most commonly used. Macrolides can be used for women with a sensitivity to penicillin although they may alter the taste of the milk and make it unpalatable to the infant [68]. Treatment should be prescribed for at least 2 weeks, and sometimes it is necessary to continue treatment for up to 6 weeks. It is important to reassure the mother that she can continue to nurse the baby while she is taking these antibiotics but the infant should be observed for gastrointestinal side effects due to ingestion of the antibiotic via the breast milk. Probiotics administration to both the mother and the baby can decrease the risk of anti-biotic associated diarrhea [136, 137].

Yeast Infection

Yeast infection on the nipple is characterized by a burning and stinging pain of the nipple is often associated with a pink nipple area, sensitivity to touch and pain described by the patient that is out of proportion to the clinical signs [138, 139]. A fissure between the nipple and areola is not infre-quently seen. While the pain in the nipple is par-ticularly intense at the beginning of nursing, stabbing pains can occur at any time without any temporal relationship to nursing. In the past, yeast infection remained a poorly defined entity because of the difficulty in culturing candida from milk, with many health professionals deny-ing its existence [140]. Culturing breast milk is difficult because of the presence of immunoglob-ulins and lactoferrin which inhibit the growth of candida [141, 142].

More recently techniques have been devel-oped to culture candida at the nipple and from breast milk, and a clear association between can-dida of the nipple/breast and its presence in the child's mouth and diaper area, and the associa-tion with breast and nipple pain has been clearly demonstrated [143]. A number of factors have been found to increase the risk of a woman suf-fering from an infection with candida. Longer duration of the second stage of labour, bottle use in the first 2 weeks postpartum, and longer dura-tion of gestation [144], as well as recent and long term use of antibiotics, nipple damage in early lactation and a history of vaginal thrush are all associated with increased risk of nipple and breast pain due to candida [145].

When Candida is restricted to the nipple, most sources recommend a topical Azole antifungal agent as treatment to nipples infected with Candida, together with topical miconazole gel for treatment of the infant's mouth. In the past topi-cal Nystatin suspension was recommended but today some Candida is resistant to it. It is noted that miconazole and Clotrimazole also inhibit growth of Staphylococcus species [116, 146].

Although triple antibiotics have not been shown in studies to be more useful that simple anti-fungal creams, it is noted that the fissures on nipples often are colonized with both S. Aureus as well as Candida. Mupirocin oint-ment is often very helpful (its greasy base is also very soothing) and in nipples that are red an inflamed a low potency steroid can be used in addition [147]. Resistant cases may require treatment with oral fluconazole. An initial dose of 200 mg is given and then 100 mg daily for 7–10 days [139].

To relieve pain in the nipples during breast-feeding when the nipples are infected with Candida it is suggested to breastfeed frequently for short periods of time, so that the infant is not extremely hungry at the initiation of the feed and will suck less vigorously. Mothers need to be encouraged to do this because the latch and unlatch of the infant's mouth is extremely painful.

It is recommended to breastfeed first on the less painful side and to break the vacuum manually after feeding (by inserting a finger between the nipple and the babies mouth) [148].

Candida can survive for up to 4 months on surfaces, especially in conditions of low temperature and high humidity [149] so infant's bottles and pacifiers and all things that come into contact with the baby's mouth should be sterilized. Breast pads should be disposed of as soon as they become wet, and nipples should be "air dried" if possible [150]. Sexual partners should be treated for Candida if there is suspicion transmission by oral or genital sexual activity (Fig. 11.20).

Viral

Herpes Simplex

Herpes Simplex virus is a commonly acquired virus in the community with 50–80%% of the population having antibodies to HSV 1 type 1 and 18–35% of adults with HSV 11. HSV 1 is generally acquired from non-sexual contact and HSV11 by sexual contact but there is considerable overlap in the epidemiology and clinical manifestations [151]. Individuals that have been infected with herpes in the past can shed the virus asymptomatically, with 70% of the population shedding asymptomatically at least once a month and many shedding up to 6 times per month [152]. The most common mode of transmission to neonates in the peripartum is during passage in the birth canal but in 10% of cases the infection is transmitted postnatally through contact with a skin lesion. Only 2% of those lesions are found on the breast. HSV infection of the nipple can result in neonatal transmission during breastfeeding and may put the infant at considerable risk for morbidity and mortality [153].

Herpes simplex infection presents exquisitely tender small blisters or punched out round erosions on an erythematous base. The infection can predate lactation or acquired on the nipple from a breastfeeding child.

Culturing the lesions for herpes is optimal, but due to the considerable risk to the newborn, if herpes is suspected then breastfeeding on that side should be stopped immediately, and the expressed milk should be discarded. When the affected breast is covered, she may continue to nurse on the other side. Breastfeeding on the affected side may be recommenced when the lesions are healed [146]. Until healing is complete on that breast the mother must express milk from that breast 8–10 times daily in order to protect milk supply (Fig. 11.21).

Herpes Zoster

Herpes Zoster may erupt on the T3–T5 dermatomes and involve the breast and nipple. Exposure to the lesions can result in chicken pox (varicella zoster) in unimmunized infants. The recommendations for treatment are the same as for herpes simplex and the child should not be fed on that side and milk should be discarded, even though the child should have passive immunity from

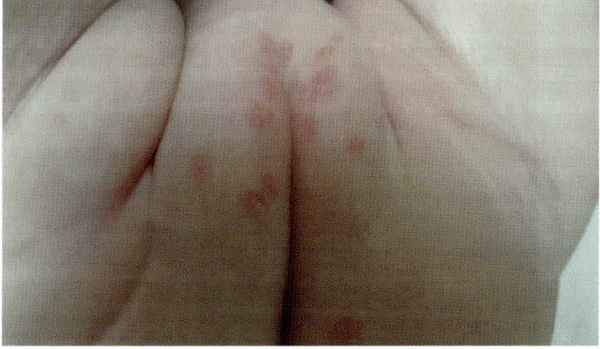
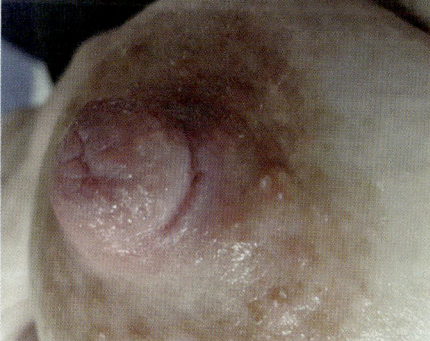

Fig. 11.20 Candida—Mother's nipple and her infant's diaper area both infected with Candida

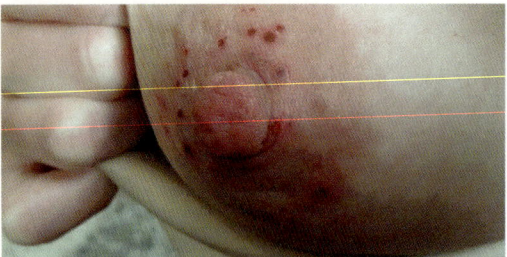

Fig. 11.21 Herpes simplex infection of the nipple. Photo credit: Rachelle Tohar, IBCLC

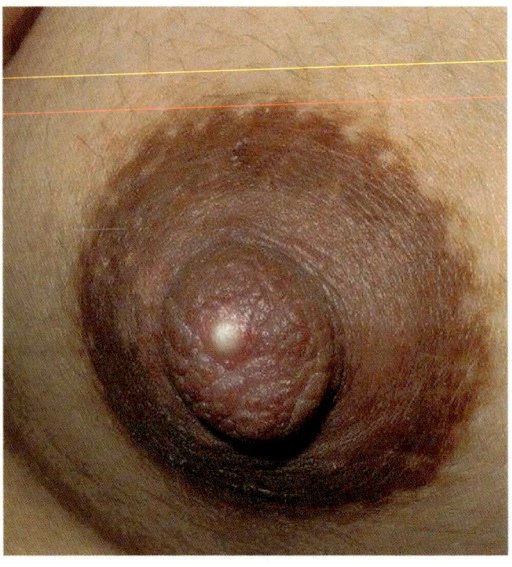

Fig. 11.22 Milk bleb. Photo credit: Dr. Gina Weissman, IBCLC

placental immunity in the first 8 months of life and the secretory IgA in breastmilk is active against the varicella virus in vitro [154]. The mother may be treated with intravenous or oral acyclovir which is considered safe for breastfeeding and the infant may be given Zoster immunoglobulin if he is immunocompromised.

11.14.1.5 Inflammation

Milk Blebs
Milk blebs, also known as Milk stones, plugged ducts or milk blisters present as extreme pinpoint pain and tenderness of the nipple when the baby nurses. On examination one can see a white subcutaneous blister or bleb. Whilst sometimes there is surrounding erythema in most occasions there is not, and the clinical findings seem unimpressive and not in correlation with the severe, unbearable pain that the nursing mother describes. The bleb appears on the surface of the nipple, usually at the opening of a duct, has a shiny, smooth surface, and is a millimetre or less in diameter. Sometimes the ducts are plugged deeper in the breast and so there is no white milk bleb to help with making the diagnosis. While most nipple pain presents early in the postpartum period, milk blebs can present after months of painless nursing. Despite treatment they can recur or may appear in subsequent pregnancies. The bleb is most likely caused by a small pressure cyst formed at the end of the duct from milk seeping under the epidermis. Nipple blebs appear to be an inflammatory response to nipple trauma in some women [13]. If there is more than one bleb it must be distinguished from Candida infection. Blebs may lead to mastitis if the tissue overgrowth causes stasis by blocking milk flow from a nipple pore that drains a larger area of the breast. Incidence and cause of this condition is unknown. It has been speculated that some people have a tendency for epithelial overgrowth due to the epithelial growth factor in the mother's milk [155] (Fig. 11.22).

Massaging the breast in the area of pain prior to and during nursing, after applying warm hot compresses, or massaging and expressing milk while directing warm water onto the breast whilst in the shower can help to open the blockage and prevent the development of mastitis. If the bleb doesn't open spontaneously gently rubbing with a towel may be helpful. If this is not effective, the bleb can be opened with a sterile needle (a procedure with minimal or no pain). Once the bleb is open a white, thick, stringy looking material is usually expressed. An alternate method of opening the bleb is to take a strand of sterile heavy suture and cannulate the duct, threading the suture up the duct until the plug is released. If attempts to open the bleb are not effective then the frequent application wet/warm compresses should be applied to the breast and nipple area. Rubbing Lecithin into the nipple after each feeding may be effective or a Lecithin supplement can be taken orally (1–2 1200 mg capsules 3 or 4 times per day) [2], O'Hara reported using a punch biopsy tool, for blebs resistant to other treatment, which resolved pain and symptoms. This study analyzed the content of the blebs and found them to contain histiocytes with foamy cytoplasmic vacuoles and fibrin deposition indicating a tissue reaction to milk that had leaked from the ducts to the surrounding tissue O'Hara recommended a short daily course of a very thin layer of mid-potency steroid under an occlusive dressing to enhance penetration of the steroid [156].

Dermatitis is Referred to in the Section on Skin Disease

11.14.1.6 Allodynia/Functional Pain

Allodynia is defined as the sensation of pain in response to a stimulus that does not usually cause pain, such as light touch of a bra or blouse causing pain in the nipple. It can occur in isolation or in the context of other pain disorders such as irritable bowel syndrome, fibromyalgia, temporomandibular pain, and vaginismus. Allodynia of the nipple can be extremely troublesome. Allodynia can also occur secondary to nerve damage from aesthetic breast surgery [157] or due to Herpes Zoster or post herpetic neuralgia. There have been 3 recorded cases of Galactorrhea secondary to Herpes Zoster of the T4 dermatome [158]. These pain disorders can lead to depression and anxiety and when these factors are present, treatment may be more resistant to medical therapies, and psychological therapies such as Cognitive Behavioral Therapy may be a useful [159]. Non-steroidal anti-inflammatory agents can bring relief, and antidepressants may also be helpful. Pressure points may also be sought and successfully treated with pectoral muscle massage [160]. Fatigue and lack of social support are other contributing factors in this condition that are more difficult to treat.

In the case of neuropathic pain Gabapentin may be helpful treatment [161] however, Gabapentin is category C for pregnancy and is secreted in breast milk so should be avoided for pregnant and breastfeeding women.

11.14.1.7 Miscellaneous and Other External Factors

Breast pumps, if used inappropriately may cause an inflammatory response in the nipple skin which may result in erythema, oedema, fissures and/or blisters [146]. Common sources of nipple damage in mothers who use breast pumps are using suction that is too strong, misfit of the flange to the nipple, and extended pumping time. Prevention of further damage requires appropriate guidance for use of breast pumps by a Lactation Consultant [112].

11.15 Treatment: General Measures

As mentioned, the treatment of nipple pain involves ascertaining the cause and treating appropriately. There are also general measures that can help to alleviate the pain of damaged nipples. A study comparing the efficacy of warm compresses, dried breast milk and lanolin in relieving nipple pain reported that women using warm water compresses reported significantly less pain than the other groups [162]. Warm water compresses have the advantage of not needing a prescription and are convenient and inexpensive. More recent studies have confirmed that while topical treatments increase women's satisfaction with treatment outcome there is no significant differences between the various topical products [163, 164].

When tissue breakdown has taken place the principles of moist wound healing is employed to increase the rate of reepithelialisation. Hydrogel dressings are very effective at providing a moist environment that facilitates healing. The dressing is placed under a nursing pad to keep it in place and it removed and replaced for each feeding it is replaced whenever it becomes moist [165, 166].

11.15.1 Breast Shells

Breast shells are plastic domes that are placed over the nipple. In the past they were used to evert flat or inverted nipples but they been shown to be ineffective for this purpose. They are however extremely helpful for short periods of time when the nipple is so sensitive that the patient complains that she cannot tolerate any contact of material on her nipples as they serve as a buffer between her breast and clothing (Table 11.1).

Table 11.1 Classification and treatment of common causes of nipple pain associated with breast feeding

	Condition	Treatment
Attributes of the mother	Nipple shape/anatomy-flat, inverted	Adjust infant's position Allow baby to suck after manually everting the nipple Use a Nipple shield Use a negative suction device to evert the nipple
	Skin disease	Psoriasis and eczema of the nipples can be treated with emollients and low dose steroid ointments twice daily immediately after breast feeding Phototherapy with UVB is safe. Each disease modifying oral agent must be considered individually
	Vasospasm of the nipple	Warm compresses Avoid triggers (nicotine, caffeine) Avoid cold on breasts and nipples Nifedipine SR 30–60 mg a day
Attributes of the infant	Palatal anomalies–high palate Receding chin	Adjustment of infant's position
	Lip tie with restriction	Supportive treatment. Frenulectomy
	Tongue tie with restricted tongue movement	Correct positioning. Improved attachment. Supportive treatments. Frenulectomy by a trained health professional
	High intraoral vacuum	Supportive treatment
The interaction between mother and infant	Poor attachment of infant to breast	Assessment and guidance of Lactation consultant
	Mismatch between mothers nipple size and infant's mouth size	Adjustment of infant's position and attachment Silicone Nipple Shield
Infections	Bacterial	Oral Antibiotics (e.g. Cephalosporin amoxicillin/clavulanate) for 2–6 weeks and probiotics
	Yeast	Topical azole antifungal ointment to nipple and oral gel to infants mouth Oral Fluconazole 200 mg stat then 100 mg daily for 10 days for resistant cases
	Herpes	Prevent contact between infant and the lesions and discard the milk pumped from that side Oral Acyclovir/Valcyclovir can be used
Inflammation	Milk blebs	Applying warm compresses, massage of the breast and rubbing the nipple Opening with a needle Cannulating with thick suture Lecithin 2400 mg 3–4 times per day
	Dermatitis	Patch test to determine allergens in topical agents, and avoid irritation to nipples. Apply emollients frequently and low dose steroids twice daily to nipples (immediately after nursing) Apply PolyMem and antibiotic ointment to fissures
Miscellaneous	Breast pump trauma	Adjust level of suction or fit of flange
	Allodynia-functional pain	Round the clock treatment with Nonsteroidal anti-inflammatory agents Cognitive Behavioural Therapy Antidepressants

Conclusion

The female nipple is a very sensitive area, both physiologically and psychologically. Perhaps due to its sexualization, conditions of the female nipple are often ignored in medical texts and women delay presenting to physicians when nipple conditions occur.

The postpartum period is a challenging time for many women and it is during this time that nipple pain associated with breastfeeding is prevalent. Breastfeeding is of utmost importance for infant and maternal health. Early diagnosis and treatment of nipple pain associated with breastfeeding is therefore critical.

Despite WHO\Unicef recommendations [167], advice on breastfeeding is unfortunately not part of the routine antenatal care and is not offered universally to postpartum women in hospital. Subsequently, many woman first present to their medical practitioners with nipple pain. The increased efficacy of a multidisciplinary approach to diagnosis and treatment of nipple pain associated with breastfeeding has been established [168]. Understanding the factors involved in nipple pain and collaboration with lactation consultants and other health professionals is essential for physicians dealing with this complex and multifactorial problem.

Acknowledgments With gratitude to the ever-generous Dr. Mei Tam for her contribution to the section on contact dermatitis. Her expert advice has helped many of my patients over the years.

And with tremendous gratitude to my brother, Associate Professor David Finkelstein for helping me with everything technical.

References

1. Montagna W, Macpherson EE. Some neglected aspects of the anatomy of human breasts. J Investig Dermatol. 1974;63(1):10–6.
2. Lawrence RA, Lawrence RM. Breastfeeding: a guide for the medical professional. Philadelphia: Elsevier; 2010.
3. Schlenz I, Kuzbari R, Gruber H, Holle J. The sensitivity of the nipple-areola complex: an anatomic study. Plast Reconstr Surg. 2000;105(3):905–9.
4. Standring S, Ellis H, Healy J, Johnson D, Williams A, Collins P, et al. Gray's anatomy: the anatomical basis of clinical practice. Am J Neuroradiol. 2005;26(10):2703.
5. Mortazavi SN, Geddes D, Hassiotou F, Hassanipour F. Mathematical analysis of mammary ducts in lactating human breast. In: 2014 36th annual international conference of the ieee engineering in medicine and biology society (EMBC). IEEE; 2014.
6. Geddes DT. Inside the lactating breast: the latest anatomy research. J Midwifery Womens Health. 2007;52(6):556–63.
7. Rusby JE, Brachtel EF, Michaelson JS, Koerner FC, Smith BL. Breast duct anatomy in the human nipple: three-dimensional patterns and clinical implications. Breast Cancer Res Treat. 2007;106(2):171–9.
8. Walker M. Breastfeeding management for the clinician. 4th ed. Burlington: Jones & Bartlett Learning; 2017.
9. Tezer M, Ozluk Y, Sanli O, Asoglu O, Kadioglu A. Nitric oxide may mediate nipple erection. J Androl. 2012;33(5):805–10.
10. Koyama S, Wu HJ, Easwaran T, Thopady S, Foley J. The nipple: a simple intersection of mammary gland and integument, but focal point of organ function. J Mammary Gland Biol Neoplasia. 2013;18(2):121–31.
11. Komisaruk BR, Wise N, Frangos E, Liu WC, Allen K, Brody S. Women's clitoris, vagina, and cervix mapped on the sensory cortex: fMRI evidence. J Sex Med. 2011;8(10):2822–30.
12. Masters WH, Johnson VE. Human sexual response. Bronx, NY: Ishi Press; 2010. xiii, 366pp.
13. Lawrence RA, Lawrence RM. Breastfeeding e-book: a guide for the medical professional. Philadelphia: Elsevier; 2015.
14. Beer T. Social construction of the body: the nipple. Sociology toolbox. 2016. https://thesocietypages.org/toolbox/social-construction-of-the-body/.
15. Battersby S. Not in public please: breastfeeding as dirty work in the UK. In: Exploring the dirty side of women's health. London: Routledge; 2007. p. 101–14.
16. Henderson L, McMillan B, Green JM, Renfrew MJ. Men and infant feeding: perceptions of embarrassment, sexuality, and social conduct in white low-income British men. Birth. 2011;38(1):61–70.
17. Wilson MG, Hall EB, Ebbin AJ. Dominant inheritance of absence of the breast. Humangenetik. 1972;15(3):268–70.
18. Finlay A, Marks R. An hereditary syndrome of lumpy scalp, odd ears, and rudimentary nipples. Br J Dermatol. 1978;99(4):423–30.
19. Pellegrino JE, Schnur RE, Boghosian-Sell L, Strathdee G, Overhauser J, Spinner NB, et al.

Ablepharon macrostomia syndrome with associated cutis laxa: possible localization to 18q. Hum Genet. 1996;97(4):532–6.

20. Evers ME, Steijlen PM, Hamel BC. Aplasia cutis congenita and associated disorders: an update. Clin Genet. 1995;47(6):295–301.

21. Martínez-Chéquer JC, Carranza-Lira S, López-Silva JD, Mainero-Ratchelous F, Zenteno JC. Congenital absence of the breasts: a case report. Am J Obstet Gynecol. 2004;191(1):372–4.

22. Javed A, Lteif A. Development of the human breast. In: Seminars in plastic surgery. New York: Thieme; 2013.

23. Robinson GW. Identification of signaling pathways in early mammary gland development by mouse genetics. Breast Cancer Res. 2004;6(3):105–8.

24. Koltuksuz U, Aydin E. Supernumerary breast tissue: a case of pseudomamma on the face. J Pediatr Surg. 1997;32(9):1377–8.

25. Conde DM, Kashimoto E, Torresan RZ, Alvarenga M. Pseudomamma on the foot: an unusual presentation of supernumerary breast tissue. Dermatol Online J. 2006;12(4):7.

26. Schmidt H. Supernumerary nipples: prevalence, size, sex and side predilection–a prospective clinical study. Eur J Pediatr. 1998;157(10):821–3.

27. Kajava Y. The proportions of supernumerary nipples in the Finnish population. Duodecim. 1915;1(1):143–70.

28. Minić S, Trpinac D, Obradović M. Incontinentia pigmenti diagnostic criteria update. Clin Genet. 2014;85(6):536–42.

29. Landauer W. Supernumerary nipples, congenital hemihypertrophy and congenital hemiatrophy. Hum Biol. 1939;11(4):447–72.

30. Gurrieri F, Cappa M, Neri G. Further delineation of the Simpson-Golabi-Behmel (SGB) syndrome. Am J Med Genet. 1992;44(2):136–7.

31. Urbani CE, Betti R. Accessory mammary tissue associated with congenital and hereditary nephrourinary malformations. Int J Dermatol. 1996;35(5):349–52.

32. Urbani CE, Betti R. Aberrant mammary tissue and nephrourinary malignancy: a man with unilateral polythelia and ipsilateral renal adenocarcinoma associated with polycystic kidney disease. Cancer Genet Cytogenet. 1996;87(1):88–9.

33. Cohen P. The significance of familial polythelia-reply. St. Louis: Mosby; 1995. p. 688.

34. Obayashi H, Tsuchida T, Ikeda S. Hyperkeratosis of the nipple and areola. Rinsho Dermatol. 1998;40:147–50.

35. Vestey JP, Bunney MH. Unilateral hyperkeratosis of the nipple: the response to cryotherapy. Arch Dermatol. 1986;122(12):1360–1.

36. Özcan M, Özüntürk E, Kahveci R. Congenital mamillary hyperkeratosis—a case report. Eur J Plast Surg. 1987;9(4):179–80.

37. Perez-Izquierdo JM, Vilata JJ, Sanchez JL, Gargallo E, Millan F, Aliaga A. Retinoic acid treatment of nipple hyperkeratosis. Arch Dermatol. 1990;126(5):687–8.

38. Bayramgurler D, Bilen N, Apaydin R, Ercin C. Nevoid hyperkeratosis of the nipple and areola: treatment of two patients with topical calcipotriol. J Am Acad Dermatol. 2002;46(1):131–3.

39. Mazzella C, Costa C, Fabbrocini G, Marangi GF, Russo D, Merolla F, et al. Nevoid hyperkeratosis of the nipple mimicking a pigmented basal cell carcinoma. JAAD Case Rep. 2016;2(6):500–1.

40. Nambi R. Hyperkeratosis of nipple and areola. 2017. http://emedicine.medscape.com/article/1107107-overview#a4.

41. Schwartz RA. Acanthosis nigricans. J Am Acad Dermatol. 1994;31(1):1–19; quiz 20-2.

42. Higgins SP, Freemark M, Prose NS. Acanthosis nigricans: a practical approach to evaluation and management. Dermatol Online J. 2008;14(9):2.

43. Ances IG. Serum concentrations of epidermal growth factor in human pregnancy. Am J Obstet Gynecol. 1973;115(3):357–62.

44. Ellis DL, Nanney LB, King LE Jr. Increased epidermal growth factor receptors in seborrheic keratoses and acrochordons of patients with the dysplastic nevus syndrome. J Am Acad Dermatol. 1990;23(6 Pt 1):1070–7.

45. Shamsadini S, Wadji MB, Shamsadini A. Surrounding ipsilateral eruptive seborrheic keratosis as a warning sign of intraductal breast carcinoma and Paget's disease (Leser Trelat sign). Dermatol Online J. 2005;12(6):27.

46. Schwartz RA. Sign of Leser-Trélat. J Am Acad Dermatol. 1996;35(1):88–95.

47. Haagensen C. Mammary-duct ectasia. A disease that may simulate carcinoma. Cancer. 1951;4(4):749–61.

48. Dixon JM, Mansel RE. ABC of breast diseases. Congenital problems and aberrations of normal breast development and involution. BMJ. 1994;309(6957):797–800.

49. Hidano A, Kobayashi T. Adnexal polyp of neonatal skin. Br J Dermatol. 1975;92(6):659–62.

50. Brownstein MH, Phelps RG, Magnin PH. Papillary adenoma of the nipple: analysis of fifteeen new cases. J Am Acad Dermatol. 1985;12(4):707–15.

51. Montemarano AD, Sau P, James WD. Superficial papillary adenomatosis of the nipple: a case report and review of the literature. J Am Acad Dermatol. 1995;33(5:871–5.

52. Van Mierlo PL, Geelen GM, Neumann HA. Mohs micrographic surgery for an erosive adenomatosis of the nipple. Dermatol Surg. 1998;24(6):681–3.

53. Kuflik EG. Erosive adenomatosis of the nipple treated with cryosurgery. J Am Acad Dermatol. 1998;38(2 Pt 1):270–1.

54. Ashikari R, Park K, Huvos AG, Urban JA. Paget's disease of the breast. Cancer. 1970;26(3):680–5.

55. Sahoo S, Green I, Rosen PP. Bilateral Paget disease of the nipple associated with lobular carcinoma in situ: application of immunohistochemistry to a rare finding. Arch Pathol Lab Med. 2002;126(1):90–2.

56. Laumann AE, Derick AJ. Tattoos and body piercings in the United States: a national data set. J Am Acad Dermatol. 2006;55(3):413–21.

57. Armstrong ML, McConnell C. Tattooing in adolescents: more common than you think—the phenomenon and risks. J Sch Nurs. 1994;10(1):26–33.

58. Carroll ST, Riffenburgh RH, Roberts TA, Myhre EB. Tattoos and body piercings as indicators of adolescent risk-taking behaviors. Pediatrics. 2002;109(6):1021–7.

59. Pugatch D, Mileno M, Rich JD. Possible transmission of human immunodeficiency virus type 1 from body piercing. Clin Infect Dis. 1998;26(3):767–8.

60. Ochsenfahrt C, Friedl R, Hannekum A, Schumacher BA. Endocarditis after nipple piercing in a patient with a bicuspid aortic valve. Ann Thorac Surg. 2001;71(4):1365–6.

61. Collins RE. Breast disease associated with tassel dancing. Br Med J (Clin Res Ed). 1981;283(6307):1660.

62. Garbin CP, Deacon JP, Rowan MK, Hartmann PE, Geddes DT. Association of nipple piercing with abnormal milk production and breastfeeding. JAMA. 2009;301(24):2550–1.

63. Muallem MM, Rubeiz NG. Physiological and biological skin changes in pregnancy. Clin Dermatol. 2006;24(2):80–3.

64. Doucet S, Soussignan R, Sagot P, Schaal B. The secretion of areolar (Montgomery's) glands from lactating women elicits selective, unconditional responses in neonates. PLoS One. 2009;4(10): e7579.

65. Skov L, Baadsgaard O. Bacterial superantigens and inflammatory skin diseases. Clin Exp Dermatol. 2000;25(1):57–61.

66. Tokura Y, Yagi H, Ohshima A, Kurokawa S, Wakita H, Yokote R, et al. Cutaneous colonization with staphylococci influences the disease activity of Sezary syndrome: a potential role for bacterial superantigens. Br J Dermatol. 1995;133(1):6–12.

67. Dodiuk-Gad R, Cohen-Barak E, Ziv M, Shani-Adir A, Shalev S, Chazan B, et al. Bacteriological aspects of Darier's disease. J Eur Acad Dermatol Venereol. 2013;27(11):1405–9.

68. Hale TW, Rowe HE. Medications and mothers' milk. Plano: Hale; 2014.

69. Atkinson AJ Jr. Pharmacokinetics of prednisolone transfer to breast milk. Clin Pharmacol Ther. 1993;53(3):324–8.

70. Chi C-C, Wang S-H, Kirtschig G, Wojnarowska F. Systematic review of the safety of topical corticosteroids in pregnancy. J Am Acad Dermatol. 2010;62:694.

71. Murase JE, Chan KK, Garite TJ, Cooper DM, Weinstein GD. Hormonal effect on psoriasis in pregnancy and post partum. Arch Dermatol. 2005;141(5):601–6.

72. Krishnan L, Guilbert LJ, Wegmann TG, Belosevic M, Mosmann TR. T helper 1 response against Leishmania major in pregnant C57BL/6 mice increases implantation failure and fetal resorptions. Correlation with increased IFN-gamma and TNF and reduced IL-10 production by placental cells. J Immunol. 1996;156(2):653–62.

73. Maes M, Ombelet W, De Jongh R, Kenis G, Bosmans E. The inflammatory response following delivery is amplified in women who previously suffered from major depression, suggesting that major depression is accompanied by a sensitization of the inflammatory response system. J Affect Disord. 2001;63(1):85–92.

74. Groer MW, Davis MW, Smith K, Casey K, Kramer V, Bukovsky E. Immunity, inflammation and infection in post-partum breast and formula feeders. Am J Reprod Immunol. 2005;54(4):222–31.

75. Hirotsu C, Rydlewski M, Araujo MS, Tufik S, Andersen ML. Sleep loss and cytokines levels in an experimental model of psoriasis. PLoS One. 2012;7(11):e51183.

76. Rademaker M, Agnew K, Andrews M, Armour K, Baker C, Foley P, et al. Psoriasis in those planning a family, pregnant or breast-feeding. The Australasian Psoriasis Collaboration. Australas J Dermatol. 2017. https://doi.org/10.1111/ajd.12641.

77. Bae YS, Van Voorhees AS, Hsu S, Korman NJ, Lebwohl MG, Young M, et al. Review of treatment options for psoriasis in pregnant or lactating women: from the Medical Board of the National Psoriasis Foundation. J Am Acad Dermatol. 2012;67(3):459–77.

78. Mahadevan U, Wolf DC, Dubinsky M, Cortot A, Lee SD, Siegel CA, et al. Placental transfer of anti-tumor necrosis factor agents in pregnant patients with inflammatory bowel disease. Clin Gastroenterol Hepatol. 2013;11(3):286–92; quiz e24.

79. Baker K, Qiao S-W, Kuo T, Kobayashi K, Yoshida M, Lencer WI, et al. Immune and non-immune functions of the (not so) neonatal Fc receptor, FcRn. Semin Immunopathol. 2009;31:223.

80. Vasiliauskas EA, Church JA, Silverman N, Barry M, Targan SR, Dubinsky MC. Case report: evidence for transplacental transfer of maternally administered infliximab to the newborn. Clin Gastroenterol Hepatol. 2006;4(10):1255–8.

81. Zelinkova Z, de Haar C, de Ridder L, Pierik MJ, Kuipers EJ, Peppelenbosch MP, et al. High intrauterine exposure to infliximab following maternal anti-TNF treatment during pregnancy. Aliment Pharmacol Ther. 2011;33(9):1053–8.

82. Cheent K, Nolan J, Shariq S, Kiho L, Pal A, Arnold J. Case report: fatal case of disseminated BCG infection in an infant born to a mother taking infliximab for Crohn's disease. J Crohns Colitis. 2010;4(5):603–5.

83. Porter ML, Lockwood SJ, Kimball AB. Update on biologic safety for patients with psoriasis during pregnancy. Int J Womens Dermatol. 2017;3(1):21–5.

84. Oz BB, Hackman R, Einarson T, Koren G. Pregnancy outcome after cyclosporine therapy

during pregnancy: a meta-analysis. Transplantation. 2001;71(8):1051–5.

85. Palmer CN, Irvine AD, Terron-Kwiatkowski A, Zhao Y, Liao H, Lee SP, et al. Common loss-of-function variants of the epidermal barrier protein filaggrin are a major predisposing factor for atopic dermatitis. Nat Genet. 2006;38(4):441–6.

86. Darwazeh AM, al-Bashir A. Oral candidal flora in healthy infants. J Oral Pathol Med. 1995;24(8):361–4.

87. McCarthy C, Snyder ML, Parker RB. The indigenous oral flora of man. I. The newborn to the 1-year-old infant. Arch Oral Biol. 1965;10(1):61–70.

88. Shaffer KK, Jaimes JP, Hordinsky MK, Zielke GR, Warshaw EM. Allergenicity and cross-reactivity of coconut oil derivatives: a double-blind randomized controlled pilot study. Dermatitis. 2006;17(2):71–6.

89. Kapur N, Goldsmith P. Nipple dermatitis–not all what it 'seams'. Contact Dermatitis. 2001;45(1):44–5.

90. Levit F. Jogger's nipples. N Engl J Med. 1977;297(20):1127.

91. Powell B. Bicyclist's nipples. JAMA. 1983;249(18):2457.

92. Bischof RO. Surf rider's dermatitis. Contact Dermatitis. 1995;32(4):247.

93. Fisher AA. Sports-related allergic dermatitis. Cutis. 1992;50(2):95–7.

94. McGforge BC, Steele MC. Allergic contact dermatitis of the nipple from Roman chamomile ointment. Contact Dermatitis. 1991;24(2):139–40.

95. Warshaw EM, Nelsen DD, Maibach HI, Marks JG, Zug KA, Taylor JS, et al. Positive patch test reactions to lanolin: cross-sectional data from the north american contact dermatitis group, 1994 to 2006. Dermatitis. 2009;20(2):79–88.

96. Garcia M, del Pozo MD, Diez J, Munoz D, de Corres LF. Allergic contact dermatitis from a beeswax nipple-protective. Contact Dermatitis. 1995;33(6):440–1.

97. Goossens A, Verhamme B. Contact allergy to permanent colorants used for tattooing a nipple after breast reconstruction. Contact Dermatitis. 2002;47(4):250.

98. Wold AE, Adlerberth I. Breast feeding and the intestinal microflora of the infant—implications for protection against infectious diseases. In: Koletzko B, Michaelsen KF, Hernell O, editors. Short and long term effects of breast feeding on child health. Boston: Springer; 2002. p. 77–93.

99. Johnston M, Landers S, Noble L, Szucs K, Viehmann L. Breastfeeding and the use of human milk. Pediatrics. 2012;129(3):e827–41.

100. The World Health Organization's infant feeding recommendation. 2002. http://www.who.int/nutrition/topics/infantfeeding_recommendation/en/.

101. Kramer MS, Aboud F, Mironova E, Vanilovich I, Platt RW, Matush L, et al. Breastfeeding and child cognitive development: new evidence from a large randomized trial. Arch Gen Psychiatry. 2008;65(5):578–84.

102. Jordan SJ, Na R, Johnatty SE, Wise LA, Adami HO, Brinton LA, et al. Breastfeeding and endometrial cancer risk: an analysis from the epidemiology of endometrial cancer consortium. Obstet Gynecol. 2017;129(6):1059–67.

103. Victora CG, Bahl R, Barros AJ, Franca GV, Horton S, Krasevec J, et al. Breastfeeding in the 21st century: epidemiology, mechanisms, and lifelong effect. Lancet. 2016;387(10017):475–90.

104. Chowdhury R, Sinha B, Sankar MJ, Taneja S, Bhandari N, Rollins N, et al. Breastfeeding and maternal health outcomes: a systematic review and meta-analysis. Acta Paediatr. 2015;104(467):96–113.

105. Kent JC, Ashton E, Hardwick CM, Rowan MK, Chia ES, Fairclough KA, et al. Nipple pain in breastfeeding mothers: incidence, causes and treatments. Int J Environ Res Public Health. 2015;12(10):12247–63.

106. Buck ML, Amir LH, Cullinane M, Donath SM, Team CS. Nipple pain, damage, and vasospasm in the first 8 weeks postpartum. Breastfeed Med. 2014;9(2):56–62.

107. Wagner EA, Chantry CJ, Dewey KG, Nommsen-Rivers LA. Breastfeeding concerns at 3 and 7 days postpartum and feeding status at 2 months. Pediatrics. 2013. https://doi.org/10.1542/peds.2013-0724.

108. McClellan HL, Hepworth AR, Garbin CP, Rowan MK, Deacon J, Hartmann PE, et al. Nipple pain during breastfeeding with or without visible trauma. J Hum Lact. 2012;28(4):511–21.

109. Brown S, Lumley J. Maternal health after childbirth: results of an Australian population based survey. Br J Obstet Gynaecol. 1998;105(2):156–61.

110. Jager S, Jacobs S, Kroger J, Fritsche A, Schienkiewitz A, Rubin D, et al. Breast-feeding and maternal risk of type 2 diabetes: a prospective study and meta-analysis. Diabetologia. 2014;57(7):1355–65.

111. Eidelman AI, Schanler RJ, Johnston M, Landers S, Noble L, Szucs K, et al. Breastfeeding and the use of human milk. Pediatrics. 2012;129(3):e827–e41.

112. Amir LH, Jones LE, Buck ML. Nipple pain associated with breastfeeding: Incorporating current neurophysiology into clinical reasoning. Aust Fam Physician. 2015;44(3):127.

113. Ardran GM, Kemp FH, Lind J. A cineradiographic study of bottle feeding. Br J Radiol. 1958;31(361):11–22.

114. Sakalidis VS, Geddes DT. Suck-swallow-breathe dynamics in breastfed infants. J Hum Lact. 2016; 32(2):201–11.

115. Park HS, Yoon CH, Kim HJ. The prevalence of congenital inverted nipple. Aesthet Plast Surg. 1999;23(2):144–6.

116. Barrett ME, Heller MM, Fullerton Stone H, Murase JE. Dermatoses of the breast in lactation. Dermatol Ther. 2013;26(4):331–6.

117. Barrett ME, Heller MM, Stone HF, Murase JE. Raynaud phenomenon of the nipple in breastfeeding mothers: an underdiagnosed cause of nipple pain. JAMA Dermatol. 2013;149(3):300–6.

118. McGuinness N, Cording V. Raynaud's phenomenon of the nipple associated with labetalol use. J Hum Lact. 2013;29(1):17–9.

119. Anderson JE, Held N, Wright K. Raynaud's phenomenon of the nipple: a treatable cause of painful breastfeeding. Pediatrics. 2004;113(4):e360–4.
120. Smith W, Erenberg A, Nowak A, Franken E Jr. Physiology of sucking in the normal term infant using real-time US. Radiology. 1985;156(2): 379–81.
121. Messner AH, Lalakea ML, Aby J, Macmahon J, Bair E. Ankyloglossia: incidence and associated feeding difficulties. Arch Otolaryngol Head Neck Surg. 2000;126(1):36–9.
122. Hazelbaker A. The assessment tool for lingual frenulum function (ATLFF): use in a lactation consultant private practice. Thesis. Pasadena, CA: Pacific Oaks College; 1993.
123. Messner AH, Lalakea ML. Ankyloglossia: controversies in management. Int J Pediatr Otorhinolaryngol. 2000;54(2-3):123–31.
124. Ballard JL, Auer CE, Khoury JC. Ankyloglossia: assessment, incidence, and effect of frenuloplasty on the breastfeeding dyad. Pediatrics. 2002;110(5):e63.
125. Masaitis NS, Kaempf JW. Developing a frenotomy policy at one medical center: a case study approach. J Hum Lact. 1996;12(3):229–32.
126. Williams WN, Waldron CM. Assessment of lingual function when ankyloglossia (tongue-tie) is suspected. J Am Dent Assoc. 1985;110(3):353–6.
127. Dollberg S, Botzer E, Grunis E, Mimouni FB. Immediate nipple pain relief after frenotomy in breast-fed infants with ankyloglossia: a randomized, prospective study. J Pediatr Surg. 2006;41(9):1598–600.
128. Kotlow LA. Diagnosing and understanding the maxillary lip-tie (superior labial, the maxillary labial frenum) as it relates to breastfeeding. J Hum Lact. 2013;29(4):458–64.
129. McClellan H, Geddes D, Kent J, Garbin C, Mitoulas L, Hartmann P. Infants of mothers with persistent nipple pain exert strong sucking vacuums. Acta Paediatr. 2008;97(9):1205–9.
130. Brimdyr K, Blair A, Cadwell K, Turner-Maffei C. The relationship between positioning, the breastfeeding dynamic, the latching process and pain in breastfeeding mothers with sore nipples. Breastfeed Rev. 2003;11(2):5.
131. Chiu IM, Heesters BA, Ghasemlou N, Von Hehn CA, Zhao F, Tran J, et al. Bacteria activate sensory neurons that modulate pain and inflammation. Nature. 2013;501(7465):52.
132. Heikkila MP, Saris PE. Inhibition of Staphylococcus aureus by the commensal bacteria of human milk. J Appl Microbiol. 2003;95(3):471–8.
133. Vuong C, Otto M. Staphylococcus epidermidis infections. Microbes Infect. 2002;4(4):481–9.
134. Delgado S, Arroyo R, Martin R, Rodriguez JM. PCR-DGGE assessment of the bacterial diversity of breast milk in women with lactational infectious mastitis. BMC Infect Dis. 2008;8(1):51.
135. Amir LH, Academy of Breastfeeding Medicine Protocol Committee. ABM clinical protocol #4: Mastitis, revised March 2014. Breastfeed Med. 2014;9(5):239–43.
136. Szajewska H, Ruszczynski M, Radzikowski A. Probiotics in the prevention of antibiotic-associated diarrhea in children: a meta-analysis of randomized controlled trials. J Pediatr. 2006;149(3):367–72.
137. D'Souza AL, Rajkumar C, Cooke J, Bulpitt CJ. Probiotics in prevention of antibiotic associated diarrhoea: meta-analysis. BMJ. 2002;324(7350):1361.
138. Moorhead AM, Amir LH, O'Brien PW, Wong S. A prospective study of fluconazole treatment for breast and nipple thrush. Breastfeed Rev. 2011;19(3):25–9.
139. Francis-Morrill J, Heinig MJ, Pappagianis D, Dewey KG. Diagnostic value of signs and symptoms of mammary candidosis among lactating women. J Hum Lact. 2004;20(3):288–95.
140. Carmichael A, Dixon J. Is lactation mastitis and shooting breast pain experienced by women during lactation caused by Candida albicans? Breast. 2002;11(1):88–90.
141. Viejo-Diaz M, Andres MT, Fierro JF. Different anti-Candida activities of two human lactoferrin-derived peptides, Lfpep and kaliocin-1. Antimicrob Agents Chemother. 2005;49(7):2583–8.
142. Montagne P, Cuilliere M, Mole C, Bene M, Faure G. Changes in lactoferrin and lysozyme levels in human milk during the first twelve weeks of lactation. In: Bioactive components of human milk. New York: Springer; 2001. p. 241–7.
143. Amir LH, Donath SM, Garland SM, Tabrizi SN, Bennett CM, Cullinane M, et al. Does Candida and/or Staphylococcus play a role in nipple and breast pain in lactation? A cohort study in Melbourne, Australia. BMJ Open. 2013;3(3):e002351.
144. Morrill JF, Heinig MJ, Pappagianis D, Dewey KG. Risk factors for mammary candidosis among lactating women. J Obstet Gynecol Neonatal Nurs. 2005;34(1):37–45.
145. Amir LH. Candida and the lactating breast: predisposing factors. J Hum Lact. 1991;7(4):177–81.
146. Berens P, Eglash A, Malloy M, Steube AM. ABM clinical protocol# 26: persistent pain with breastfeeding. Breastfeed Med. 2016;11(2):46–53.
147. Wiener S. Diagnosis and management of Candida of the nipple and breast. J Midwifery Womens Health. 2006;51(2):125–8.
148. Wambach K, Riordan J. Breastfeeding and human lactation. Burlington: Jones & Bartlett Publishers; 2014.
149. Kramer A, Schwebke I, Kampf G. How long do nosocomial pathogens persist on inanimate surfaces? A systematic review. BMC Infect Dis. 2006;6(1):130.
150. Wilson-Clay B, Hoover K. The breastfeeding atlas. Manchaca: LactNews Press; 2008.
151. Whitley RJ, Kimberlin DW, Roizman B. Herpes simplex viruses. Clin Infect Dis. 1998;26(3):541–53; quiz 54-5.
152. Miller CS, Danaher RJ. Asymptomatic shedding of herpes simplex virus (HSV) in the oral cavity.

Oral Surg Oral Med Oral Pathol Oral Radiol Endod. 2008;105(1):43–50.

153. Parra J, Cneude F, Huin N, Bru CB, Debillon T. Mammary herpes: a little known mode of neonatal herpes contamination. J Perinatol. 2013;33(9):736–7.

154. Sabin AB, Fieldsteel AH. Antipoliomyelitic activity of human and bovine colostrum and milk. Pediatrics. 1962;29(1):105–15.

155. Noble R. Milk under the skin (milk blister). A simple problem causing other breast conditions. Breastfeed Rev J. 1991;2:118–9.

156. O'Hara M. Bleb histology reveals inflammatory infiltrate that regresses with topical steroids; a case series [platform abstract]. Breastfeed Med. 2012;7(Suppl 1):2.

157. Ducic I, Zakaria HM, Felder JM 3rd, Fantus S. Nerve Injuries in aesthetic breast surgery: systematic review and treatment options. Aesthet Surg J. 2014;34(6):841–56.

158. Jindal N, Jain VK, Aggarwal S, Kaur S. Ipsilateral galactorrhea following zoster of the T4 dermatome. Indian J Dermatol Venereol Leprol. 2014;80(6):540–2.

159. Eccleston C, Williams AC, Morley S. Psychological therapies for the management of chronic pain (excluding headache) in adults. Cochrane Database Syst Rev. 2009;2:CD007407.

160. Kernerman E, Park E. Severe breast pain resolved with pectoral muscle massage. J Hum Lact. 2014;30(3):287–91.

161. Rowbotham M, Harden N, Stacey B, Bernstein P, Magnus-Miller L. Gabapentin for the treatment of postherpetic neuralgia: a randomized controlled trial. JAMA. 1998;280(21):1837–42.

162. Pugh LC, Buchko BL, Bishop BA, Cochran JF, Smith LR, Lerew DJ. A comparison of topical agents to relieve nipple pain and enhance breastfeeding. Birth. 1996;23(2):88–93.

163. Shanazi M, Farshbaf Khalili A, Kamalifard M, Asghari Jafarabadi M, Masoudin K, Esmaeli F. Comparison of the effects of lanolin, peppermint, and dexpanthenol creams on treatment of traumatic nipples in breastfeeding mothers. J Caring Sci. 2015;4(4):297–307.

164. Jackson KT, Dennis CL. Lanolin for the treatment of nipple pain in breastfeeding women: a randomized controlled trial. Matern Child Nutr. 2016;13:e12357.

165. Cable B, Stewart M, Davis J. Nipple wound care: a new approach to an old problem. J Hum Lact. 1997;13(4):313–8.

166. Tait P. Nipple pain in breastfeeding women: causes, treatment, and prevention strategies. J Midwifery Womens Health. 2000;45(3):212–5.

167. WHO. Protecting, promoting and supporting breastfeeding: the special role of maternity services. 1989.

168. Huggins KE, Billon SF. Twenty cases of persistent sore nipples: collaboration between lactation consultant and dermatologist. J Hum Lact. 1993;9(3):155–60.

Acne Vulgaris

12

Gila Isman Nelkenbaum

12.1 Introduction

Acne Vulgaris is a skin disorder of the pilosebaceous unit influenced by androgenic hormones and therefore there are many variances in its appearance between genders. As a result, physical examination, workup and management should be distinct for each gender.

The pathogenesis of acne is multifactorial and it involves four main pathways: excess sebum production, comedogenesis, *Propionibacterium acnes* and complex inflammatory mechanisms involving both innate and acquired immunity. Excess Sebum production and comedogenesis are known to be induced by androgen secretion.

12.2 Hormonal Influence on Acne Pathogenesis

Hormonal effects on sebum secretion are key to the pathogenesis of acne.

Androgens are produced primarily from the gonads and adrenal glands as well as within the sebaceous gland via the action of androgen-metabolizing enzymes such as 3β-hydroxysteroid dehydrogenase (HSD), 17β-HSD and 5α-reductase.

Androgen receptors found in the cells of the basal layer of the sebaceous gland and the outer root sheath of the hair follicle are responsive to testosterone and 5α-dihydrotestosterone (DHT), the most potent androgens. DHT is also thought to be the principal androgen mediating sebum production [1].

Exessive sebum production as well as alternations in sebum composition leed to follicular hyperkeratinization by activating the innate immune system and forming anaerobic environment that promotes *proprionibacterium acne* to thrive. This inflammatory process induces toll like receptors (TLRs) 2 and 4 to increase production of interleukins 1β and promotes activation of IL-6, IL-8, IL-12. As a consequence, activator protein −1 activates metalloproteinase which may cause scar formation [2].

The sebaceous gland is controlled primarily by hormonal stimulation which changes throughout life. During the first 6 months of life, sebum production is relatively high, then its production rate decreases and remains stable during childhood. At adrenarche (typically at 7–8 years of age) circulating levels of DHEAS begin to rise and as a result sebum production dramatically increases, which leads to the initial development of comedonal acne in prepubescent children [3].

Estrogen, whether given systemically or as in contraceptive pill, has a role in acne treatment. However its role in the physiology of acne is not

G. I. Nelkenbaum
Department of Dermatology, Tel Aviv Sourasky
Medical Center, Tel Aviv, Israel

clear. Acne may response to low dose contraceptive, even though higher doses of estrogen are often required to demonstrate a reduction in sebum secretion [4]. There are several hypothesis regarding estrogen influence in acne treatment, it may be directly opposing effects of androgens locally within the sebaceous gland or by inhibiting the production of androgens by gonadal tissue. Another possible mechanism is via regulating genes that negatively influence sebaceous gland growth or lipid production.

12.3 Clinical Features of Adolescent Acne

Acne affects more than 80% of the teenage population. Classic acne begins earlier in females close to the menarche (10–14 years) and reaches its peak at the ages of 14–17 years. On the other hand, males will present with acne usually at the age of 14 and will reach acne peak at the ages of 16 to 19.

Hormonal surges before and during puberty are often related to the onset of typical acne vulgaris. Teenaged boys are more frequently affected than teenaged girls. Adrenal maturation and gonadal development cause androgen production and subsequent sebaceous gland enlargement. Both sebum production and the levels of DHEAS increase during puberty. During physical examination, the main findings will be comedones, papules, pustules and cysts on face and upper trunk.

Non inflammatory acne is characterized by open (white heads) and closed (black heads) comedones, while inflammatory acne is characterized by erythematous papules, pustules and in more severe cases nodules, cysts and sinus tracts. Males are more prone to suffer from severe acne during adolescence and acne fulminans is more prevalent in this population. Consequently, severe scars are more prevalent among males and therefore topical and systemic therapies based on retinoid may be preferred in males because of their direct effect on sebaceous gland activity. In the case of moderate to severe acne, treatment should be initiated early to avoid scar formation.

Scarring occurs early in acne and may affect some 95 percent of patients [5], relating to both its severity and delay before treatment.

Approximately 40% of all acne patients have clinically relevant scars [6].

For both genders, acne can affect self esteem, body image, social life and may cause depression, frustration and anger. Levels of social and emotional problems in acne patients is comparable with those in people with severe chronic disabling diseases such as arthritis and epilepsy. Females usually experience more embarrassment due to acne than their male counterparts [7].

12.4 Pathogenesis of Acne in Males

Sebum production is higher in males [8] and has a significant role in the pathogenesis of acne. Even though elevated sebum production alone does not induce acne, alterations in sebum composition have been demonstrated to cause follicular hyper cornification through stimulation of the innate immune system. Sebum also promotes an anaerobic environment for *propionibacterium acne* to thrive which drive an inflammatory process that in its end metalloproteinase are released which may increase scar formation.

Trans epidermal water loss (TEWL) in males has been shown to be lower than in females however, moderate to severe acne impair stratum cornea and TEWL [9]. Therefore, male patients suffering from severe acne may deviate farther from corneocytes and TEWL physiologic state and are prone to more side effects with acne therapies that augment barrier function.

Another physiologic difference between genders is the skin pH. For males the pH is lower than 5.0 due to high sebum production causing higher levels of free fatty acid in the skin while in females it is usually above 5.0 [10]. These pH levels have not yet been associated with acne pathogenesis [11], however it may have implications on future treatment.

Consuming proteins and other supplements by athletes became very popular in recent years. This consumption has been shown to trigger acne by increasing insulin growth factor-1, stimulating sterol response binding protein-1 that can induce sebaceous gland lipogenesis, comedogenesis, follicular inflammation and androgenic stimulation [12]. Acne fulminans which is more prevalent in males was also associated with anabolic steroid consumption [13].

12.4.1 Acne Conglobata

Acne Conglobata is a severe form of nodular cystic acne seen mostly in teenage males. This type of acne may appear on the back, buttocks, chest, shoulders and face. Acne Conglobata shows multi opening comedones, large tender nodules and cysts with a foul smelling purulent discharge and sinus tracts are characteristic. After healing, depressed and keloidal scars may be evident (Fig. 12.1). Therapy comprises intensive high-dose therapy with antibiotics, intralesional glucocorticoids, systemic glucocorticoids, surgical debridement, surgical incision, and surgical excision. Isotretinoin initial dose should be 0.5 mg/kg/day or less, and systemic glucocorticoids are often required either before initiating therapy or as concomitant therapy, in severe cases dosages as high as 2 mg/kg/day for a 20-week course may be necessary.

12.4.2 Acne Fulminans

Acne fulminans (AF) is a severe form of acne that appears primarily in adolescent males. The direct age group affected is between 13–22 years of age. There have been rare reported cases of Acne fulminans in females [14].

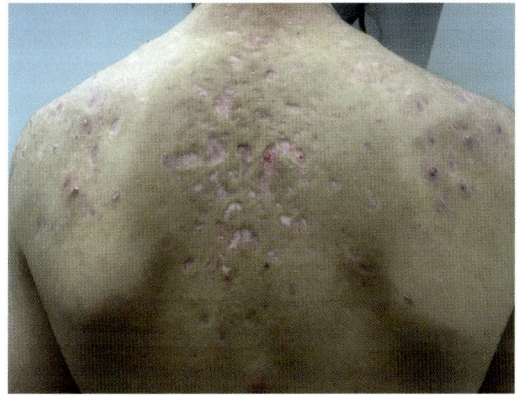

Fig. 12.1 Ulcerated and depressed atrophic scars on the trunk of a 14 year old male as a sequelae of nodulocystic acne

This type of acne has an acute presentation with a sudden onset of nodulocystic inflammatory lesions mainly affecting the trunk. Ulcerative lesions covered with hemorrhagic crusts are common and comedones are rare. Systemic symptoms include fever, myalgia, arthralgia, bone pain and anorexia. Laboratory investigations demonstrate systemic involvement with leukocytosis often with leukomoid reaction, elevation of erythrocyte sedimentation rate, anemia, proteinuria, and microscopic hematuria. Bone involvement is commonly located at the sternum and clavicle but may occur at other sites. Generally, 50% of patients have lytic bone lesions. Less commonly, these patients may also present with erythema nodosum. It can be the dermatologic manifestation of the synovitis-acne-pustulosis-hyperostosis-osteitis (SAPHO) syndrome.

The pathophysiliogy is still unclear. The triggering antigen is believed to be *p acne*. However, as AF is more frequently seen in young males, it may be that high levels of testosterone may play a role. There are also reports of acne fulminans cases after receiving high levels of testosterone due to high stature [15, 16]. Other cases of acne fulminans were attributed to anabolic steroids consumption [17]. There is usually a history of mild to moderate acne years before the onset of AF [14]. Genetic factors may play an important roll in AF.

Therapy is mainly systemic steroids. Prednisolone 0.5–1.0 mg/kg/day should be commenced and decreased gradually over 2–3 months. Low dose Isotretinoin should be introduced after 3–4 weeks of prednisolone initiation with increasing doses according to clinical response. Oral Isotertinoin should be used cautiously due to paradoxical effect it may cause as was reported in some cases [18].

Acne scarring is a frequent complication due to the inflammatory nodules healing with residual scars.

12.5 Infantile Acne

Acne lesions appear typically between 3 and 12 months of age. Infantile acne has male predominance and usually affects the face and specially the cheeks. The acne may include comedones (whiteheads and blackheads), inflamed papules and pustules, nodules and cysts that may result in scarring. Most cases of infantile acne are resolved by 4 or 5 years of age but in some cases they remain active into puberty. Patients with a history of infantile acne have an increased incidence of acne vulgaris during adolescence compared to their peers, with greater severity and enhanced risk for scarring [19]. The pathogenesis is unclear. It may reflect the androgen production intrinsic to this stage of development including elevated levels of LH stimulating testicular production of testosterone in boys during the first 6–12 months of life (with levels transiently equivalent to those during puberty) and elevated levels of DHEA produced by the infantile adrenal gland in both boys and girls. These androgen levels normally decrease substantially by 12 months of age and remain at nadir levels until adrenarche. [20]

12.6 Female Acne

12.6.1 Pregnancy and Lactation

The effect of acne during pregnancy is unpredictable and can vary from mild comedonal disease to severe inflammatory scarring acne. During pregnancy there may be an increase in sebaceous gland activity [21] as a result of hormonal imbalance. Circulating testosterone level is also increased slightly throughout pregnancy while dehydroepiandrosterone sulphate level decreases in the second and in the third trimester [22] during pregnancy. Progesterone and estradiol levels are found to be 100 fold and 10–50 folds higher respectively [23]. These findings however can not solely explain acne flares at the second [24] and third [25] trimesters that are most prominent during this time.

Treatment during pregnancy is limited due to safety profile concerns and lack of clinical studies and pharmacokinetic data in this patient population [26]. However, topical agents as clindamycin, erythromycin, azelaic acid (category B) and benzoyl peroxide (category C) are commonly used for mild to moderate acne. For severe acne, systemic therapy is limited to erythromycin or penicillin based antibiotics however, its efficacy is limited. Isotretinoin is teratogenic and contraindicated (category x), medications from tetracyclin family (category D) should be avoided during pregnancy because they affect teeth calcification if taken after the fourth month of pregnancy and causes permanent teeth discoloration. Hormonal therapy should be avoided during pregnancy and lactation, as they have been associated with hypospadias and feminization of the male fetus [27]. Other possible treatments are alfa hydroxyl peels, salycilic acid acne products and comedo extraction. No recommendation was ever made in the past regarding light based therapies for acne, with the exception of PDT which should be avoided due to lack of studies with aminoleuvulonic acid and methyl aminoleuvulinat in pregnant women.

12.6.2 Breastfeeding

Taking medications during the lactation period may change breast milk composition and supply, thus therapy during this period is limited.

Topical tretinoin [28] is considered safe during lactation. Because vitamin A is a normal component of breast milk, tretinoin is likely to be excreted in breast milk. However, the topical formulation is unlikely to be absorbed in significant quantities and therefore it will be safe during the lactation period.

By contrast, the use of systemic isotretinoin is contraindicated during lactation because isotretinoin is extremely lipid soluble and concentrations in milk would be significant. The risk of retinoid toxicity in the infant is too high to use in a breastfeeding woman [29].

Hormonal therapy should be avoided in lactation for two reasons: (1) The estrogen content in OCPs has been reported to decrease milk production and (2) There is a theoretical risk of infant feminization, especially in neonates who might be less capable of metabolizing the additional hormones [30].

Tetracycline are compatible with lactation. Infant absorption is low as the drug binds to calcium in the maternal milk. The medication should not be used for more than 3 weeks because when consumed over an extended period the absorption of even small amounts over a prolonged period could result in dental staining [29].

12.6.3 Adult Onset Acne

Adult onset acne is defined as a chronic inflammatory disease of the pilosabeceous unit beyond the age of 25 years [31], and it's prevalence is 12% [32]. It is subdivided to "persistent acne" which is the adolescent classic acne that continues to adult life or middle age and "late onset acne" with first onset after 25 years. The first one considered more common than the latter [33].

While adolescent acne is more prevalent among males, adult onset acne is more prevalent in women who present classically with papules nodules and cysts in jawline in the lower third face area (Fig. 12.2). Hormonal imbalance and premenstrual flares are more common in this type of acne and it is more resistant to therapy [34].

The pathophysiology in AOA is considered to be due to higher androgen levels. Studies [35] have shown raised levels of 5α reductase enzyme levels, 3α-androstanediol glucuronide, and androsterone glucuronide (tissue derived androgens). Association between PCOS and AOA was

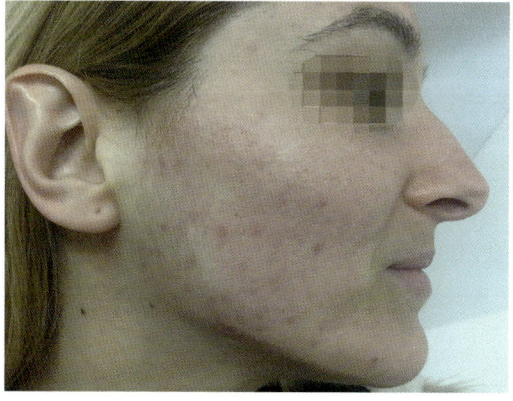

Fig. 12.2 Adult onset acne in a 30 year old female, erythemic papules in the mandibular area, no comedones are seen

found in 52–82% and association with late onset adrenal hyperlasia was found in 11.8% of cases.

12.6.4 PCOS

Polycystic ovary syndrome (PCOS) occurs in roughly 3 to 6% of the general population. PCOS has been defined using various criteria, including menstrual irregularity, hyperandrogenism, and polycystic ovary morphology (PCOM) [36]. Diagnosis of PCOS requires 2 of the 3 following criteria: androgen excess (clinical or biochemical), ovulatory dysfunction (oligo- or anovulation), or polycystic ovaries (based on ultrasonographic findings). Patients with androgen excess frequently have a history of irregular menses and present with obesity, androgenic alopecia, hirsutism and acne. In adolescent females, the diagnosis of PCOS can be made based on hyperandrogenism (clinical or biochemical) in the presence of persistent oligomenorrhea [37]. In adolescent girls, large, multicystic ovaries are a common finding, so ultrasound is not a first-line investigation in women <17 years of age. There is an increased risk of diabetes mellitus and endometrial carcinoma in patients with PCOS [38].

Girls with severe acne or acne resistant to oral and topical agents, including isotretinoin (Accutane) may have a 40% likelihood of developing PCOS. Oral contraceptives (OCPs) can effectively lower androgens and block the effect of androgens via suppression of ovarian androgen production and by increasing sex hormone-binding globulin. Physiologic doses of dexamethasone or prednisone can directly lower adrenal androgen output. Anti-androgens can be used to block the effects of androgen in the pilosebaceous unit or in the hair follicle. Anti-androgen therapy works through competitive antagonism of the androgen receptor (spironolactone, cyproterone acetate, flutamide) or inhibition of 5α-reductase (finasteride) to prevent the conversion of testosterone to its more potent form, 5α-dihydrotestosterone.

While PCOS is the most common hormonal related acne, thyroid dysfunction, prolactin excess and congenital adrenal hyperplasia must also be considered in any case of acne resistant to therapy.

Lab studies for evaluation of hyperandrogenism should be done at day 1–3 of the menstrual cycle and if on oral contraceptive it should be discontinued 4 to 6 weeks before hormone evaluation. The studies should include free testosterone levels, dehydroepiandrosterone sulfate (DHEA-S), androstenedione, luteinizing hormone and follicle-stimulating hormone, TSH, estrogen, progesterone, sex hormone binding globuline, prolactin, 21 alfa hydroxyclase level, 17-hydroxyprogesterone and anti-Müllerian hormone for the diagnosis of PCOS.

In many cases hormones levels are found to be in normal range, thus it is suggested that end organ hypersensitivity or local production of androgens are the causes in those cases.

Endocrine, inflammatory diseases and drugs such as anti epileptics, anti psycotics, anti depressants, anti tubercular, cortoicosteroids (systemic and topical) anti neoplastics and halogens are known to cause acne. Therefore, a thorough history taking is important in any case of AOA. Questions directed to hirsutism, hair loss, menstrual irregularities and previous treatment are essential in the diagnosis of AOA.

12.6.5 Psychological Effect of Adults Onset Acne

This type of acne imposes an emotional and social burden on women by impairing self-perception and behaviors [39], health related quality of life (HRQoL), psychological status, and work productivity [40]. It affects self-perceptions and emotions, as evidenced by reports of dissatisfaction with appearance, lack of confidence, and need to use coping methods.

12.6.6 Treatment

The general principles of treatment in adult onset acne is alike those for adolescent acne. However, as many cases where the acne is resistant to conventional systemic, therapy with antibiotics and

retinoides, hormonal therapy should be considered also when blood tests are normal [41].

Hormonal therapy is divided to drugs blocking androgen receptors and drugs acting by decreasing androgen synthesis.

Combined oral contraceptive usually used for the treatment of acne are ethinyl estradiol/norgestimate, ethinyl estradiol/norethindrone acetate/ferrous fumarate, ethinyl estradiol/drospirenone, and ethinyl estradiol/drospirenone/levomefolate [42].

Combined oral contraceptive (COC) block androgen synthesis in the level of the ovary, increase sex hormone binding globulin production, binding free circulating testosterone and rendering it unavailable to bind and activate the androgen receptor. In addition, oral contraceptives inhibit 5 alfa reductase activity. Numerous randomized controlled clinical trials have assessed the efficacy of OCs in the management of acne [43–45].

The risks of COCs must be weighed against the risks of acne. COC's increase risk for thromboembolism, myocardial infarction, breast and cervical cancer [46, 47]. Common side effects are weight gain, breast tenderness, inter menstrual bleeding, hypercoagulability, melasma and mood changes. Acne improvement with COCs occurs frequently after 2–3 months therefore a combined therapy with other acne medication early in the treatment is recommended.

Corticosteroids block androgen synthesis and are used in cases of congenital or late onset adrenal hyperplasia. It is sometimes used for a short duration in severe flare ups of inflammatory cystic acne.

Cyproterone acetate acts by blocking androgen receptors. It is commonly prescribed in combination with OCP. Doses ranging from 50 to 100 mg daily. Its Common side effects include menstrual abnormalities, breast tenderness, nausea, vomiting, fluid retention, leg edema, headache, and liver dysfunction.

Spironolactone is an aldosterone and 5α receptor antagonist. It exhibits potent anti androgen activity by decreasing testosterone production and by competitively inhibiting binding of testosterone and dihydrotestosterone to androgen receptors in the skin. Doses ranges from 50 to 100 mg twice daily. Spironolactone is well tolerated overall, and its side effects are dose-related. Therefore, recommended initial therapy is 25–50 mg daily. Common side effects include diuresis, hyperkalemia, menstrual irregularities, breast tenderness, breast enlargement, fatigue, headache, and dizziness. It can be combined with COC.

Flutamide is a nonsteroidal selective androgen receptor blocker used in the treatment of prostate cancer. Common side effects associated with flutamide include gastrointestinal distress, breast tenderness, hot flashes, headache, xerosis and decreased libido. Severe dose-related hepatotoxicity occasionally occurs, high rates of side effects among users may decrease compliance with use.

12.6.7 Acne Cosmetica

Acne cosmetica is most commonly found in women between the ages of 20 to 40 years and is associated with the use of cosmetics containing comedogenic substances. It is characterized by persistent, low-grade, and closed comedones and slowly resolves with the cessation of use of the causative agent. Pomade acne is a variation of acne cosmetica seen almost exclusively in African Americans and is associated with the use of greases and oils applied to the scalp and face. Lesions are closely packed closed comedones found only at the site of pomade application.

12.6.8 Acne Excoriee

Acné excoriee is a psycho dermatological disorder that occurs mainly in young women. It is characterized by picking of the face, with minimal acne and significant scarring and linear erosions. Bodily focused anxiety and even body disfigurement disorder can be participated in the pathophysiology of acne excoriee [48]. Early treatment for acne excoriee is essential for the prevention of lasting cosmetic disfigurement due to scarring.

12.7 Treatment

Acne scars may negatively impact on an affected person's psychosocial and physical well-being and though acne lesions disappear typically at the end of the second decade, scars become more prominent as fat tissue decrease. Post inflammatory hyperpigmentation and erythema usually fade over months, however pigmentation changes may stay predominantly in darker skin types.

Treatment should be initiated after a thorough history and physical examination. In female patients, a menstrual and oral contraceptive history is important in determining hormonal influences on acne. Future pregnancies should be discussed in order to tailor a suitable therapy. In the case of male patients, these should be questioned on food supplement intake and the use of anabolic steroids. Psychological and social effects should be assessed in both females and males but emphasize must be on the adult female group. On Physical examination lesion morphology should be evaluated and the existence of comedones, papules, pustules, cyst and nodules should be determined. Secondary changes such as ice picked, rolling scars, box scars and hypertrophic scars should be carefully noted as well as post inflammatory hyperpigmentation.

12.7.1 Topical Therapy

Topical retinoids for acne are adapelene, tretioin and tarazotene. They have anti acne activity and are used as first line therapy alone or in combination with clindamycin or benzoyl peroxide. Topical retinoids allow for maintenance of clearance after discontinuation of oral therapy and are ideal for comedonal acne, when used in combination with other agents, for all acne variants. Benzoyl peroxide can be used as a monotherapy or in combination with topical antibiotic or retinoids. Other commonly used topical acne therapies include salicylic acid, antibiotics, azelaic acid, and sulfone agents. Monotherapy with topical antibiotics in the management of acne is not recommended because of the development of antibiotic resistance.

12.7.2 Systemic Therapy

Systemic antibiotics have been a mainstay of acne treatment for years. They are indicated for use in moderate to severe inflammatory acne and should be used in combination with a topical retinoid and BP [40]. The tetracycline class of antibiotics should be considered first-line therapy in moderate to severe acne, except when contraindicated because of other circumstances (i.e., pregnancy, <8 years of age or allergy). Adverse events with the tetracycline class will vary with each medication. Photosensitivity can be seen with the tetracycline class, doxycycline being more photosensitizing than minocycline. However, pigment deposition of the skin, mucous membranes and teeth is associated with minocycline and is common in patients taking higher doses for longer periods of time. Other minocycline known side effects are tinnitus and dizziness. Doxycycline is more frequently associated with gastrointestinal disturbances [49]. A rare complication of the tetracycline class is pseudotumor cerebri. Other antibiotics used for acne treatments are trimethoprim/sulfamethoxazole (TMP/SMX), erythromycin, azithromycin, amoxicillin, and cephalexin.

When prescribing systemic antibiotics, the issue of bacterial resistance remains a major concern. Limiting antibiotic use to the shortest possible duration, ideally 3–4 months can be accomplished with the concomitant use of topical treatment.

Oral contraceptives may improve acne for many women. They may be used alone or in combination with other acne treatments. While some women present with signs or symptoms suggestive of a hormonally induced worsening of acne, the use of combined oral contraceptives (COCs) is not limited to these individuals. Any woman with signs or symptoms of hyperandrogenism should be evaluated appropriately for an underlying cause. However, COCs may be beneficial to women with clinical and laboratory findings of hyperandrogenism and in women without these findings. Other hormonal therapies have already been discussed in adult onset acne section.

Oral isotretinoin is the first line of therapy for severe acne. It may also be used in the treatment of moderate acne that is either treatment-resistant or that relapses quickly after the discontinuation of oral antibiotic therapy. In patients with severe acne, isotretinoin should be initiated in doses of 0.5 mg/kg/day and subsequently increased to a full dose of 1 mg/kg/day after the first month with a cumulative goal dose between 120 and 150 mg/kg. Common side effects are cheilitis, xerosis, conjunctivitis, epistaxis, pruritus, irritation, photosensitivity, hypertriglyceridemia, myalgia, arthralgia [50]. The teratogenic effects of isotretinoin are well documented (class x) hence all women of child bearing age should be instructed to use two methods of contraception. Serum cholesterol and triglycerides, as well as transaminases must be followed routinely while taking the drug.

Chemical peels as salicylic acid and glycolic acid may be helpful in noninflammatory acne [51, 52] but multiple treatments are needed.

Light device therapies include pulse dye laser, fractional CO_2 laser, phototherapy with red and blue light, radiofrequency and photodynamic therapy are used to treat acne, but there is very limited evidence to recommend their use.

12.7.2.1 Hidradradenitis Suppurativae: Acné Inversa

Hidradenitis suppurativa (HS) is a chronic, recurrent, inflammatory disorder of hair follicles in apocrine gland-bearing sites resulting in abscesses and potentially fistula formation [53]. HS is associated with smoking, obesity, and inflammatory bowel disease. Several observations imply that sex hormones may play a role in its pathogenesis [54]. Hidradenitis suppurativae is more common in women [55], and the disease severity appears to vary in intensity according to the menstrual cycle. Peak incidence of HS occur during the third decade with sharp decline after the fifth decade likely due to onset of menopause in women [56]. Axillary and upper torso involvement are more common in women while men are significantly more likely to have perianal or perineal disease [57]. Men are more likely to have more severe disease than women.

	Female	Male
Infantile acne	+	+++
Adolescent acne	Peak 14–17 years	Peak 16–19 years More severe More scarring
Acne fulminans	Very rare	+
Acne conglabata	Very rare	+
Adult onset acne	+ Mandibular area, papules, pustules No comedones	–
Acne cosmetica	+ 20–40 years localized comedones	–
Acne excoree	+ Linear erosions, scarring	–

References

1. Bolognia JL, Jorizzo JJ, Schaffer JV, Callen JP, Cerroni L, Heymann WR, et al. Dermatology. 3rd ed. London: Elsevier; 2012.
2. McCarty M. Evaluation and management of refractory acne vulgaris in adolescent and adult men. Dermatol Clin. 2016;34(2):203–6.
3. Lucky AW, et al. Acne vulgaris in premenarchal girls: an early sign of puberty associated with rising levels of dehydroepiandrosterone. Arch Dermatol. 1994;130(3):308–14.
4. Strauss JS, Pochi PE. Effect of cyclic progestin-estrogen therapy on sebum and acne in women. JAMA. 1964;190(9):815–9.
5. Fabbrocini G, et al. Acne scars: pathogenesis, classification and treatment. Dermatol Res Pract. 2010;2010:893080.
6. Layton AM, Henderson CA, Cunliffe WJ. A clinical evaluation of acne scarring and its incidence. Clin Exp Dermatol. 1994;19(4):303–8.
7. Kellett SC, Gawkrodger DJ. The psychological and emotional impact of acne and the effect of treatment with isotretinoin. Br J Dermatol. 1999;140:273–82.
8. Del Rosso JQ, Levin J. The clinical relevance of maintaining the functional integrity of the stratum corneum in both healthy and disease-affected skin. J Clin Aesthet Dermatol. 2011;4(9):22.
9. Yamamoto A, Takenouchi K, Ito M. Impaired water barrier function in acne vulgaris. Arch Dermatol Res. 1995;287(2):214–8.
10. Luebbering S, Krueger N, Kerscher M. Skin physiology in men and women: in vivo evaluation of 300 people including TEWL, SC hydration, sebum content and skin surface pH. Int J Cosmet Sci. 2013;35(5):477–83.
11. Youn SH, et al. The skin surface pH and its different influence on the development of acne lesion according to gender and age. Skin Res Technol. 2013;19(2):131–6.
12. Silverberg NB. Whey protein precipitating moderate to severe acne flares in 5 teenaged athletes. Cutis. 2012;90(2):70–2.
13. Kraus SL, et al. The dark side of beauty: acne fulminans induced by anabolic steroids in a male bodybuilder. Arch Dermatol. 2012;148(10):1210–2.
14. Karvonen S-L. Acne fulminans: report of clinical findings and treatment of twenty-four patients. J Am Acad Dermatol. 1993;28(4):572–9.
15. Fyrand O, Fiskaadal HJ, Trygstad O. Acne in pubertal boys undergoing treatment with androgens. Acta Derm Venereol. 1991;72(2):148–9.
16. Traupe H, et al. Acne of the fulminans type following testosterone therapy in three excessively tall boys. Arch Dermatol. 1988;124(3):414–7.
17. Heydenreich G. Testosterone and anabolic steroids and acne fulminans. Arch Dermatol. 1989;125(4):571–2.
18. Hartmann RR, Plewing G. Acne fulminans: tratamento de 11 pacientes com o acido 13-cis-retinoico. An Bras Dermatol. 1983;58(1):3–10.
19. Chew EW, Bingham A, Burrows D. Incidence of acne vulgaris in patients with infantile acne. Clin Exp Dermatol. 1990;15(5):376–7.
20. Bolognia L. Dermatology. 3rd ed. London: Elsevier; 2012. p. 545–55.
21. Elling SV, Powell FC. Physiological changes in the skin during pregnancy. Clin Dermatol. 1997;15(1):35–43.
22. Tagawa N, et al. Serum concentrations of dehydroepiandrosterone and dehydroepiandrosterone sulfate and their relation to cytokine production during and after normal pregnancy. Clin Chim Acta. 2004;340(1):187–93.
23. Mesiano S. Roles of estrogen and progesterone in human parturition. Front Horm Res. 2001;27:86–104.
24. Yang C-C, et al. Inflammatory facial acne during uncomplicated pregnancy and post-partum in adult women: a preliminary hospital-based prospective observational study of 35 cases from Taiwan. J Eur Acad Dermatol Venereol. 2016;30(10):1787–9.
25. Wong RC, Ellis CN. Physiologic skin changes in pregnancy. J Am Acad Dermatol. 1984;10(6):929–40.
26. Meredith FM, Ormerod AD. The management of acne vulgaris in pregnancy. Am J Clin Dermatol. 2013;14(5):351–8.
27. Kong YL, Tey HL. Treatment of acne vulgaris during pregnancy and lactation. Drugs. 2013;73(8):779–87.
28. Butler DC, Heller MM, Murase JE. Safety of dermatologic medications in pregnancy and lactation: part II. Lactation. J Am Acad Dermatol. 2014;70(3):417–e1.
29. Hale TW, Hartmann PE. Hale & Hartmann's textbook of human lactation. 1st ed. Amarillo: Hale; 2007.

30. Tankeyoon M, et al. Effects of hormonal contraceptives on milk volume and infant growth: WHO special programme of research and development and research training in human reproduction. Contraception. 1984;30(6):505–22.

31. Williams C, Layton AM. Persistent acne in women. Am J Clin Dermatol. 2006;7(5):281–90.

32. Goulden V, Stables GI, Cunliffe WJ. Prevalence of facial acne in adults. J Am Acad Dermatol. 1999;41(4):577–80.

33. Preneau S, Dreno B. Female acne–a different subtype of teenager acne? J Eur Acad Dermatol Venereol. 2012;26(3):277–82.

34. Kaur S, et al. Etiopathogenesis and therapeutic approach to adult onset acne. Indian J Dermatol. 2016;61(4):403–7.

35. Seirafi H, et al. Assessment of androgens in women with adult-onset acne. Int J Dermatol. 2007;46(11):1188–91.

36. Goodman NF, et al. American Association of Clinical Endocrinologists, American College of Endocrinology, and androgen excess and PCOS society disease state clinical review: guide to the best practices in the evaluation and treatment of polycystic ovary syndrome-part 1. Endocr Pract. 2015;21(11):1291–300.

37. Legro RS, et al. Diagnosis and treatment of polycystic ovary syndrome: an Endocrine Society clinical practice guideline. J Clin Endocrinol Metabol. 2013;98(12):4565–92.

38. Lane DE. Polycystic ovary syndrome and its differential diagnosis. Obstet Gynecol Surv. 2006;61(2):125–35.

39. Kokandi A. Evaluation of acne quality of life and clinical severity in acne female adults. Dermatol Res Pract. 2010;2010:410809.

40. Tan JKL, Vasey K, Fung KY. Beliefs and perceptions of patients with acne. J Am Acad Dermatol. 2001;44(3):439–45.

41. Lakshmi C. Hormone therapy in acne. Indian J Dermatol Venereol Leprol. 2013;79(3):322.

42. Zaenglein AL, et al. Guidelines of care for the manageent of acne vulgaris. J Am Acad Dermatol. 2016;74(5):945–73.

43. Lucky AW, et al. A combined oral contraceptive containing 3-mg drospirenone/20-microg ethinyl estradiol in the treatment of acne vulgaris: a randomized, double-blind, placebo-controlled study evaluating lesion counts and participant self-assessment. Cutis. 2008;82(2):143–50.

44. Maloney JM, et al. Treatment of acne using a 3-milligram drospirenone/20-microgram ethinyl estradiol oral contraceptive administered in a 24/4 regimen: a randomized controlled trial. Obstet Gynecol. 2008;112(4):773–81.

45. Maloney JM, et al. A randomized controlled trial of a low-dose combined oral contraceptive containing 3 mg drospirenone plus 20 microg ethinylestradiol in the treatment of acne vulgaris: lesion counts, investigator ratings and subject self-assessment. J Drugs Dermatol. 2009;8(9):837–44.

46. Gierisch JM, et al. Oral contraceptive use and risk of breast, cervical, colorectal, and endometrial cancers: a systematic review. Cancer Epidemiol Prev Biomarkers. 2013;22(11):1931–43.

47. International Collaboration of Epidemiological Studies of Cervical Cancer. Cervical cancer and hormonal contraceptives: collaborative reanalysis of individual data for 16 573 women with cervical cancer and 35 509 women without cervical cancer from 24 epidemiological studies. Lancet. 2007;370(9599): 1609–21.

48. Gieler U, et al. Self-inflicted lesions in dermatology: terminology and classification–a position paper from the European Society for Dermatology and Psychiatry (ESDaP). Acta Derm Venereol. 2013;93(1):4–12.

49. Leyden JJ, et al. A randomized, phase 2, dose-ranging study in the treatment of moderate to severe inflammatory facial acne vulgaris with doxycycline calcium. J Drugs Dermatol. 2013;12(6):658–63.

50. Strauss JS, et al. Guidelines of care for acne vulgaris management. J Am Acad Dermatol. 2007;56(4): 651–63.

51. Grover C, Reddu BS. The therapeutic value of glycolic acid peels in dermatology. Indian J Dermatol Venereol Leprol. 2003;69(2):148.

52. Dreno B, et al. Expert opinion: efficacy of superficial chemical peels in active acne management–what can we learn from the literature today? Evidence-based recommendations. J Eur Acad Dermatol Venereol. 2011;25(6):695–704.

53. Alikhan A, Lynch PJ, Eisen DB. Hidradenitis suppurativa: a comprehensive review. J Am Acad Dermatol. 2009;60(4):539–61.

54. Riis PT, et al. The role of androgens and estrogens in hidradenitis suppurativa–a systematic review. Acta Dermatovenerol Croat. 2016;24(4):239.

55. Vazquez BG, et al. Incidence of hidradenitis suppurativa and associated factors: a population-based study of Olmsted County, Minnesota. J Investig Dermatol. 2013;133(1):97–103.

56. Revuz JE, et al. Prevalence and factors associated with hidradenitis suppurativa: results from two case-control studies. J Am Acad Dermatol. 2008;59(4): 596–601.

57. Canoui-Poitrine F, et al. Clinical characteristics of a series of 302 French patients with hidradenitis suppurativa, with an analysis of factors associated with disease severity. J Am Acad Dermatol. 2009;61(1): 51–7.

Miryam Kerner

Abbreviations

AMN   Acquired melanocytic nevi
AMNGT   Atypical melanocytic nevi of the genital type
CMN   Congenital melanocytic nevus
DEJ   Dermo-epidermal junction
ERbeta   Estrogen receptor beta
SONIC   The study of nevi in children

13.1 Melanocytic Nevi

Melanocytic nevi encompass a variety of lesions including congenital melanocytic nevi, acquired nevi, blue nevi, and Spitz nevi. These nevi can occasionally manifest gender differences depending on the different life cycles of the women versus the men and the unique anatomic differences.

M. Kerner
Department of Dermatology, HaEmek Medical Center, Afula, Israel

Rappaport Faculty of Medicine, Technion – Israel Institute of Technology, Haifa, Israel
e-mail: kerneram@netvision.net.il

13.1.1 Congenital Melanocytic Nevi (CMN)

CMN result from errors in migration and proliferation of melanocytic progenitor cells during embryogenesis. They are found in 1–6% of newborns [1]. Most CMN are present at birth, but a subset termed "tardive nevi" may appear after birth [2]. Clinically, CMN are symmetrical lesions with well-demarcated borders and a smooth to mammillated surface. Their color varies from light to dark-brown and may darken or lighten and acquire coarse hairs. CMN are usually classified by size into small (<1.5 cm), medium (1.5–19.9 cm), and large (>20 cm) [3]. Very large CMN (>40 cm), also known as giant CMN or "garment" nevi, are frequently accompanied by scattered smaller satellite congenital nevi. Recent data suggests that very large CMN and patients with many satellite nevi are at greatest risk for developing cutaneous and extracutaneous melanoma, and neurocutaneous melanocytosis [4, 5].

The dermoscopic structures found in CMN are pigment network and aggregated globules, which can present individually or as a combination of the two.

Other dermoscopic structures frequently observed in CMN include milia-like cysts, perifollicular pigment changes, and hypertrichosis. In addition, almost 70% of CMN will reveal vascular structures under dermoscopy, in particular comma vessels, dotted vessels, serpentine vessels, and target network with vessels [6, 7]. CMN manifest one of the benign dermoscopic patterns including reticular diffuse, reticular patchy, peripheral reticular with central hypopigmentation, peripheral reticular with central hyperpigmentation, globular, peripheral reticular with central globules, peripheral globules with central network or homogeneous area, homogeneous brown, tan, or blue pigmentation, two-component, multi-component, or a starburst pattern.

CMN with a reticular pattern are usually found on the lower extremities, whereas those with a globular pattern are most often located on the head, neck, and torso. This variation of patterns as a function of anatomic location might be due to the embryonic migration route taken by melanoblasts [7]. There is no difference between women and men in the anatomic location pattern variation. In addition to the patterns mentioned, acral CMN commonly present additional patterns consisting of crista dotted or the parallel furrow pattern. CMN on volar skin can also manifest a combination of the two aforementioned patterns, which is known as the "peas in the pod" pattern [8]. The predominant dermoscopic pattern of CMN doesn't vary based on sex [7].

Nevus spilus is a hyperpigmented patch studded with numerous discrete macules and/or papules, which give the appearance of speckling. These lesions are usually evident at birth and thus can be considered a variant of a CMN [9].

13.1.2 Acquired Melanocytic Nevi (AMN)

AMN (includes both common and atypical/dysplastic nevi) start appearing in early childhood and increase in numbers during adolescence [10]. They predominate on sun exposed skin above the waist. AMN appear to be at least threefold less common in blacks and Asians than in whites [11]. Dermoscopically, AMN usually manifest a reticular pattern (diffuse or patchy), peripheral reticular network with central hyperpigmentation, peripheral reticular network with central hypopigmentation, peripheral reticular with central globules, or

homogeneous pattern [12–15]. The most common dermoscopic nevus pattern in childhood is the globular pattern [9, 16]. The peripheral globular pattern is seen in a subgroup of growing nevi. A cross-sectional analysis of the dermoscopic patterns and structures of melanocytic nevi on the back and legs of adolescents found that the globular nevi are significantly more likely to be found on the back than on the legs, whereas reticular nevi predominate on the legs compared with other dermoscopic patterns [17].

13.1.3 Blue Nevi

Blue nevi are composed of dermal melanocytes that became arrested in the dermis during migration to the DEJ during fetal life [18]. They typically become apparent during childhood or adolescence. The common blue nevus presents as a symmetrical blue to black macule or papule, usually less than 1 cm in diameter, located on the head, neck, sacrum, or dorsum of the hands and feet. Cellular blue nevi are blue to black nodules generally 1–3 cm in diameter [18]. They are usually located on the buttocks or sacrum, but may also be found on the scalp, face, and feet. Women have cellular blue nevi 2.5 times as frequently as men. A histologic subtype known as epithelioid blue nevus is almost exclusively associated with the Carney complex [19].

The dermoscopic pattern of common blue nevi is a homogenous blue-grey to steel–blue pattern, with well-circumscribed pigmentation, which is diffuse and devoid of any other structures such as network, dots, globules, and vessels [6].

13.1.4 Halo Nevi (Sutton's Nevi)

Halo nevi are benign melanocytic nevi that have a peripheral zone of depigmentation. They are commonly encountered in the pediatric population with a prevalence of about 1% [20]. These nevi are in the process of undergoing involution via an immune-mediated reaction [21]. Once the nevus has completely regressed, the depigmented halo tends to re-pigment back to normal skin color. Although most halo nevi are inconsequential isolated lesions, the sudden appearance of multiple halo nevi can be associated with melanoma [19]. Approximately 80% of halo nevi exhibit a dermoscopic globular and/or homogenous pattern in the center of the lesion with a surrounding halo of de-pigmentation [9, 22].

13.1.5 Spitz Nevus

Typical Spitz nevi are well-circumscribed, dome-shaped papules less than 10 mm in diameter. They are benign melanocytic nevi with characteristic histological features that often overlap with melanoma [23]. Spitz nevi may take on different morphologies, some lesions presenting as pink-red papules and others as darkly pigmented papules; they may occur anywhere on the body but have a predilection for the head and neck [18]. Several series documented predominance of females of any age with lower extremity more affected, whereas the trunk was more frequently involved in men over 40 [24].

Spitz nevi display at least one of the dermoscopic melanoma-specific structures. The most common melanoma-specific structures seen in Spitz nevi are atypical network, negative network, crystalline structures, atypical dots and globules, streaks, blue white veil overlying a palpable portion of the lesion, atypical blotch, and atypical vascular structures [23]. There are several dermoscopic patterns that can be appreciated in Spitz nevi including starburst, globular, homogeneous (pink or black lamella), negative network, atypical (thick) reticular, and atypical (also known as multi-component) [6, 25, 26]. The patterns that reveal dermoscopic symmetry of structures and colors are likely to be found in typical Spitz nevi, whereas the disorganized patterns are likely present in atypical Spitz nevi.

Melanocytic nevi are a strong phenotypic marker of cutaneous melanoma risk [27]. Common and atypical nevi are both independent risk factors for melanoma [28]. Constitutional factors, such as hair, eye, and skin color, are known to be associated with the number of nevi [29].

Gender differences were also found to be associated with nevi count. The study of nevi in children (SONIC), a longitudinal study of nevi in a US cohort of children using digital photography over a 4-year follow up found that male students had 38% more nevi on their back than females did [29].

In multivariate analysis, male gender was associated with increased number of nevi. Other studies have also suggested that male children have more nevi than female children [30]. In an analysis of nevi in 2552 Australian schoolchildren aged 5–14 years, males had more nevi at all ages than did females; median total body nevi counts ranged from 40 at 5-years-of-age to 96 at 14-years-of-age in females, and from 51 to 120 in males, respectively [30]. High number of nevi is a high risk nevus phenotype. The etiologic fraction of melanoma attributable to high risk nevus phenotype may exceed 50% [29]. Atypia of nevi is another high risk nevus phenotype of melanoma. Along the SONIC study no significant differences were detected between boys and girls regarding the clinical phenotypic parameters of asymmetry of nevi, clinical borders of nevi, color, median and mean diameter of nevi [11], and mean surface area of nevi [17]. Nevi appear to share a common casual pathway with melanoma that involves interplay between constitutional factors and environmental factors of sun exposure [31]. Environmental factors including hours spent in the sun, sporadic use of sunscreen [11], and wearing a shirt or hat were associated with increased number of nevi [29]. Identifying predictors of nevi counts can assist in improving potential primary and secondary prevention by focusing relevant public health campaigns and clinical efforts to reduce melanoma deaths to the relevant subgroups.

13.2 Melanocytic Nevi and Pregnancy

Pregnancy is a unique period in the life cycle of women. Pregnancy influences melanocytic nevi of the women's body. Pregnancy-associated changes in melanocytic nevi are represented clinically in color changes: darkening and whitening [32], and symmetrical growth of the lesion [33]. Changes in the size of nevi most often occur on the front of the body, likely because of stretching of the skin during pregnancy [34].

Dermoscopically: the network becomes thicker and irregular, brown globules and black dots increase in number and size and become darker [35].

On the molecular level: as melanocytes are estrogen responsive, and estrogen levels increase during pregnancy, enhanced positivity for estrogen receptor beta (ERbeta) in common acquired nevi during pregnancy was noted (compared with non-pregnant controls) [36], including nevocytes in the epidermis and in the dermis. Acquired nevi (of non-pregnant women) with increased melanocytic atypia showed increased ERbeta in the nest of melanocytes in the epidermis. No additional increase in ERbeta in acquired atypical nevi was observed during pregnancy.

In biopsy samples of CMN of non-pregnant women, dermally associated nevocytes tended to have greater ERbeta immunoreactivity. Significant decrease in ERbeta immunoreactivity was observed in CMN from pregnant women compared with typical and atypical AMN of pregnant women. In melanocytic nevi excised from women who were taking oral contraceptives markedly increased numbers of estrogen- and progesterone-binding cells were documented [37]. This result raises a question regarding the correlation between oral contraceptive and melanoma risk. No official contraindication is reported by the pharmaceutical industry.

Pregnancy-associated changes in melanocytic nevi are transient in the clinical, dermoscopic, and molecular basis [35]. These changes were not associated with histologic atypia during pregnancy or after delivery [32] and there is no substantiated evidence of increased risk of malignant transformation of melanocytic nevi in gestation [35]. Factors of pregnancy, taking oral contraceptives, and degree of atypia are associated with enhanced ERbeta with the exception of CMN, where the melanocytes were unique in their response to pregnancy. These data support previous findings suggesting that AMN and CMN are biologically distinct, which may have strong implications for the progression of nevi to melanoma.

A gender-specific advantage for women versus men diagnosed with melanoma is seen for characteristics such as stage at presentation, site of primary tumor, and better prognosis: longer disease-free interval and longer survival time [38]. Post-menopausal women, however, do not enjoy such benefits of melanoma prognosis [38].

Recurrent comparisons between pregnant women diagnosed with melanoma to non-pregnant women diagnosed with melanoma of the same age at diagnosis, histological type and tumor thickness, stage of disease, and surgical management show there was no significant difference in outcome and survival rate between pregnant and non-pregnant women with melanoma [39].

Pregnancy-related changes in mole size or color during pregnancy can be normal, but all changing moles warrant careful examination, and irregular or asymmetric change is suspicious for melanoma [33]. There is no need to delay obtaining a biopsy specimen from a suspicious melanocytic lesion during pregnancy [34]. Future studies of the molecular changes and the potential influences on the progression of nevi to melanoma may provide future insight into the biological basis on the unique period of pregnancy.

13.3 Melanocytic Nevi of Special Sites

13.3.1 Breast Nevi

Melanocytic nevi as well as melanomas were reported in women's and men's breasts. The breast melanocytic nevi represent clinical, dermoscopic, and histologic atypical features that can be difficult to distinguish from melanoma and are site related. This atypia was documented in women as well in men [39].

Other special anatomical locations also representing site-related atypia are ear, the milk lines (axillary, breast, periumbilical, and inguinal regions), palms, soles, and flexural regions [40].

The clinical atypia that can be manifested in benign breast nevi include asymmetry, border irregularity, color variegation, and large diameter (>6 mm).

Dermoscopically, benign breast nevi as well as breast melanomas display atypical network and irregular dots and globules. Therefore, compared to melanomas from other sites, atypical networks and irregular dots and globules are poor indicators for breast melanoma. Presence of irregular blotches, nonuniform radial streak, blue-gray veil, and regression are highly specific for melanoma and should heighten clinical suspicion for melanoma arising on the breast [41].

Breast nevi present more atypical histologic features than the nevi from other sites: absence of demarcation of melanocytes at lateral margins, nest and discohesive pattern, and melanocytic atypia [40]. It is imperative for dermatologists and pathologists to distinguish benign melanocytic nevi with site-related atypia from malignant melanoma to avoid unnecessary surgical intervention [42].

Nevi on the nipple and areola are infrequent [43]. CMN are documented on the nipple and areola with a special variant sparing nipple and areola in large CMN involving the breast known as the Bork–Baykal phenomenon [44, 45].

13.3.2 Melanocytic Nevi of the Genitalia

Melanocytic nevi of the genital area are uncommon. They arise mainly in the vulva, although they can also occur less frequently in the perineum, mons pubis, and male genitalia: documented on penis and prepuce [46]. Genital nevi totaled only four (0.5%) in a series of 780 nevi [47].

The largest group of melanocytic genital nevi is females' vulvar nevi. Approximately 2% of adult females have vulvar nevi, accounting for 23% of all pigmented vulvar lesions. There is a small subset of benign nevi termed atypical melanocytic nevi of the genital type (AMNGT) that occur in young women. This subgroup isn't documented in the male genitalia and represents approximately 5% of vulvar nevi [48]. Vulvar nevi may present during childhood [48]. The incidental melanocytic nevi observed in the prepuce were detected in adults. This is probably because of the different ages at which genitalia are subjected to medical examination in the different genders. In a series of 372 consecutive circumcisions for phimosis, incidental preputial melanocytic nevi were detected in four (1.1%) patients [47].

The clinical presentation of the common vulvar nevi varies from symmetrical macules to symmetrical papules, ranging in color from pink to dark brown-black, or, rarely, blue. Their diameter is typically less than 1 cm. They are most often located on the labia majora, labia minora, and clitoral hood. AMNGT can present as asymmetric dark macules-papules larger than 1 cm in diameter. Compared with common vulvar nevi, AMNGT are more frequently located on the labia minora and have equal distribution between mucosal surfaces and hair-bearing skin of the external genitalia in adults [48]. Melanocytic nevi of the male genitalia vary from symmetrical lesions to unapparent [47]. Dermoscopically—according to a multicenter study by the International Dermoscopy Society, the combination of blue, gray, or white color with structureless zones are the strongest indicators when differentiating between benign and malignant mucosal lesions in dermoscopy [49]. The presence of white colors within vulvar lesions has a reported sensitivity of 100% for melanoma [50]. These described criteria don't have high sensitivity for early melanoma [50]. In common vulvar nevi globular and homogenous patterns predominate. In AMNGT a mixed pattern is observed most frequently [48].

Histopathologically, the common genital nevi exhibit regularly sized, evenly distributed nests of melanocytes without cytologic atypia [48]. AMNGT show histologic features overlapping with melanoma such as architectural disorder, cellular atypia growth as single cells with focal pagetoid spread and dense fibrosis in the papillary dermis [46]. Genital nevi including the AMNGT are believed to follow a benign clinical course [48].

Vulvar melanoma accounts for approximately 10% of vulvar malignancies. Two percent of all melanomas in females occur on the vulvar mucosa and represent about 2.6% of all melanomas [48]. Affected women are generally Caucasian between the ages of 40–70. It has an aggressive clinical course and is most often detected after metastasis to the groin has occurred [48].

Penile melanoma makes up about 0.1% of all primary and mucosal melanomas; it is more common in whites, and usually occurs between the ages of 50 and 70 years. Pre-existing or co-existing melanocytic nevi are occasionally found in this location [47].

Although the risk of transformation of genital lesions into melanoma is low, dermatologists should have a low threshold for biopsy of genital lesions with any clinical or dermoscopic features of melanoma.

Conflict of Interest The author has no conflict of interest to declare.

References

1. Price HN, Schaffer JV. Congenital melanocytic nevi-when to worry and how to treat: facts and controversies. Clin Dermatol. 2010;28:293–302.
2. Rhodes AR, Albert LS, Weinstock MA. Congenital nevomelanocytic nevi: proportionate area expansion during infancy and early childhood. J Am Acad Dermatol. 1996;34:51–62.
3. Consensus conference: precursors to malignant melanoma. JAMA. 1984;251:1864–66.
4. Slutsky JB, Barr JM, Femia AN, Marghoob AA. Large congenital melanocytic nevi: associated risks and management considerations. Semin Cutan Med Surg. 2010;29:79–84.
5. Kovalyshyn I, Braun R, Marghoob A. Congenital melanocytic naevi. Australas J Dermatol. 2009;50:231–40; quiz 241-232.
6. Marghoob AA, Braun RP, Kopf AW. Atlas of dermoscopy. Abingdon: Taylor and Francis; 2005.
7. Changchien L, Dusza SW, Agero AL, Korzenko AJ, Braun RP, Sachs D, et al. Age- and site-specific variation in the dermoscopic patterns of congenital melanocytic nevi: an aid to accurate classification and assessment of melanocytic nevi. Arch Dermatol. 2007;143:1007–14.
8. Minagawa A, Koga H, Saida T. Dermoscopic characteristics of congenital melanocytic nevi affecting acral volar skin. Arch Dermatol. 2011;147:809–13.
9. Haliasos EC, Kerner M, Jaimes N, Zalaudek I, Malvehy J, Hofmann-Wellenhof R, et al. Dermoscopy for the pediatric dermatologist part III: dermoscopy of melanocytic lesions. Pediatr Dermatol. 2013;30(3):281–93.
10. Stinco G, Argenziano G, Favot F, Valent F, Patrone P. Absence of clinical and dermoscopic differences between congenital and noncongenital melanocytic naevi in a cohort of 2-year-old children. Br J Dermatol. 2011;165:1303–7.
11. Oliveria SA, Geller AC, Dusza SW, Marghoob AA, Sachs D, Weinstock MA, et al. The Framingham school nevus study: a pilot study. Arch Dermatol. 2004;140(5):545–51.
12. Zalaudek I, Grinschgl S, Argenziano G, Marghoob AA, Blum A, Richtig E, et al. Age-related prevalence of dermoscopy patterns in acquired melanocytic naevi. Br J Dermatol. 2006;154:299–304.
13. Zalaudek I, Hofmann-Wellenhof R, Kittler H, Argenziano G, Ferrara G, Petrillo L, et al. A dual concept of nevogenesis: theoretical considerations based on dermoscopic features of melanocytic nevi. J Dtsch Dermatol Ges. 2007;5:985–92.
14. Scope A, Marghoob AA, Dusza SW, Satagopan JM, Agero AL, Benvenuto-Andrade C, et al. Dermoscopic patterns of naevi in fifth grade children of the Framingham school system. Br J Dermatol. 2008;158:1041–9.
15. Aguilera P, Puig S, Guilabert A, Julia M, Romero D, Vicente A, et al. Prevalence study of nevi in children from Barcelona. Dermoscopy, constitutional and environmental factors. Dermatology. 2009;218:203–14.
16. Zalaudek I, Schmid K, Marghoob AA, Scope A, Manzo M, Moscarella E, et al. Frequency of dermoscopic nevus subtypes by age and body site: a cross-sectional study. Arch Dermatol. 2011;147:663–70.
17. Fonseca M, Marchetti MA, Chung E, Dusza SW, Burnett ME, Marghoob AA, et al. Cross-sectional analysis of the dermoscopic patterns and structures of melanocytic naevi on the back and legs of adolescents. Br J Dermatol. 2015;173(6):1486–93.
18. Barnhill RL, Rabinovitz HS. Benign melanocytic neoplasms. In: Bolognia JL, Jorizzo JL, Rapini RP, editors. Dermatology. Basel: Mosby; 2007. p. 1722–3.
19. Schaffer JV. Pigmented lesions in children: when to worry. Curr Opin Pediatr. 2007;19:430–40.
20. Larsson PA, Liden S. Prevalence of skin diseases among adolescents 12–16 years of age. Acta Derm Venereol. 1980;60:415–23.
21. Zeff RA, Freitag A, Grin CM, Grant-Kels JM. The immune response in halo nevi. J Am Acad Dermatol. 1997;37:620–4.
22. Kolm I, Di Stefani A, Hofmann-Wellenhof R, Fink-Puches R, Wolf IH, Richtig E, et al. Dermoscopy patterns of halo nevi. Arch Dermatol. 2006;142:1627–32.
23. Kerner M, Jaimes N, Scope A, Marghoob AA. Spitz nevi: a bridge between dermoscopic morphology and histopathology. Dermatol Clin. 2013;31(2):327–35.
24. Cesinaro AM, Foroni M, Sighinolfi P, Migaldi M, Trentini GP. Spitz nevus is relatively frequent

in adults: a clinico-pathologic study of 247 cases related to patient's age. Am J Dermatopathol. 2005;27(6):469–75.

25. Soyer HP, Argenziano G, Hofmann-Wellenhof R, Johr RH. Color atlas of melanocytic lesions of the skin. New York: Springer; 2007.

26. Pellacani G, Longo C, Ferrara G, Cesinaro AM, Bassoli S, Guitera P, et al. Spitz nevi: in vivo confocal microscopic features, dermatoscopic aspects, histopathologic correlates, and diagnostic significance. J Am Acad Dermatol. 2009;60:236–47.

27. Scope A, Marchetti MA, Marghoob AA, Dusza SW, Geller AC, Satagopan JM, et al. The study of nevi in children: principles learned and implications for melanoma diagnosis. J Am Acad Dermatol. 2016;75(4):813–23.

28. Gandini S, Sera F, Cattaruzza MS, Pasquini P, Abeni D, Boyle P, et al. Meta-analysis of risk factors for cutaneous melanoma: I. Common and atypical naevi. Eur J Cancer. 2005;41(1):28–44.

29. Oliveria SA, Satagopan JM, Geller AC, Dusza SW, Weinstock MA, Berwick M, et al. Study of nevi in children (SONIC): baseline findings and predictors of nevus count. Am J Epidemiol. 2009;169(1):41–53.

30. English DR, Armstrong BK. Melanocytic nevi in children. I. Anatomic sites and demographic and host factors. Am J Epidemiol. 1994;139(4):390–401.

31. Dwyer T, Blizzard L, Ashbolt R. Sunburn associated with increased number of nevi in darker as well as lighter skinned adolescents of northern European descent. Cancer epidemiology and prevention. Biomarkers. 1995;4(8):825–30.

32. Nading MA, Nanney LB, Ellis DL. Pregnancy and estrogen receptor beta expression in a large congenital nevus. Arch Dermatol. 2009;145(6):691–4.

33. Wrone DA, Duncan LM, Sober AJ. Melanoma and pregnancy: eight questions with discussion. J Gend Specif Med. 1999;2(4):52–4.

34. Bieber AK, Martires KJ, Driscoll MS, Grant-Kels JM, Pomeranz MK, Stein JA. Nevi and pregnancy. J Am Acad Dermatol. 2016;75(4):661–6.

35. Rubegni P, Sbano P, Burroni M, Cevenini G, Bocchi C, Severi FM, et al. Melanocytic skin lesions and pregnancy: digital dermoscopy analysis. Skin Res Technol. 2007;13(2):143–7.

36. Nading MA, Nanney LB, Boyd AS, Ellis DL. Estrogen receptor beta expression in nevi during pregnancy. Exp Dermatol. 2008;17(6):489–97.

37. Ellis DL, Wheeland RG. Increased nevus estrogen and progesterone ligand binding related to oral contraceptives or pregnancy. J Am Acad Dermatol. 1986;14(1):25–31.

38. Travers RL, Sober AJ, Berwick M, Mihm MC Jr, Barnhill RL, Duncan LM. Increased thickness of pregnancy-associated melanoma. Br J Dermatol. 1995;132(6):876–83.

39. Rongioletti F, Urso C, Batolo D, Chimenti S, Fanti PA, Filotico R, et al. Melanocytic nevi of the breast: a histologic case-control study. J Cutan Pathol. 2004;31(2):137–40.

40. Nicolau AA, Aşchie M. Morphologic and immunohistochemical features of breast nevi. Rom J Morphol Embryol. 2013;54(2):371–5.

41. Merkel EA, Martini MC, Amin SM, Lee CY, Gerami P. Evaluation of dermoscopic features for distinguishing melanoma from special site nevi of the breast. J Am Acad Dermatol. 2016;75(2):364–70.

42. Ahn CS, Guerra A, Sangüeza OP. Melanocytic nevi of special sites. Am J Dermatopathol. 2016;38(12):867–81. Review

43. Kolm I, Kamarashev J, Kerl K, Mainetti C, Giovanoli P, French LE, et al. Diagnostic pitfall: pigmented lesion of the nipple—correlation between dermoscopy, reflectance confocal microscopy and histopathology. Dermatology. 2011;222(1):1–4.

44. Happle R. The Bork-Baykal phenomenon: a revised eponymic designation for the sparing of nipple and areola in large melanocytic nevi involving the breast. J Eur Acad Dermatol Venereol. 2017; 31:e214.

45. Baykal C, Solakoğlu S, Polat Ekinci A, Yazganoğlu KD. Large congenital melanocytic nevus on the breast sparing the nipple and areola. Pediatr Dermatol. 2015;32(4):514–7.

46. Ribé A. Melanocytic lesions of the genital area with attention given to atypical genital nevi. J Cutan Pathol. 2008;35(s2):24–7.

47. Val-Bernal JF, Val D, Garijo MF. Clinically unapparent melanocytic nevi on the prepuce. J Cutan Pathol. 2009;36(4):444–7.

48. Murzaku EC, Penn LA, Hale CS, Pomeranz MK, Polsky D. Vulvar nevi, melanosis, and melanoma: an epidemiologic, clinical, and histopathologic review. J Am Acad Dermatol. 2014;71(6):1241–9.

49. Blum A, Simionescu O, Argenziano G, Braun R, Cabo H, Eichhorn A, et al. Dermoscopy of pigmented lesions of the mucosa and the mucocutaneous junction: results of a multicenter study by the International Dermoscopy Society (IDS). Arch Dermatol. 2011;147(10):1181–7.

50. Rogers T, Pulitzer M, Marino ML, Marghoob AA, Zivanovic O, Marchetti MA. Early diagnosis of genital mucosal melanoma: how good are our dermoscopic criteria? Dermatol Pract Concept. 2016;6(4):43–6.

Clinical and Therapeutic Considerations of Acquired Melanocytic Nevi

14

Baruch Kaplan

The common mole can be referred to by various names. These include: typical acquired nevomelanocytic nevus, nevus cell, nevocytic nevus, and cellular nevus. They represent a benign proliferation of nevomelanocytes characterized by regularly shaped hyperpigmented macules or papules of a uniform color. Nevus cells, like melanocytes, are derived from the neural crest precursor cells. However, nevus cells differ from melanocytes in that they are found in aggregations and are devoid of dendritic processes. They typically appear after birth and most commonly increase in number over the course of the second and third decades of life and after that the numbers start to decline. The prevalence of nevi in females and males is similar. It is important to differentiate them from malignant lesions and to follow up for any changes in lesions over the course of years. During pregnancy nevi may darken in color or enlarge in size. Treatment is usually performed for cosmetic reasons. Females have a greater tendency to seek removal than males.

14.1 Epidemiology

Numerous studies have attempted to quantify the number of nevi in various ages groups. In one European study, the maximum number of nevi were found in the third decade in females and males at median numbers of 16 and 24 respectively [1]. In Australia, these numbers seem to be much higher peaking at 43 for males and 27 for females [2]. Whites have more nevi than blacks as well as individuals with a light complexion have more nevi than those with dark complexions [3]. It is not clear whether there is a difference in frequency according to gender. Most series have shown equal prevalence in males and female.

Sun exposure seems to increase number of nevi in exposed areas. The use of ultraviolet radiation sunscreens have been shown to decrease the number of nevi developing in children [4].

Genetic factors seemingly play a role in the development of nevi as well as the size, frequency and distribution.

14.2 Clinical Features

Nevi vary in clinical appearance. They usually have a homogenous surface and coloration with regular outlines and borders. *Junctional nevi* are light to dark brown flat macules varying in size from 1 to 6 mm in diameter. They are composed of nests of uniform nevus cells located com-

B. Kaplan
Mohs Micrographic Surgery Unit, Assuta Medical Center, Tel Aviv, Israel
e-mail: drbkaplan@gmail.com

© Springer International Publishing AG, part of Springer Nature 2018
E. Tur, H. I. Maibach (eds.), *Gender and Dermatology*,
https://doi.org/10.1007/978-3-319-72156-9_14

pletely within the lower epidermeis. Following their appearance they may persist as such and remain flat or may extend into the dermis and thus become *compound* (with junctional and intradermal components). They may be papillomatous, dome shaped or pedunculated skin colored, brown or pink. With further evolution, they lose their junctional melanocytic component and evolve into a *dermal nevus* with all the nevus cell lying in the dermis. The dermal nevus is usually larger than the junctional or compound nevus and appear as domed shaped or papillomatous lesions. Although, they are mostly tan or brown, at times they lack clinically evident pigmentation. The nevus cells of intradermal nevi are found in the deeper papillary and reticular dermis. In addition, the production of melanin by nevus cells is most prominent in the cells located in or near the epidermis and decreases with increasing depth. The nevus cells located deeply in the dermis usually do not contain melanin.

14.3   Diagnosis and Follow Up

Lesions are usually diagnosed easily by clinical examination. Clinical judgment along with the rule of "ABCDE "serves as the cornerstone of diagnosis [5]. Dermascopy is a useful tool to aid in the differentiation of pigmented lesions from non pigmented lesions as well as diagnosing malignant lesions [6]. The dermoscopic features of a junctional nevus show a uniform pigment network thinning out towards the periphery. Compound nevi, have various degrees of elevation and a somewhat lighter shade of brown than junctional nevi and are dermoscopically characterized by a globular architecture with multiple round to ovoid globules, sometimes forming a cobblestone pattern. Dermal nevi which are usually more elevated and are a lighter shade of brown or even skin-colored compared with compound nevi demonstrate dermoscopic features consisting of focal globules or globular-like structures. In addition, there may be pale to whitish structureless areas and fine linear or comma vessels.

Any changes in existing nevi should cause an increase in suspicion and warrant further investigation. The "ugly duckling" sign, referring to a nevus that stands out from other nevi should be considered for a biopsy.

Biopsies should be obtained for histopathologic examination of any suspicious lesions. It is advisable to perform excisional biopsies when possible. Immunostaining is routinely used in the pathology labs with very high specificity and sensitivity. Patients are recommended to undergo self- examinations and periodic Dermatological examinations. Digital photography and mapping is advisable for patients with numerous nevi.

14.4   Nevi and Pregnancy

Changes in the moles of pregnant women are frequently attributed to pregnancy such as an increase in size or darken in color, but recent studies suggest that pregnancy does not cause significant physiologic changes in nevi. Although, it is common for nevi on the breasts and abdomen to grow with normal skin expansion, studies that have examined melanocytic nevi on the backs or lower extremities have found no significant changes in size during pregnancy. Several studies have also investigated the belief that moles darken during pregnancy and have found insufficient evidence to support this idea [7]. In any case of aberrant changes or any clinical suspicion a biopsy should be taken.

14.5   Treatment

The great majority of nevi require no treatment. In the event of suspicion for malignancy a biopsy should be obtained for histopathologic examination. Removal of nevi for cosmetic reasons is very common. In the experience of the author, females seek elective removal of nevi, especially on the face, more often than males. The lesions can be removed under local anesthesia either by a shave biopsy or a fusiform excision (see Table 14.1) with excellent cosmetic results (Figs. 14.1 and 14.2). All lesions removed should

Table 14.1 Comparison of types of biopsies

Type of biopsy	Advantages	Disadvantages
Shave biopsy	Fast	Chance of incomplete removal
	Easily performed	Increased chance of recurrence
	Minimal scar	
	No sutures	
	Inexpensive	
Fusiform excisional biopsy		Time consuming
	Adequate biopsy specimen	Learning curve
	Decreased chance of recurrence	Elongated suture line scar
		Expense of consumables
		Requires surgical instrumentation

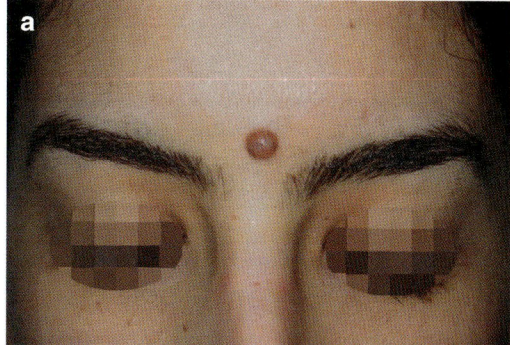

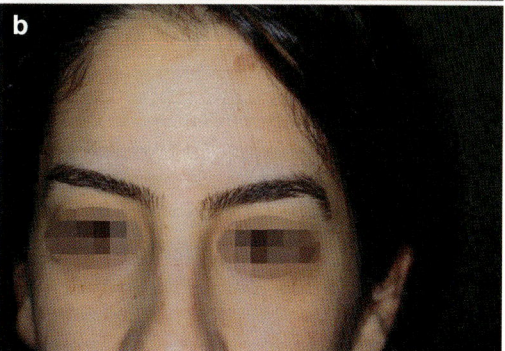

Fig. 14.2 Shave removal. (**a**) Compound nevus glabella. (**b**) Following removal of nevus

be sent for histopathologic examination for medical-legal reasons. In one study, 2.3% of clinically diagnosed benign nevi were microscopically diagnosed as malignant tumors, either melanomas or basal or squamous cell carcinomas [8]. Therefore, even when clinically there is no suspicion of malignancy the removed specimen should be submitted for pathologic evaluation.

Summary Acquired melanocytic nevi are commonly found in equal frequency in females and males. They appear following birth and increase in number over the course of several decades. They can be of various types correlating to the involvement of various levels in the epidermis and dermis. They must be distinguished from malignant lesions such as malignant melanoma. During pregnancy nevi may darken in color or enlarge in size. In general any suspicious lesions should be removed for histopathologic examination; however, removal is usually for cosmetic reasons.

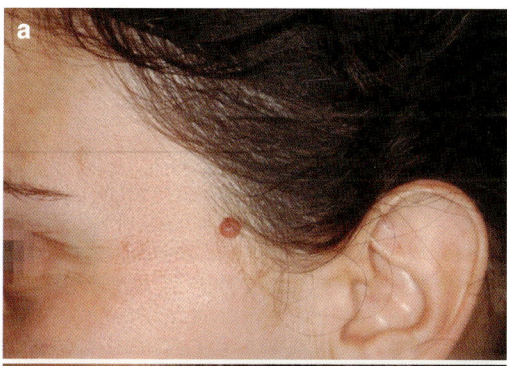

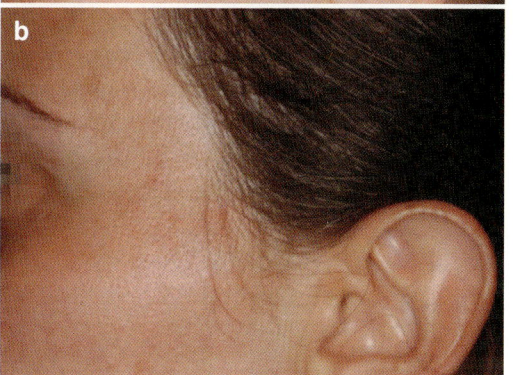

Fig. 14.1 Shave removal. (**a**) Compound nevus near hair line. (**b**) Following removal of nevus

References

1. MacKie RM, et al. The number and distribution of benign pigmented moles (melanocytic naevi) in a healthy British population. Br J Dermatol. 1985;113:167.
2. Nicholls EM. Development and elimination of pigmented moles, and the anatomical distribution of primary malignant melanoma. Cancer. 1973;32:191.
3. Coleman WP, et al. Nevi, lentigines, and melanomas in blacks. Arch Dermatol. 1980;116:548.
4. Gallagher RP, et al. Broad-spectrum sunscreen use and the development of new nevi in white children: a randomized controlled trial. JAMA. 2000;283:2955.
5. Tsao H, Olazagasti JM, Cordoro KM, et al. Early detection of melanoma: reviewing the ABCDEs. J Am Acad Dermatol. 2015;72(4):717–23.
6. Lucas CR, et al. Early melanoma detection: nonuniform dermoscopic features and growth. J Am Acad Dermatol. 2003;48:663.
7. Bieber AK, Martires KJ, Driscoll MS, et al. Nevi and pregnancy. J Am Acad Dermatol. 2016;75(4):661–6.
8. Reeck MC, Chuang T-Y, Eads TJ, et al. The diagnostic yield in submitting nevi for histologic examination. J Am Acad Dermatol. 1999;40:567–71.

Biology and Sex Disparities in Melanoma Outcomes

15

Adi Nosrati and Maria L. Wei

Abbreviations

8-OG	8-Oxo-deoxyguanosine
AR	Androgen receptor
DSS	Disease-specific survival
E2	17-βeta-estradiol
ERα	Estrogen receptor alpha
ERβ	Estrogen receptor beta
HCC	Hepatocellular cancer
NAC	N-acetylcysteine
ROS	Reactive oxygen species
PD-1	Programmed cell death protein-1
Xm	Maternal X chromosome
Xp	Paternal X chromosome

15.1 Introduction

The incidence of cutaneous melanoma in most developed countries has risen faster than any other cancer type since the mid-1950s [1–4]. While the outcome for thin, localized melanomas is excellent, the prognosis for advanced metastatic cases remains poor [5, 6]. Many prognostic factors have been proposed for melanoma: age,

A. Nosrati (✉) · M. L. Wei
Department of Dermatology, University of California, San Francisco, San Francisco, CA, USA

Dermatology Service, Veterans Affairs Medical Center, San Francisco, CA, USA
e-mail: maria.wei@ucsf.edu

sex, lesion thickness, anatomic location, ulceration, mitotic rate, lymph node involvement, tumor vascularity, elevated serum lactic dehydrogenase and presence and location of metastasis [7]. One of the most intriguing prognostic factors is sex. Significant differences exist in both melanoma incidence and mortality between men and women. Women present more frequently with early stage tumors, experience longer survival and have a better outcome compared with men [8–14].

In the United States in 2016, there were an estimated 76,380 new cases of invasive cutaneous melanoma, of which 61% (46,870) occurred in men, whereas the sex ratio of the total population was 0.97 M:F. In addition, of the 10,130 melanoma-related deaths, 67% (6750 deaths) occurred in men compared to 33% (3380 deaths) in women [15].

Furthermore, the probability of developing an invasive melanoma from birth to death was found to be 1.5 times higher in men compared with women [3% (1 in 33) vs. 1.9% (1 in 52)] [15]. In a large population-based setting with a total of 10,538 patients diagnosed with melanoma from 1993 to 2004 in The Netherlands, de Vries et al. studied sex differences in melanoma survival after adjusting for tumor-related variables (Breslow thickness, histology, body site and metastatic and nodal status) and found relative excess risk (RER) of dying of 2.70 (95% CI 2.38, 3.06) in males vs. females. The superior

© Springer International Publishing AG, part of Springer Nature 2018
E. Tur, H. I. Maibach (eds.), *Gender and Dermatology*,
https://doi.org/10.1007/978-3-319-72156-9_15

survival for women compared with men persisted after adjusting for multiple confounding variables including tumor thickness [12]. Most recently, a population-based study by Gamba et al. focused on 26,107 individuals from the US National Cancer Institute's Surveillance, Epidemiology, and End Results registry ages 15–39 years. They reported that young men had a 55% decrease in melanoma survival compared with age-matched young women, and concluded that male sex within all specific age groups and across all tumor thickness categories, histologic subtypes, and anatomic sites is associated with a disproportionate burden of melanoma deaths [14].

Stage specific survival was examined in a recent pooled analysis of 2672 patients with clinically localized (stage I/II) melanoma enrolled into four European Organization for Research and Treatment of Cancer prospective trials. In this analysis women were observed to have advantages in overall survival, melanoma-specific survival, and time to lymph node and distant metastases even when adjusted for prognostic factors such as age, Breslow thickness, body site, ulceration, performed lymph node dissection, and for treatment. These advantages were consistently in the 30% range. This study concluded that these differences are most likely caused by an underlying fundamental biologic sex differences, either tumor or host-related [10]. In another analysis by the same group, survival differences were studies in females and males with stage III and IV metastatic melanoma. In this study, in stage III patients, women had a superior 5-year disease-specific survival (DSS) rate compared with men (51.5% vs. 43.3%). In stage IV patients, women also exhibited an advantage in DSS (2 years survival rate 19.0% vs. 14.1%). This advantage was consistent across pre- and postmenopausal age categories and across different prognostic subgroups [16].

Gupta et al. recently studied gender disparity and mutation burden in metastatic melanoma patients. In the study, 266 metastatic melanomas were analyzed from The Cancer Genome Atlas

(TCGA) with a goal of finding genetically distinct differences between male and female. Interestingly, male tumors were found to harbor a higher mutation burden than female tumors (male median 298 vs. female median 211.5, male to female ratio [M:F] = 1.85, 95% CI 1.44, 2.39). They hypothesized that men exhibit less effective anti-tumor immune surveillance, and are thus less able to clear the mutation-rich population of tumor cells compared with women, leading to a higher mutation burden [17].

More broadly, women have an outcome advantage compared to men in many different cancer types, suggesting that shared molecular mechanisms may be responsible for the sex differences in a wide variety of malignancies. Micheli et al. examined the role of sex in determining cancer survival by analyzing 1.6 million population based EUROCARE-4 cancer cases and reported that women have a significant survival advantage for most cancers, including cancers of the salivary glands, head and neck, esophagus, stomach, colon and rectum, pancreas, lung, pleura, bone, kidney, brain, thyroid, Hodgkin disease and non-Hodgkin's lymphoma, as well as cutaneous melanoma [18]. This group reported that women had an estimated overall 2% lower relative risk of dying from melanoma compared to men. In addition, melanoma survival was 50% higher in women compared with men [19]. In the US, from 2009 to 2013, the Centers for Disease Control and Prevention report a higher incidence and mortality for men vs. women for almost all cancers, including melanoma, with the exception of thyroid cancer (http://www.cdc.gov/cancer/skin/statistics/race.htm, http://seer.cancer.gov/faststats/selections.php? –Output) (Table 15.1, Figs. 15.3 and 15.4).

While studies clearly indicate that women with melanoma have a better prognosis than men with melanoma, the basis for this phenomenon remains poorly understood. Several biological mechanisms have been proposed in the literature, e.g. differences in sex hormones levels, estrogen and androgen receptor expression, immune homeostasis and function, oxidative

Table 15.1 Age adjusted SEER incidence (2009–2013), U.S. death rates (2009–2013) and 5-year relative survival, percent (2009–2012)

Cancer type	Total	Incidence[a]		Total	Mortality[b]		Total	Survival[c]	
		Males	Females		Males	Females		Males	Females
Lung and bronchus	57.3	67.9	49.4	46.0	57.8	37.0	17.7	14.9	20.8
Colon and rectum	41.0	47.1	36.0	15.1	18.1	12.7	65.1	64.9	65.2
Melanoma of the skin	21.8	28.5	16.9	2.7	4.1	1.7	91.5	89.5	94.0
Bladder	20.1	35.3	8.6	4.4	7.7	2.2	77.5	78.9	73.0
Non-Hodgkin lymphoma	19.5	23.7	16.1	6.0	7.7	4.7	70.7	69.2	72.4
Kidney and renal pelvis	15.6	21.4	10.7	3.9	5.7	2.5	73.7	73.0	75.0
Thyroid	13.9	6.9	20.6	0.5	0.5	0.5	98.1	95.7	98.7
Leukemia	13.5	17.3	10.5	6.9	9.3	5.2	59.7	60.7	58.3
Pancreas	12.4	14.1	11.0	10.9	12.5	9.5	7.7	7.6	7.8
Oral cavity and pharynx	11.1	16.7	6.2	2.4	3.8	1.3	64.0	63.0	66.3
Liver and intrahepatic bile duct	8.4	13.0	4.4	6.1	9.1	3.6	17.5	17.1	18.5
Stomach	7.4	10.0	5.3	3.3	4.5	2.4	30.4	28.5	33.2
Myeloma	6.5	8.2	5.2	3.3	4.2	2.7	48.5	49.4	47.4
Brain and other nervous system	6.4	7.6	5.4	4.3	5.3	3.5	33.8	32.8	35.1
Esophagus	4.3	7.4	1.7	4.1	7.4	1.5	18.4	18.3	18.5
Larynx	3.2	5.6	1.1	1.1	1.9	0.4	60.7	61.5	57.4
Hodgkin lymphoma	2.6	3.0	2.3	0.4	0.5	0.3	86.2	85.4	87.3

Note: Incidence and death rates are per 100,000 and are age-adjusted to the 2000 US Std Population (19 age groups—Census P25–1130), https://seer.cancer.gov/
[a]Incidence source: SEER 2009–2013, 18 areas (San Francisco, Connecticut, Detroit, Hawaii, Iowa, New Mexico, Seattle, Utah, Atlanta, Sann Jose Monterrey, Los Angeles, Alaska Native Registry, Rural Georgia, California excluding SF/SJM/LA, Kentucky, Louisiana, New Jeresy and Georgia excluding ATL/RG)
[b]Mortality source: US Mortality Files, National Center for Health Statistics, 2009–2013, CDC. http://seer.cancer.gov/
[c]SEER 18 areas, 2009–2013. Based on follow-up of patients into 2013

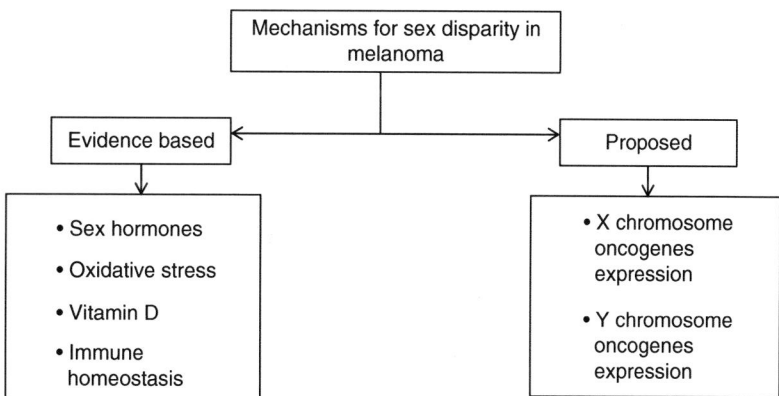

Fig. 15.1 Summary of the main biological etiologies for sex disparity in melanoma

stress response and X chromosome linked genes (Fig. 15.1). Behavioral differences between the sexes have also been proposed, such as differences health maintenance behaviors or in ultraviolet light exposure [13, 14, 20]. This chapter reviews the current state of knowledge of biological factors underlying sex disparities in melanoma outcomes (Table 15.2).

Table 15.2 Women survival advantage vs. men survival disadvantage in melanoma

	Women survival advantage	Men survival disadvantage
Sex hormones	High estrogen levels *Direct effect* • Inhibit the growth of human melanoma cell by inhibiting the expression of IL8 [21] *Indirect effect* • Induce B cell activation and prolong B cell survival by up regulating expression of CD22, SHP-1, and Bcl-2 [22–26] • Protect isolated primary B cells from B cell receptor-mediated apoptosis [22] • Act as a direct anti-oxidant by inhibiting iron-induced lipid peroxidation in liver cells [27] • Protect cells from oxidative damage [28]	High androgen levels *Direct effect* • Stimulate melanoma cell proliferation and tumor growth in a dose-dependent manner [29] *Indirect effect* • Increase T cell apoptosis [30] • Inhibit B cells differentiation [31] • Diminish protection against oxidative stress [32] • Increase vitamin D receptor expression and translocation to the nucleus [33–35]
Immune homeostasis	Increased B cell activation, proliferation and survival (via estrogen) [22–26] Increased T lymphocytes activation and proliferation [36]	Humeral and cell mediated suppression: • Decreased B cell activation, differentiation and survival [31] • Low CD$_3$ + cells-T lymphocytes [36] • Increased T cell apoptosis [30] • Low IL2 and TH1 responses and thus suppression of T and B-lymphocytes development [36]
Oxidative processes	Decreased oxidative damage to mitochondrial DNA [28] Estrogen protects cells against oxidative stress and acts as a direct antioxidant [28] High level of anti-oxidant enzymes [37]	High oxidative damage to mitochondrial DNA (fourfold higher compared with women) [28] Androgens diminish protection against oxidative stress [32] Decreased number of anti-oxidants and anti-oxidant enzymes [37] Elevated ROS cellular environment promote tumor metastasis [37–39]
Sex chromosomes	X chromosome inactivation process: [40–42] • Decreased tissue X chromosome oncogenes expression. [mi-RNAs, cancer/testis antigens (CT-X)] [43–47] • Tissue mosaicism in X chromosome associated oncogenes Lack of Y chromosome associated oncogenes	No X chromosome inactivation process: [40–42] • Monosomic expression of X chromosome specific oncogenes • Increased tissue expression of X chromosome oncogenes Y chromosome associated oncogene expression [TSPY] [48–52]

15.2 Female Sex Hormones

A frequently advanced hypothesis to explain the difference in survival between men and women involves the difference in the cellular hormonal environments. Although the influence of endogenous estrogen on the incidence and outcome of melanoma in women had been suggested by earlier studies [53] more recent large clinical studies did not find this association to be significant [10, 12, 18]. Exogenous estrogens such as oral contraceptives and hormone-replacement therapy have been studied for many years for their potential to influence risk of melanoma and although some studies supported an effect of exogenous estrogen on melanoma incidence and outcome [54, 55], other studies did not find this associations to be significant [56–59].

Parity (i.e. number of past pregnancies) was found to be inversely associated with the risk of developing melanoma in case controls studies and population based cohorts [60–62], but the underlying factors for this phenomenon remain unclear. Studies with smaller sample sizes found that women diagnosed with melanoma during pregnancy have increased risk of recurrence and mortality [63–66], but more recent large population based studies did not find any association between pregnancy and melanoma outcome [61, 67, 68].

It is likely that the conflicting nature of the observational clinical studies in aggregate is due in part to the difficulty in controlling for estrogen levels, which will vary due to ovarian cycling, age of onset of menopause, history of oophorectomy, use of oral contraceptives and hormone replacement therapy. In addition, the hormonal effects of estrogen and its metabolites are complex, since they can affect both the tumor directly and the tumor microenvironment as well as influence immune function, vitamin D metabolism and oxidative stress response. However, laboratory studies with cultured cells and animal models support a role for estrogens in contributing to the survival advantage for women vs. men with melanoma, either directly, discussed below, or indirectly via influencing immune cells, vitamin D metabolism or protecting against oxidative stress, as discussed in subsequent sections.

The effects of estrogens are mediated by the estrogen receptors α (ERα) and β (ERβ), which are members of the nuclear steroid receptor superfamily. ERα and ERβ classically mediate their action by ligand-dependent binding of the receptor to the estrogen response element of target genes, resulting in transcriptional regulation [69]. ERβ was found to be the predominant ER type in melanocytic lesions (both benign and malignant) suggesting that estrogen and estrogen like ligands might play roles in melanocyte physiology via ERβ [70]. de Giorgi et al. found a decrease in ER expression with the progression of melanoma invasiveness. ERβ protein levels were inversely correlated with Breslow thickness, with lower ERβ protein levels found in thicker tumors. The authors suggested that progression to metastasis in melanoma might involve a step in which melanomas become independent

of estrogen via loss of the ERβ receptor [70]. In agreement with those findings, when dysplastic nevi, lentigo malignas and melanomas were assessed for ERβ expression, the most intense immunostaining was found in melanocytes in dysplastic nevi with severe cytological atypia and in lentigo malignas. ERβ expression levels varied with the tumor microenvironment; i.e., melanocytes in proximity with keratinocytes > deeper dermal melanocytes in contact with stroma > minimally invasive melanomas > Clark Level III/IV or thick melanomas [71].

Kanda and Watanabe found that incubation of 17-βeta-estradiol (E2, the predominant estrogen during reproductive years) inhibited the growth of human metastatic melanoma cells in vitro with a concomitant reduction in constitutive interleukin-8 (IL-8) mRNA and secretion. In addition, the growth inhibition by E2 was counteracted by exogenously added IL-8, suggesting that estrogen can act as a growth suppressor in melanoma cells by inhibiting the expression of IL-8, which is transcriptionally regulated by ER binding. This effect was only observed in ER (+) cells and not ER (−) cells, indicating that, at least in vitro, estrogen mediates an inhibitory effect on melanomas via the ER and IL8 [21]. Richardson et al. [72] reported that E2 inhibited the invasiveness of cultured human melanoma cells grown on fibronectin. However, E2 was not found have antitumor activity in C57BL/6 mice inoculated with syngeneic B16 tumors [73]. 2-methoxyestradiol (2ME$_2$), an endogenous metabolite of 17-βeta-estradiol, inhibited the growth of a series of human melanoma cell lines in vitro [74, 75]. In vivo, 2ME$_2$ also inhibited growth of implanted murine B16 tumors, which was attributed to the anti-angiogenic effects of 2ME$_2$, although a direct effect on tumor cells was not excluded [76]. Cho et al. found that implanted B16 murine melanoma cells grew more rapidly in ERβ knockout mice than in congenic C56BL/6 mice with intact ERβ, suggesting that the presence of ERβ in the tumor microenvironment was protective against tumor growth [77]. Thus estrogen and its metabolites appear able to exert a direct inhibitory activity on melanoma cells and can have an indirect inhibitory effect via influencing the tumor microenvironment.

15.3 Male Sex Hormones

Androgen receptors have a similar mechanism of action as the estrogen receptors, binding ligand (testosterone/5α-dihydroxytestosterone), then translocating to the nucleus and interacting with DNA binding sites to elicit transcriptional regulation of target genes. Studies from androgen receptor knockout mouse models demonstrate that androgens influence the promotion of tumorigenesis in liver and prostate cancer and promote both tumorigenesis and metastasis in bladder, lung, kidney cancers [78], which have sex dis-

parities in incidence and outcome favoring women (Table 15.1, Figs. 15.2, 15.3, and 15.4), suggesting that androgen driven tumorigenesis is a shared mechanism for sex-based differences in cancer incidences and outcomes.

In 1980 Rampen and Mulder found that the interval to progression in women with melanoma was longer compared to in men, survival after metastasis was longer in women, tumor-volume doubling time of metastatic lesions was increased in women and there was no difference in survival between pre- and postmenopausal women with melanoma. This group proposed that androgens could explain the shorter survival time in men with melanoma, irrespective of the hormonal status of women [79]. In support of this, a retrospective study by Brinton et al. assessed cancer risk

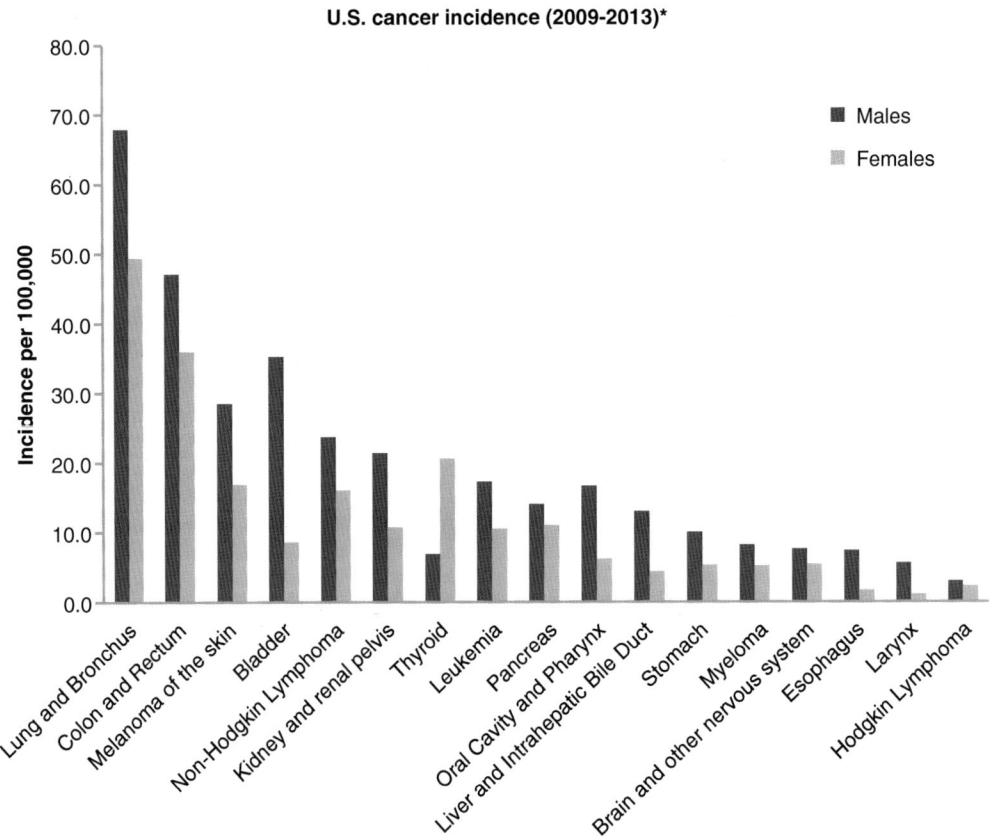

Fig. 15.2 U.S. cancer incidence rates, 2009–2013. SEER 18 areas (San Francisco, Connecticut, Detroit, Hawaii, Iowa, New Mexico, Seattle, Utah, Atlanta, San Jose-Monterey, Los Angeles, Alaska Native Registry, Rural Georgia, California excluding SF/SJM/LA, Kentucky, Louisiana, New Jersey and Georgia excluding ATL/RG). http://seer.cancer.gov/. *Ordered by the total incidence of each cancer

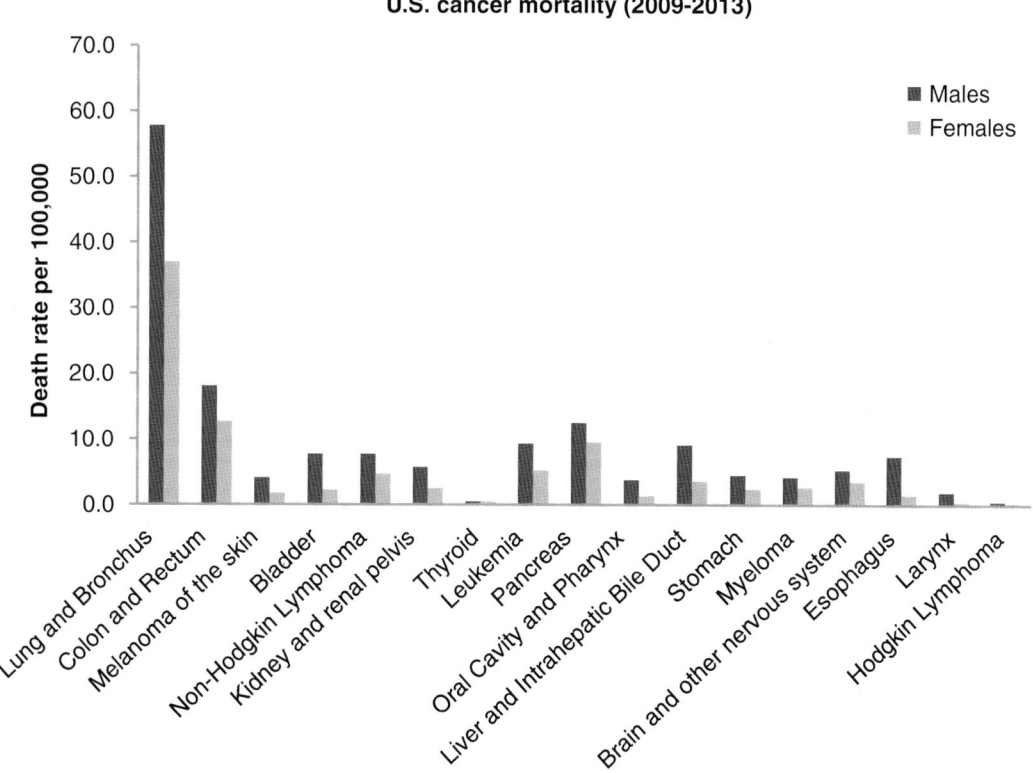

Fig. 15.3 U.S. cancer mortality rates, 2009–2013. US Mortality Files, National Center for Health Statistics, CDC. http://seer.cancer.gov/

among 2560 infertile women with androgen excess disorders and found that the standardized incidence ratio was statistically significant for breast cancer (1.31, 95% CI 1.05, 1.62), uterine cancer (2.02, 95% CI 1.13, 3.34) and melanoma (1.96, 95% CI 1.12, 3.18). An alternative analysis by the authors comparing cancer risks among women with different androgen excess disorders to those without these disorders also showed a twofold increase in melanoma incidence, and while this result did not reach significance, the results suggest the possible association between androgen excess and the risk of developing melanoma and other cancers [80].

Morvillo and colleagues demonstrated the existence of androgen receptors (ARs) in human melanoma cell lines and found that the incubation of these cells in the presence of an androgen significantly stimulated cell proliferation; this stimulation could be reversed by the anti-androgen flutamide (or its active metabolite hydroxyflutamide). Flutamide was also found to be effective in diminishing tumor growth and increasing the survival rate of the animals when administered to nude mice inoculated with human melanoma [81]. Allil et al. investigated the in vivo and in vitro effect of testosterone on tumor growth and melanogenesis on cultured murine melanoma cells. Testosterone was found to increase cell proliferation in vitro in a dose-dependent manner; in vivo assays demonstrated increasing tumor sizes in castrated mice receiving increasing concentrations of testosterone [29].

In another in vivo study, Hsueh et al. demonstrated that treatment with an anti-androgen influences the immune response to melanoma tumors. Administration of flutamide increased murine splenocyte proliferation and interferon secretion in response to irradiated murine B16

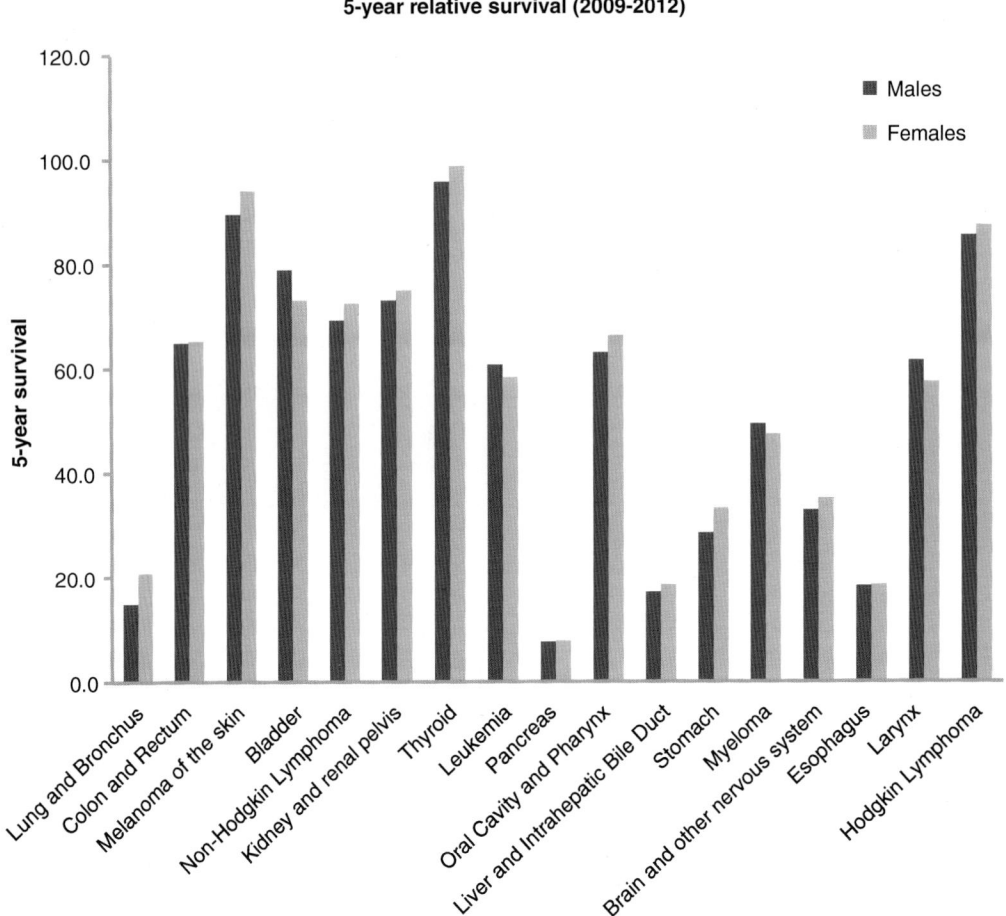

Fig. 15.4 U.S. cancer survival; 5-year relative survival, 2009–2012. SEER 18 areas. Based on follow-up of patients into 2013

melanoma cells, and when flutamide was administered with an irradiated B16 vaccine, this combination improved the survival of mice implanted with non-irradiated B16 tumor cells, compared with non-flutamide treated mice, suggesting that androgen blockade with flutamide enhanced the immune response to the tumor [82].

Together, the clinical and laboratory studies suggest that estrogens are directly and indirectly inhibitory for melanoma tumorigenesis while androgens can directly promote melanoma tumorigenesis and indirectly inhibit melanoma immunotherapy. These opposing actions and the differing hormonal milieu in men vs. women likely contribute to the survival disparities seen in melanoma.

15.4   Immune Homeostasis

Studies in immunocompromised patients indicate that competency and function of the immune system has a significant influence on melanoma outcomes. Patients with chronic lymphocytic leukemia or non-Hodgkins lymphoma have a 2.8-fold increased risk of dying from melanoma [83], and patients with a history of a solid organ transplant had a decreased melanoma specific survival rate for thicker tumors [84, 85].

There are baseline differences in the immune systems of men and women, both measured and observed functionally. For example, women on average have a higher measured IgG and IgM levels compared with men [86]. The total lymphocyte count in men was found to be similar to that in women [87], but the percentage of CD3+ cells-T lymphocytes in men is slightly lower compared to in women, by 5%, and men were found to have a reduced TH1 response, with 50% reduced IL-2 production in men compared with women [86]. IL-2 is a major cytokine responsible for the T lymphocyte activation and proliferation and has important growth promoting function in relation to B lymphocyte development. These studies suggest a relative attenuation of the adaptive immune response in men as compared with women [36].

15.4.1 Sex Hormones and Their Effect on the Immune System

The sex hormones can potentially exert additional differential effects on immune cells since the ERα and ERβ receptors are expressed by many types of immune cell, including T cytotoxic cells, B cells, dendritic cells (DCs), macrophages, neutrophils and murine NK cells [88], and the AR is expressed by B cells and murine macrophages [86]. However, the data reported are complex, due to biphasic responses to hormones, cell type specific responses and technical differences in experimental protocols; studies are reviewed by Fish [40]; a few salient results are summarized below.

Estrogen stimulates monocytes to produce IL-10, which in return triggers IgG and IgM secretion in human peripheral blood monocytes [89]. Grimaldi et al. identified genes that are differentially regulated by estrogen in mouse B cells [22]. They found that binding of estrogen directly upregulated expression of CD22, SHP-1, and Bcl-2, proteins known to play a role in B cell survival and activation [23–25]. They also observed an expansion of Bcl-2+ B cell progenitors in the bone marrow of the 17-βeta-estradiol treated mice. Furthermore, estrogen treatment protected isolated primary B cells from B cell receptor-mediated apoptosis, suggesting that estrogen influences the immune system by inducing a genetic program that alters the survival and activation of B cells. The same group also showed that E2 administration rescues a population of naive autoreactive B cells in mice that would normally be deleted at an immature stage of B cell development, altering the process of self-tolerance, which may have implications for tumor surveillance capacity [26]. Normal female mice have a higher baseline incidence of autoantibodies, and estrogen administration increases the frequency of those antibodies in non-immunized mice [90, 91], again suggestive of an increased tumor surveillance capacity. And E2 significantly stimulated B cell differentiation in response to pokeweed antigen [31]. Interestingly, estrogen was also found to be a potent driver of regulatory T cells (T-reg cells) that play a significant role in the maintenance of self-tolerance mechanism [92]. These results implicate the probable contribution of estrogen to the development of autoimmune diseases, which are significantly more prevalent in women compared with men [92].

Testosterone, in contrast, is reported to have opposing effects on immune cells compared with estrogen, however, the mechanism was found to be different compared with estrogen [92]. Testosterone directly inhibits the secretion of IgG and IgM by human peripheral blood mononuclear cells [93], and indirectly reduces the production of IL-6 by monocytes [93]. It was also found to exert significant inhibitory effect on human B cell differentiation in response to pokeweed mitogen [31]. The inhibitory effects of testosterone are found in other species as well. In an in-vivo study by Duffy and colleagues, male and female starlings were wild-caught, housed in the laboratory, and implanted with either empty silastic capsules or capsules containing testosterone and found that antibody responses in both sexes to antigenic challenge were significantly suppressed. Cell-mediated responses to phytohemagglutinin stimulation were also significantly suppressed in testosterone-treated males, but not in females, compared to same-sex controls [94].

15.4.2 Immunotherapies

In the recent years, new immunomodulatory therapies for melanoma have shown promising results, with higher response rates and more durable responses in patients with advanced melanoma [95–98]. One approach targets the PD-1 signaling pathway, which modulates the activity of T-cells that have become nonresponsive after encountering PD-1 ligands in the tumor microenvironment. B7-H1, also known as PD-L1, is a ligand for PD-1 and is expressed aberrantly on melanoma cells [99]. Since estradiol has been shown to upregulate the expression of PD-1 in several types of immune cells, including regulatory T cells [100, 101], it could have been expected that anti-PD-L1 therapies would be more effective in females. However, a recent study conducted by Lin et al. presents opposite results; they report differential melanoma tumor growth suppression in male vs. female mice after treatment with anti-B7-H1 antibody. In male mice, tumor growth was reduced by 91% vs. 68% reduction in female mice. This marked differential response was attributed to the finding that T-regs in females were rescued from PDL-1 engagement more than in males since male T-regs expressed less PD-1 due to a low exposure to estradiol [92, 102]. A recent clinical study have found similar results reporting a lower response to anti-PD-1 monotherapy in women compared with men [103].

In summary, there are baseline differences in the immune systems of men vs. women and there is interplay between the hormonal milieu and immune function. Given the novelty of this field, however, sex-dependent immune differences in response to immunotherapy require further research with a special focus on identifying the nature of these differences in immunoregulatory pathways [104]. Additionally, in order to optimize the response to immunotherapies, clinical trials will need to take into account the differences in the immune response between the genders [92].

15.5   Reactive Oxygen Species

By-products of oxygen metabolism lead to the production of reactive oxygen species (ROS), which can damage a wide range of molecules leading to oxidative stress [105] and increased

melanoma tumorigenesis [106]. Joosse et al. proposed that sex difference in ability to neutralize oxidative stress caused by ROS is a possible biological mechanism underlying the melanoma survival advantage in females [38], since the primary melanoma tumor environment is understood to be one of high levels of oxidative stress: melanoma cells generate large amounts of ROS compared with surrounding tissues or melanocytes [38, 107, 108], tumor associated immune cells secrete ROS [109] and ultraviolet (UV) radiation further increases oxidative stress in the skin and melanocytes [38, 106, 110]. This hypothesis is supported by the findings of Sander et al. who compared skin biopsies of melanoma with age-matched benign melanocytic nevi and young healthy controls, analyzed the expression of the antioxidant enzymes copper–zinc superoxide dismutase, manganese superoxide dismutase and catalase by immunohistochemical techniques and found a significant overexpression of the antioxidant enzymes in human melanoma biopsies compared with surrounding non-tumor tissue, benign melanocytic nevi, and skin from control subjects, suggesting that the melanoma cells were responding to increased oxidative stress [107].

There appear to be baseline differences in the oxidative environment in the skin of males vs. females, which are amplified by UV-induced oxidative stress. The skin of male hairless mice was found to have a lower baseline level of anti-oxidant enzyme, and approximately a tenfold lower anti-oxidant functional capacity compared to in females. After UVB radiation, the skin of females exhibited a markedly greater induction of anti-oxidant level, greater anti-oxidant functional capacity and lower levels of 8-oxo-deoxyguanosine (8-OG, the most common type of DNA damage caused by ROS), compared to male skin [111].

Other tissue types in addition to skin exhibit differences in oxidative capacity when female vs. male cells are compared. Malorni et al. found that rat vascular smooth muscle cells demonstrate sexual dimorphism in their oxidative state: female cells have less ROS and higher levels of antioxidant enzymes; in response to oxidative stress induced by ultraviolet B (UVB) radiation, the male cells produce more ROS compared to female cells, and the levels of antioxidant enzyme activity in male cells are reduced to below those of control non-UV irradiated male cells [112]. Borrás et al. found differences in inherent mitochondrial oxidative stress between males and females rat liver cells. They found that male liver cells express lower levels of anti-oxidant enzymes, higher levels of reactive oxygen species (ROS) such as peroxides, and that oxidative damage to mitochondrial DNA in males was threefold higher than that in females [28]. Ovariectomy in female rats increased peroxide production in liver cells to male cell levels, decreased levels of anti-oxidant enzymes to male levels, and both peroxide and anti-oxidant enzymes levels in female cells were restored to control female levels by estrogen replacement therapy [28]. This group found that 17-βeta-estradiol incubated with isolated mitochondrion also reduced hydrogen peroxide (an ROS) production in a dose dependent manner [113]. Ruiz-Larrea et al., found that addition of 17-βeta-estradiol to isolated rat hepatocytes efficiently prevented cellular lipid oxidation induced by the Fe(III)/ADP complex [27].

Bokov et al. found that ovariectomy induced menopause in mice increased vulnerability to oxidative damage and attendant mortality. They administered low yet physiologically effective dose of E2 using subcutaneous time-release pellets to ovariectomized mice. Two weeks after E2 pellet implantation, sham-operated female mice, ovariectomized mice, and ovariectomized + E2-supplemented mice were injected with a paraquat, a ROS catalyzer, and survival was monitored. They found that ovariectomy resulted in a small increase in paraquat-induced mortality and this could be rescued by E2 supplementation. An equivalent experiment was performed on sham-operated, orchidectomized male mice and the survival of male mice was improved by orchidectomy suggesting that testosterone diminishes protection against oxidative stress [32].

Modifying the anti-oxidant cellular environment has been shown to influence the onset of UV induced melanomas. The exogenously added anti-oxidant N-acetylcysteine (NAC) reduced the level of UV induced ROS in cultured immortalized mouse melanocytes and protected treated melanocytes from the formation of the UV-induced oxidative products 8-OG and cyclobutane pyrimidine dimers. Supplementing the diet of pregnant mice with NAC delayed the onset of UV induced melanomas in neonatal mice [106]. Thus it is clear that the anti-oxidant microenvironment affects melanoma biology, but the effect on survival has not been determined.

In summary, male cells of various tissue types have an elevated ROS cellular environment, due to the expression of lower levels of anti-oxidant enzymes compared with females [37, 39]; estrogen appears to have a direct antioxidant and protective effects, while testosterone may potentiate oxidative stress and this difference may contribute to disparities in melanoma outcomes [38].

15.6 Vitamin D

Vitamin D, 1,25-dihydroxyvitamin D3 [1,25(OH)$_2$ D$_3$], has been suggested to have a protective effect on melanoma outcomes [114]. There are sex differences in vitamin D plasma levels, with the level in young adult and older female rats significantly lower than males of the same ages [115] and estrogens modulate 1,25(OH)$_2$ D$_3$ activity by upregulating vitamin D receptor (VDR) expression in several cell types and by causing translocation of the VDR from the cytoplasm to the nucleus, shown in cultured human fibroblasts [33–35]. The vitamin D receptor is expressed at a variety of levels on cultured human melanoma cell lines and 1,25(OH)$_2$ D$_3$ inhibited both DNA synthesis and cell growth and induced apoptosis in many but not all melanoma cell lines [116–121]. 1,25-(OH)$_2$ D$_3$ inhibited human melanoma cell doubling time [122] and decreased the number of invading mouse B16 melanoma cells in vitro and the number metastases in vivo [123].

While the in vitro studies indicate an inhibitory effect of 1,25-(OH)$_2$ D$_3$ on cultured melanoma cells lines, definitive randomized controlled clinical studies are lacking. In an observational study, Newton-Bishop and colleagues correlated a higher vitamin D serum level with thinner Breslow depth at diagnosis; these patients were less likely to relapse or die of any cause [114, 124]. However, a recent large meta-analysis which examined the evidence for a relation between high vitamin D concentrations or vitamin D supplementation and clinical outcomes found that no conclusion could be drawn from currently existing studies for an effect on melanoma prognosis [125].

15.7 X Chromosome Gene Expression

There is sexual dimorphism in gene expression throughout the human genome. A microarray analysis of 23,574 transcripts revealed that the extent of sexual dimorphism in gene expression ranges from 14% (in the brain) to 70% (in the liver) of active genes. These genes display highly tissue-specific patterns of expression and are enriched for distinct pathways [126, 127]. Thus autosomal genes demonstrate a sex-biased expression pattern [128], and likely play a role in the mechanisms described in the preceding sections. In addition, the differential expression of X chromosome genes in women vs. men has been proposed to influence the sex disparity in cancer [129] and will be the focus of the discussion here.

The X chromosome encodes approximately 1500 genes. Many of the X-linked genes encode key metabolic and regulatory proteins, including hormone homeostasis proteins such as the androgen receptor, members of the apoptotic cascade, glucose metabolic enzymes, superoxide-producing machinery. In contrast, the Y chromosome has approximately 344 genes, highlighting the greater X chromosome genetic repertoire. A role for X linked genes in contributing to the sex disparity observed for melanoma outcomes has been suggested but no direct or indirect evidence specifically links this mechanism with melanoma disparities. However, several studies provide intriguing findings that suggest a role for X linked genes in sex based melanoma outcome differences.

15.7.1 X Inactivation Process

Cells in women carry both paternal (Xp) and maternal X (Xm) chromosomes, whereas men carry only the maternal chromosome (Xm). However, women are tissue mosaics for the X-linked genes, due to the inactivation of one copy of the X chromosome in each cell, so that approximately half of the female cells express either Xm or Xp [41] and in each tissue type, there is X chromosome heterogeneity. X chromosome inactivation likely has profound but somewhat unpredictable effects on tumorigenesis in women compared with in men. The inactivation process is not entirely understood and until recently was thought to be a random process; however, recent studies suggest otherwise [42, 130]. Approximately 15% of X chromosomes escape inactivation and another 10% show variable patterns of inactivation [131]. Skewing of X inactivation can lead to a selection of wild-type cells over mutant cells, giving women an advantage on a cellular basis [40]. In addition, Indsto et al. found that 35% of metastatic melanomas from women had loss of heterozygosity; this group noted that since in each individual cell in women the X chromosome is functionally monosomic, each observation of LOH has a 50% probability of causing a complete knockout of local gene functions in the absence of other compensatory changes in copy number or gene activation [132].

In men, every organ and tissue type is identically monosomic for the maternal X chromosome. The potential deleterious effects of X chromosome monosomy is illustrated by findings in the Turner syndrome, in which women inherit only one X chromosome (complete X-chromosome monosomy) or only part of a second X chromosome (partial X-chromosome monosomy) [133]. Schoemaker et al. compared the risk of cancer in women with Turner syndrome with that of the general population. They followed a national cohort of 3425 women who were cytogenetically diagnosed with Turner syndrome in Great Britain between 1959 and 2002 for cancer incidence. A total of 86 malignant neoplasms were recorded during the follow up. The standardized incidence ratio for cutaneous melanoma was increased at 2.2 (95% CI 1.0, 4.4; n = 8) compared to the general population but did not reach significance; risks were significantly increased for others tumors: tumors of the CNS (n = 13; 4.3, 95% CI 2.3, 7.4), cancers of the bladder and urethra (n = 5; 4.0, 95% CI 1.3, 9.2) and eye (n = 2; 10.5, 95% CI 1.3, 37.9). While the results were not adjusted for any growth factor or estrogen replacement therapy received by the study subjects, and the numbers were small, they do suggest that X monosomy carries an elevated risk of tumorigenesis [134].

15.7.2 X Chromosome Oncogenes

Several loci located on the X chromosome have been associated with cancer progression and oncogenic protein expression. MicroRNAs (miR-NAs) are small non-coding RNAs important for a diverse range of biological functions in both normal and pathological settings, are encoded on the X chromosome at a 2-fold higher density than on autosomes, and are absent on the Y chromosome [135]. Significant data have accumulated showing that dysregulated miRNAs act as oncogenes (onco-miRs) or tumor suppressors (TS-miRs) through their effects on various pathways critical to the cancer phenotype [43, 136].

Streicher et al. studied the role of miRNA in the pathogenesis of malignant melanoma. They compared miRNA expression profiles in skin punches from 33 metastatic melanoma patients and 14 normal healthy donors and identified a cluster of 14 miRNAs on the X chromosome, termed the miR-506-514 cluster, which was consistently overexpressed in nearly all melanomas tested (30–60 fold, P < 0.001), regardless of mutations in *NRAS* or *BRAF*. Interestingly, inhibition of the expression of this cluster as a whole, or one of its sub-clusters consisting of six miRNAs, led to significant inhibition of cell growth, induction of apoptosis, decreased invasiveness and decreased colony formation in soft agar across multiple melanoma cell lines, suggesting a role for the X chromosome miRNA cluster in promoting melanoma growth and progression [44].

Cancer/testis (CT) antigens are proteins that are normally tissue-restricted in expression but are also expressed by some cancer cell types and can be recognized by T cells and antibodies in cancer patients, and are the focus of intensive cancer vaccine research. Melanoma has been classified as a high CT expresser tumor type and some of the genes encoding CT antigens are located on the X chromosome [45, 46]. Organized clusters of multigene families, between Xq24 and Xq28, encode many of these genes. Caballero and group demonstrated that CT-X genes encoding members of the MAGE protein family on Xq28 influence melanomagenesis. Depletion of GAGE, SSX or XAGE1 by small interfering RNA inhibited melanoma cell migration and invasion and decreased the clonogenic survival of melanoma cells [47].

15.7.3 X Chromosome Tumor Suppressors

The X chromosome also encodes tumor suppressor genes. The initiation of X inactivation depends on the action of X inactive-specific transcript (Xist), a long non-coding RNA [137]. Xist is located on the X chromosome and is a potent suppressor of hematologic cancer in mice. When Xist is deleted from the blood compartment of mice, mutant females develop a highly aggressive myeloproliferative neoplasm and myelodysplastic syndrome with 100% penetrance, suggesting that Xist loss results in X reactivation and consequent genome-wide changes that lead to cancer, illustrating the importance of Xist and the X inactivation process in suppressing cancer in women [138].

Another tumor suppressor gene, the Wilms' tumor gene on X chromosome (WTX) promotes the ubiquitination and degradation of β-catenin, a protein that alters cell adhesion that plays an important role in the tumorigenesis of melanoma [139]. β-catenin stimulates proliferation and clonogenic growth in melanoma cells and dysregulation of β-catenin is reported in a substantial fraction of melanoma cells [140, 141]. Given its location on the X chromosome, "one hit" somatic mutations involving either the single X chromosome in males or the active X chromosome in females can lead to inactivation of WTX [142].

The X-linked TSPX (also called TSPYL2, CDA1 and DENTT) functions as a tumor suppressor by activating the tumor suppressor p53 and inhibiting cyclin B-CDK1 activity (a mitotic cyclin). TSPX and its homologue the testis-specific protein Y-encoded (TSPY) are members of the SET/NAP1 superfamily of proteins [143]. Over-expression of TSPX retards cell cycle progression and promotes cell death [144]. Kandalaft et al. found that human primary lung tumors and breast cancer cells have significant downregulation of DENTT/TSPX mRNA when compared with their normal matching counterpart tissue (~sixfold decrease), and exogenously introduced DENTT/TSPX inhibited the growth of cultured lung and breast cancer cells in vitro, demonstrating a function for DENTT/TSPX as a tumor suppressor [144]. FoxP3 is an X-linked tumor suppressor found to be expressed in melanomas; when FoxP3 is overexpressed in a melanoma cell line, proliferation and clonogeniticity in vitro were reduced, apoptosis was increased and tumor growth in vivo was reduced as well [145, 146]. It remains to be determined whether perturbations in the function of FoxP3 contribute to the sexual dimorphism of melanoma outcomes. It was found that no mutations of FoxP3 were detected in melanoma cell lines, no expression of FoxP3 was detected in normal melanocytes and the expression of FoxP3 was found infrequently on staining of melanoma tumor samples, leading Tan to conclude that FoxP3 does not play a significant role as a tumor suppressor in melanomas; however the results were not adjusted for sex [147].

Thus the X chromosome encodes molecules that are tumor promoting and tumor suppressing and the process of X inactivation undoubtedly plays a complex role in moderating the function of these genes, by rendering any given tissue in women mosaic for gene expression, by skewed inactivation and by the potential absence of inactivation. In contrast, cells in men are homogeneous for X encoded genes and are susceptible to X-linked oncogene activation or tumor suppressor inactivation. How this difference affects tumorigenesis in general and melanoma specifically awaits further investigation.

15.8   Y Chromosome Gene Expression

While X-linked genes have been suggested to contribute to melanoma sex disparities, the contribution of Y-linked genes has not been suggested or speculated upon to date, however since Y chromosome genetic material is expressed in a male biased manner, this preferential expression pattern could also contribute to the poor prognosis of melanoma in men compared to women.

TSPY is a repeated gene mapped to the critical region harboring the gonadoblastoma locus on the Y chromosome (*GBY*), and is expressed in testis [48, 49]. It plays a role in cell cycle regulation by interacting with cyclin B-CDK1 complex, stimulating its kinase activities and accelerating G2/M transition of the host cells [50, 51]. In addition, it also binds the translation elongation factor eEF1A and promotes cellular protein synthesis [148].

When ectopically expressed, TSPY accelerates the tumor growth of human HeLa cervical cancer cells in vivo and transforms murine NIH-3 T3 cells from non-tumorigenic to tumorigenic [48]. TSPY transcription was found to be upregulated in human hepatocellular carcinoma, another cancer with male biased increased incidence and poorer outcomes [149]. TSPY is also found in melanoma cell lines [52] and is reported to be mutated in melanoma tumor samples [150], although the significance of the mutations remains to be determined. Interestingly, TSPY is a homologue of TSPX, the tumor suppressor found on the X chromosome, which has an opposing role in the regulation of cell proliferation and tumorigenesis, as discussed above. Such contrasting functions of a pair of sex chromosome homologues likely play important roles in the sexual dimorphisms in certain somatic cancers [151].

The male germ cell-specific RNA binding protein (RBMY), encoded on the Y chromosome, functions as a male germ cell-specific splicing regulator by modulating the activity of constitutively expressed splicing factors [152, 153]. Its deletion causes the arrest of germ cells at the meiotic stage of spermatogenesis [154]. Its aberrant activation was detected in about 1/3 of male hepatocellular cancer (HCC) and hepatoblastoma tumor tissues, but not in paired non-tumor liver tissues, female HCC, or other types of cancers [155]. Depletion of RBMY expression in HepG2 cells by RNA interference reduced the transformation and anti-apoptotic efficiency of HepG2 cells and liver-specific RBMY expressing transgenic mice developed hepatic pre-cancerous lesions, adenoma, and HCC at rates increased above control levels, in both male and female transgenic mice, but caused a more rapid rate of tumor growth in the male mice [156]. These studies suggest that oncogenes on the Y chromosome that could contribute to the male predominance and worse outcomes in cancer, however their influence and specific effects on melanomas remain to be determined.

Conclusion

In this review we highlighted the current state of knowledge of biological factors underlying sex disparities in melanoma outcomes. It seems clear that sexual dimorphism in melanoma outcomes is the result of a complex interaction of a number of influencing factors, including hormonal milieu, immune homeostasis and function, oxidative environment and stress response, and sexual dimorphism in gene expression, including X- and Y-linked genes.

Sex hormones can have an effect on melanoma biology via several different mechanisms. Estrogen was found to exert a direct inhibitory effect on tumor cells, to play an indirect role by having a stimulatory effect on the immune system and acts as an antioxidant. Male sex hormones, on the contrary, were found to promote melanoma progression and carcinogenesis. Differences in the hormone milieu between males and females are likely to influence differences in melanoma outcomes.

Differences in immune homeostasis and function between males and females are another likely contributor to the female survival advantage. In addition to baseline differences in male vs. female immune homeostasis, the sex hormones also influence immune cell function. While estrogen seems to be stimulatory to the immune system by inducing a genetic program that alters the survival and activation of B cells, testosterone has been found to be an immune repressor by increasing the apoptosis of T cells and also exerting an inhibitory effect on human B cell differentiation. Generally, men appear to have reduced cell mediated and humeral immunity compared to women, a fact that might explain the higher rate of autoimmune disease in females but also offer an advantage for women in tumor surveillance. The differences in the immune responses to tumor cells between women and men also have implications for targeted immunotherapeutic approaches. However, this is still poorly explored and future research is necessary.

Several cell types and tissues demonstrate sex dependent differences in anti-oxidant capacity. The oxidative environment in the skin differs between males and females; female skin responds to UV induced oxidative stress by producing higher levels of anti-oxidant enzymes, resulting in lower levels of UV mediated DNA damage compared with in male skin. Moderating the oxidative microenvironment has been shown to influence melanoma onset, but the effect on melanoma outcomes remains to be determined; identifying sex dependent differences in oxidative stress response in melanocytes and melanoma cells awaits future studies.

There are sex differences in vitamin D regulation; studies in melanoma cell lines indicate a clear inhibitory effect of vitamin D on cell growth; and observational clinical studies suggest a survival benefit with higher levels of vitamin D, however further studies are clearly needed to determine whether or not this result will be confirmed in large randomized controlled studies.

Finally, the sex disparity in melanoma biology is mediated ultimately by sexual dimorphisms in autosomal and sex chromosome gene expression and RNA activity. The complexity of the X chromosome gene expression, mediated by non-random X chromosome inactivation, escape from inactivation, and skewed expression is anticipated to result in complex effects on the function of tumor suppressors and oncogenes and on melanoma biology; newly identified oncogenes on the Y chromosome are candidates for influencing melanoma tumorigenesis.

Both behavioral and biological processes are likely to contribute to disparities in melanoma outcomes. Future investigations into the molecular basis for disparities in melanoma outcomes will provide insights into shared mechanisms underlying sex disparities in other cancers, lead to better stratification of patients for counseling and provide the basis for developing novel sex based management strategies for malignant melanoma.

Acknowledgments Many thanks to Jerelyn Magnusson for technical assistance.

References

1. Erdei E, Torres SM. A new understanding in the epidemiology of melanoma. Expert Rev Anticancer Ther. 2010;10(11):1811 23.
2. MacKie RM, Hauschild A, Eggermont AM. Epidemiology of invasive cutaneous melanoma. Ann Oncol. 2009;20(Suppl 6):vi1–7.
3. Siegel R, Naishadham D, Jemal A. Cancer statistics, 2013. CA Cancer J Clin. 2013;63(1):11–30.
4. Lasithiotakis KG, Leiter U, Gorkievicz R, Eigentler T, Breuninger H, Metzler G, et al. The incidence and mortality of cutaneous melanoma in southern Germany: trends by anatomic site and pathologic characteristics, 1976 to 2003. Cancer. 2006;107(6):1331–9.
5. Coit DG, Andtbacka R, Anker CJ, Bichakjian CK, Carson WE 3rd, Daud A, et al. Melanoma, version 2.2013: featured updates to the NCCN guidelines. J Natl Compr Cancer Netw. 2013;11(4):395–407.
6. Balch CM, Gershenwald JE, Soong SJ, Thompson JF, Atkins MB, Byrd DR, et al. Final version of 2009 AJCC melanoma staging and classification. J Clin Oncol. 2009;27(36):6199–206.
7. Homsi J, Kashani-Sabet M, Messina JL, Daud A. Cutaneous melanoma: prognostic factors. Cancer Control. 2005;12(4):223–9.
8. Scoggins CR, Ross MI, Reintgen DS, Noyes RD, Goydos JS, Beitsch PD, et al. Gender-related differences in outcome for melanoma patients. Ann Surg. 2006;243(5):693–8; discussion 8-700.
9. Lasithiotakis K, Leiter U, Meier F, Eigentler T, Metzler G, Moehrle M, et al. Age and gender are significant independent predictors of survival in primary cutaneous melanoma. Cancer. 2008;112(8):1795–804.
10. Joosse A, Collette S, Suciu S, Nijsten T, Lejeune F, Kleeberg UR, et al. Superior outcome of women with stage I/II cutaneous melanoma: pooled analysis of four European Organisation for Research and Treatment of Cancer phase III trials. J Clin Oncol. 2012;30(18):2240–7.
11. Joosse A, de Vries E, Eckel R, Nijsten T, Eggermont AM, Holzel D, et al. Gender differences in melanoma survival: female patients have a decreased risk of metastasis. J Invest Dermatol. 2011;131(3):719–26.
12. de Vries E, Nijsten TE, Visser O, Bastiaannet E, van Hattem S, Janssen-Heijnen ML, et al. Superior survival of females among 10,538 Dutch melanoma patients is independent of Breslow thickness, histologic type and tumor site. Ann Oncol. 2008;19(3):583–9.
13. Sondak VK, Swetter SM, Berwick MA. Gender disparities in patients with melanoma: breaking the glass ceiling. J Clin Oncol. 2012;30(18):2177–8.
14. Gamba CS, Clarke CA, Keegan TH, Tao L, Swetter SM. Melanoma survival disadvantage in young, non-Hispanic white males compared with females. JAMA Dermatol. 2013;149(8):912–20.
15. American Cancer Society. Cancer facts and figures 2016. 2016. http://www.cancer.org/acs/groups/content/@research/documents/document/acspc-047079.pdf. 6 June 2016.
16. Joosse A, Collette S, Suciu S, Nijsten T, Patel PM, Keilholz U, et al. Sex is an independent prognostic indicator for survival and relapse/progression-free survival in metastasized stage III to IV melanoma: a pooled analysis of five European Organisation for Research and Treatment of Cancer randomized controlled trials. J Clin Oncol. 2013;31(18):2337–46.
17. Gupta S, Artomov M, Goggins W, Daly M, Tsao H. Gender disparity and mutation burden in metastatic melanoma. J Natl Cancer Inst. 2015;107(11):djv221.
18. Micheli A, Ciampichini R, Oberaigner W, Ciccolallo L, de Vries E, Izarzugaza I, et al. The advantage of women in cancer survival: an analysis of EUROCARE-4 data. Eur J Cancer. 2009;45(6):1017–27.
19. Micheli A, Mariotto A, Giorgi Rossi A, Gatta G, Muti P. The prognostic role of gender in survival of adult cancer patients. EUROCARE Working Group. Eur J Cancer. 1998;34(14 Spec No):2271–8.

20. Fisher DE, Geller AC. Disproportionate burden of melanoma mortality in young U.S. men: the possible role of biology and behavior. JAMA Dermatol. 2013;149(8):903–4.

21. Kanda N, Watanabe S. 17beta-estradiol, progesterone, and dihydrotestosterone suppress the growth of human melanoma by inhibiting interleukin-8 production. J Invest Dermatol. 2001;117(2):274–83.

22. Grimaldi CM, Cleary J, Dagtas AS, Moussai D, Diamond B. Estrogen alters thresholds for B cell apoptosis and activation. J Clin Invest. 2002;109(12):1625–33.

23. Merino R, Ding L, Veis DJ, Korsmeyer SJ, Nunez G. Developmental regulation of the Bcl-2 protein and susceptibility to cell death in B lymphocytes. EMBO J. 1994;13(3):683–91.

24. Sato S, Tuscano JM, Inaoki M, Tedder TF. CD22 negatively and positively regulates signal transduction through the B lymphocyte antigen receptor. Semin Immunol. 1998;10(4):287–97.

25. Cyster JG, Goodnow CC. Protein tyrosine phosphatase 1C negatively regulates antigen receptor signaling in B lymphocytes and determines thresholds for negative selection. Immunity. 1995;2(1):13–24.

26. Bynoe MS, Grimaldi CM, Diamond B. Estrogen up-regulates Bcl-2 and blocks tolerance induction of naive B cells. Proc Natl Acad Sci U S A. 2000;97(6):2703–8.

27. Ruiz-Larrea MB, Leal AM, Martin C, Martinez R, Lacort M. Antioxidant action of estrogens in rat hepatocytes. Rev Esp Fisiol. 1997;53(2):225–9.

28. Borrás C, Sastre J, Garcia-Sala D, Lloret A, Pallardo FV, Vina J. Mitochondria from females exhibit higher antioxidant gene expression and lower oxidative damage than males. Free Radic Biol Med. 2003;34(5):546–52.

29. Allil PA, Visconti MA, Castrucci AM, Isoldi MC. Photoperiod and testosterone modulate growth and melanogenesis of s91 murine melanoma. Med Chem. 2008;4(2):100–5.

30. McMurray RW, Suwannaroj S, Ndebele K, Jenkins JK. Differential effects of sex steroids on T and B cells: modulation of cell cycle phase distribution, apoptosis and bcl-2 protein levels. Pathobiology. 2001;69(1):44–58.

31. Sthoeger ZM, Chiorazzi N, Lahita RG. Regulation of the immune response by sex hormones. I. In vitro effects of estradiol and testosterone on pokeweed mitogen-induced human B cell differentiation. J Immunol. 1988;141(1):91–8.

32. Bokov AF, Ko D, Richardson A. The effect of gonadectomy and estradiol on sensitivity to oxidative stress. Endocr Res. 2009;34(1-2):43–58.

33. Barsony J, Pike JW, DeLuca HF, Marx SJ. Immunocytology with microwave-fixed fibroblasts shows 1 alpha,25-dihydroxyvitamin D3-dependent rapid and estrogen-dependent slow reorganization of vitamin D receptors. J Cell Biol. 1990;111(6 Pt 1):2385–95.

34. Liel Y, Kraus S, Levy J, Shany S. Evidence that estrogens modulate activity and increase the number of 1,25-dihydroxyvitamin D receptors in osteoblast-like cells (ROS 17/2.8). Endocrinology. 1992;130(5):2597–601.

35. Schwartz B, Smirnoff P, Shany S, Liel Y. Estrogen controls expression and bioresponse of 1,25-dihydroxyvitamin D receptors in the rat colon. Mol Cell Biochem. 2000;203(1-2):87–93.

36. Bouman A, Schipper M, Heineman MJ, Faas MM. Gender difference in the non-specific and specific immune response in humans. Am J Reprod Immunol. 2004;52(1):19–26.

37. Pinto RE, Bartley W. The effect of age and sex on glutathione reductase and glutathione peroxidase activities and on aerobic glutathione oxidation in rat liver homogenates. Biochem J. 1969;112(1):109–15.

38. Joosse A, De Vries E, van Eijck CH, Eggermont AM, Nijsten T, Coebergh JW. Reactive oxygen species and melanoma: an explanation for gender differences in survival? Pigment Cell Melanoma Res. 2010;23(3):352–64.

39. Vina J, Borras C, Gambini J, Sastre J, Pallardo FV. Why females live longer than males? Importance of the upregulation of longevity-associated genes by oestrogenic compounds. FEBS Lett. 2005;579(12):2541–5.

40. Fish EN. The X-files in immunity: sex-based differences predispose immune responses. Nat Rev Immunol. 2008;8(9):737–44.

41. Spolarics Z. The X-files of inflammation: cellular mosaicism of X-linked polymorphic genes and the female advantage in the host response to injury and infection. Shock. 2007;27(6):597–604.

42. Renault NK, Pritchett SM, Howell RE, Greer WL, Sapienza C, Orstavik KH, et al. Human X-chromosome inactivation pattern distributions fit a model of genetically influenced choice better than models of completely random choice. Eur J Hum Genet. 2013;21(12):1396–402.

43. Segura MF, Belitskaya-Levy I, Rose AE, Zakrzewski J, Gaziel A, Hanniford D, et al. Melanoma microRNA signature predicts post-recurrence survival. Clin Cancer Res. 2010;16(5):1577–86.

44. Streicher KL, Zhu W, Lehmann KP, Georgantas RW, Morehouse CA, Brohawn P, et al. A novel oncogenic role for the miRNA-506-514 cluster in initiating melanocyte transformation and promoting melanoma growth. Oncogene. 2012;31(12):1558–70.

45. Simpson AJ, Caballero OL, Jungbluth A, Chen YT, Old LJ. Cancer/testis antigens, gametogenesis and cancer. Nat Rev Cancer. 2005;5(8):615–25.

46. Scanlan MJ. The cancer/testis genes: review, standardization, and commentary. Cancer Immun. 2004;4:1.

47. Caballero OL, Cohen T, Gurung S, Chua R, Lee P, Chen YT, et al. Effects of CT-Xp gene knock down in melanoma cell lines. Oncotarget. 2013;4(4):531–41.

48. Oram SW, Liu XX, Lee TL, Chan WY, Lau YF. TSPY potentiates cell proliferation and tumorigenesis by promoting cell cycle progression in HeLa and NIH3T3 cells. BMC Cancer. 2006;6:154.

49. Zhang JS, Yang-Feng TL, Muller U, Mohandas TK, de Jong PJ, Lau YF. Molecular isolation and characterization of an expressed gene from the human Y chromosome. Hum Mol Genet. 1992;1(9):717–26.

50. Lau YF, Li Y, Kido T. Role of the Y-located putative gonadoblastoma gene in human spermatogenesis. Syst Biol Reprod Med. 2011;57(1-2):27–34.

51. Li Y, Lau YF. TSPY and its X-encoded homologue interact with cyclin B but exert contrasting functions on cyclin-dependent kinase 1 activities. Oncogene. 2008;27(47):6141–50.

52. Gallagher WM, Bergin OE, Rafferty M, Kelly ZD, Nolan IM, Fox EJ, et al. Multiple markers for melanoma progression regulated by DNA methylation: insights from transcriptomic studies. Carcinogenesis. 2005;26(11):1856–67.

53. Kemeny MM, Busch E, Stewart AK, Menck HR. Superior survival of young women with malignant melanoma. Am J Surg. 1998;175(6):437–44; discussion 44-5.

54. Koomen ER, Joosse A, Herings RM, Casparie MK, Guchelaar HJ, Nijsten T. Estrogens, oral contraceptives and hormonal replacement therapy increase the incidence of cutaneous melanoma: a population-based case-control study. Ann Oncol. 2009;20(2):358–64.

55. MacKie RM, Bray CA. Hormone replacement therapy after surgery for stage 1 or 2 cutaneous melanoma. Br J Cancer. 2004;90(4):770–2.

56. Naldi L, Altieri A, Imberti GL, Giordano L, Gallus S, La Vecchia C. Cutaneous malignant melanoma in women. Phenotypic characteristics, sun exposure, and hormonal factors: a case-control study from Italy. Ann Epidemiol. 2005;15(7):545–50.

57. Karagas MR, Stukel TA, Dykes J, Miglionico J, Greene MA, Carey M, et al. A pooled analysis of 10 case-control studies of melanoma and oral contraceptive use. Br J Cancer. 2002;86(7):1085–92.

58. Grin CM, Driscoll MS, Grant-Kels JM. The relationship of pregnancy, hormones, and melanoma. Semin Cutan Med Surg. 1998;17(3):167–71.

59. Gefeller O, Hassan K, Wille L. Cutaneous malignant melanoma in women and the role of oral contraceptives. Br J Dermatol. 1998;138(1):122–4.

60. Lambe M, Thorn M, Sparen P, Bergstrom R, Adami HO. Malignant melanoma: reduced risk associated with early childbearing and multiparity. Melanoma Res. 1996;6(2):147–53.

61. Lens M, Bataille V. Melanoma in relation to reproductive and hormonal factors in women: current review on controversial issues. Cancer Causes Control. 2008;19(5):437–42.

62. Kvale G, Heuch I, Nilssen S. Parity in relation to mortality and cancer incidence: a prospective study of Norwegian women. Int J Epidemiol. 1994;23(4):691–9.

63. Smith MA, Fine JA, Barnhill RL, Berwick M. Hormonal and reproductive influences and risk of melanoma in women. Int J Epidemiol. 1998;27(5):751–7.

64. Sutherland CM, Loutfi A, Mather FJ, Carter RD, Krementz ET. Effect of pregnancy upon malignant melanoma. Surg Gynecol Obstet. 1983;157(5):443–6.

65. Trapeznikov NN, Khasanov ShR, Iavorskii VV. [Melanoma of the skin and pregnancy]. Vopr Onkol. 1987;33(6):40–6.

66. Pack GT, Scharnagel IM. The prognosis for malignant melanoma in the pregnant woman. Cancer. 1951;4(2):324–34.

67. Lens MB, Rosdahl I, Ahlbom A, Farahmand BY, Synnerstad I, Boeryd B, et al. Effect of pregnancy on survival in women with cutaneous malignant melanoma. J Clin Oncol. 2004;22(21):4369–75.

68. O'Meara AT, Cress R, Xing G, Danielsen B, Smith LH. Malignant melanoma in pregnancy. A population-based evaluation. Cancer. 2005;103(6):1217–26.

69. Green S, Walter P, Kumar V, Krust A, Bornert JM, Argos P, et al. Human oestrogen receptor cDNA: sequence, expression and homology to v-erb-A. Nature. 1986;320(6058):134–9.

70. de Giorgi V, Mavilia C, Massi D, Gozzini A, Aragona P, Tanini A, et al. Estrogen receptor expression in cutaneous melanoma: a real-time reverse transcriptase-polymerase chain reaction and immunohistochemical study. Arch Dermatol. 2009;145(1):30–6.

71. Schmidt AN, Nanney LB, Boyd AS, King LE Jr, Ellis DL. Oestrogen receptor-beta expression in melanocytic lesions. Exp Dermatol. 2006;15(12):971–80.

72. Richardson B, Price A, Wagner M, Williams V, Lorigan P, Browne S, et al. Investigation of female survival benefit in metastatic melanoma. Br J Cancer. 1999;80(12):2025–33.

73. Roy S, Reddy BS, Sudhakar G, Kumar JM, Banerjee R. 17beta-estradiol-linked nitro-L-arginine as simultaneous inducer of apoptosis in melanoma and tumor-angiogenic vascular endothelial cells. Mol Pharm. 2011;8(2):350–9.

74. Dobos J, Timar J, Bocsi J, Burian Z, Nagy K, Barna G, et al. In vitro and in vivo antitumor effect of 2-methoxyestradiol on human melanoma. Int J Cancer. 2004;112(5):771–6.

75. Ghosh R, Ott AM, Seetharam D, Slaga TJ, Kumar AP. Cell cycle block and apoptosis induction in a human melanoma cell line following treatment with 2-methoxyoestradiol: therapeutic implications? Melanoma Res. 2003;13(2):119–27.

76. Fotsis T, Zhang Y, Pepper MS, Adlercreutz H, Montesano R, Nawroth PP, et al. The endogenous oestrogen metabolite 2-methoxyoestradiol inhibits angiogenesis and suppresses tumour growth. Nature. 1994;368(6468):237–9.

77. Cho JL, Allanson M, Reeve VE. Oestrogen receptor-beta signalling protects against transplanted skin

tumour growth in the mouse. Photochem Photobiol Sci. 2010;9(4):608–14.

78. Chang C, Lee SO, Yeh S, Chang TM. Androgen receptor (AR) differential roles in hormone-related tumors including prostate, bladder, kidney, lung, breast and liver. Oncogene. 2014;33:3225.

79. Rampen FH, Mulder JH. Malignant melanoma: an androgen-dependent tumour? Lancet. 1980;1(8168 Pt 1):562–4.

80. Brinton LA, Moghissi KS, Westhoff CL, Lamb EJ, Scoccia B. Cancer risk among infertile women with androgen excess or menstrual disorders (including polycystic ovary syndrome). Fertil Steril. 2010;94(5):1787–92.

81. Morvillo V, Luthy IA, Bravo AI, Capurro MI, Donaldson M, Quintans C, et al. Atypical androgen receptor in the human melanoma cell line IIB-MEL-J. Pigment Cell Res. 1995;8(3):135–41.

82. Hsueh EC, Gupta RK, Lefor A, Reyzin G, Ye W, Morton DL. Androgen blockade enhances response to melanoma vaccine. J Surg Res. 2003;110(2):393–8.

83. Brewer JD, Shanafelt TD, Otley CC, Roenigk RK, Cerhan JR, Kay NE, et al. Chronic lymphocytic leukemia is associated with decreased survival of patients with malignant melanoma and Merkel cell carcinoma in a SEER population-based study. J Clin Oncol. 2012;30(8):843–9.

84. Brewer JD, Christenson LJ, Weaver AL, Dapprich DC, Weenig RH, Lim KK, et al. Malignant melanoma in solid transplant recipients: collection of database cases and comparison with surveillance, epidemiology, and end results data for outcome analysis. Arch Dermatol. 2011;147(7):790–6.

85. Matin RN, Mesher D, Proby CM, McGregor JM, Bouwes Bavinck JN, del Marmol V, et al. Melanoma in organ transplant recipients: clinicopathological features and outcome in 100 cases. Am J Transplant Off J Am Soc Transplant Am Soc Transplant Surg. 2008;8(9):1891–900.

86. Bouman A, Heineman MJ, Faas MM. Sex hormones and the immune response in humans. Hum Reprod Update. 2005;11(4):411–23.

87. Giltay EJ, Fonk JC, von Blomberg BM, Drexhage HA, Schalkwijk C, Gooren LJ. In vivo effects of sex steroids on lymphocyte responsiveness and immunoglobulin levels in humans. J Clin Endocrinol Metab. 2000;85(4):1648–57.

88. McDonnell DP, Norris JD. Connections and regulation of the human estrogen receptor. Science. 2002;296(5573):1642–4.

89. Kanda N, Tamaki K. Estrogen enhances immunoglobulin production by human PBMCs. J Allergy Clin Immunol. 1999;103(2 Pt 1):282–8.

90. Verthelyi D. Sex hormones as immunomodulators in health and disease. Int Immunopharmacol. 2001;1(6):983–93.

91. Verthelyi D, Ansar AS. Characterization of estrogen-induced autoantibodies to cardiolipin in non-autoimmune mice. J Autoimmun. 1997;10(2): 115–25.

92. Mirandola L, Wade R, Verma R, Pena C, Hosiriluck N, Figueroa JA, et al. Sex-driven differences in immunological responses: challenges and opportunities for the immunotherapies of the third millennium. Int Rev Immunol. 2015;34(2):134–42.

93. Kanda N, Tsuchida T, Tamaki K. Testosterone inhibits immunoglobulin production by human peripheral blood mononuclear cells. Clin Exp Immunol. 1996;106(2):410–5.

94. Duffy DL, Bentley GE, Drazen DL, Ball GF. Effects of testerone on cell-mediated and humoral immunity in non-breeding adult European starlings. Behav Ecol. 2000;11(6):654–62.

95. Hamid O, Carvajal RD. Anti-programmed death-1 and anti-programmed death-ligand 1 antibodies in cancer therapy. Expert Opin Biol Ther. 2013;13(6):847–61.

96. Hamid O, Robert C, Daud A, Hodi FS, Hwu WJ, Kefford R, et al. Safety and tumor responses with lambrolizumab (anti-PD-1) in melanoma. N Engl J Med. 2013;369(2):134–44.

97. Ribas A, Hamid O, Daud A, Hodi FS, Wolchok JD, Kefford R, et al. Association of pembrolizumab with tumor response and survival among patients with advanced melanoma. JAMA. 2016;315(15):1600–9.

98. Ribas A, Puzanov I, Dummer R, Schadendorf D, Hamid O, Robert C, et al. Pembrolizumab versus investigator-choice chemotherapy for ipilimumab-refractory melanoma (KEYNOTE-002): a randomised, controlled, phase 2 trial. Lancet Oncol. 2015;16(8):908–18.

99. Hino R, Kabashima K, Kato Y, Yagi H, Nakamura M, Honjo T, et al. Tumor cell expression of programmed cell death-1 ligand 1 is a prognostic factor for malignant melanoma. Cancer. 2010;116(7):1757–66.

100. Polanczyk MJ, Hopke C, Vandenbark AA, Offner H. Estrogen-mediated immunomodulation involves reduced activation of effector T cells, potentiation of Treg cells, and enhanced expression of the PD-1 costimulatory pathway. J Neurosci Res. 2006;84(2):370–8.

101. Polanczyk MJ, Hopke C, Vandenbark AA, Offner H. Treg suppressive activity involves estrogen-dependent expression of programmed death-1 (PD-1). Int Immunol. 2007;19(3):337–43.

102. Lin PY, Sun L, Thibodeaux SR, Ludwig SM, Vadlamudi RK, Hurez VJ, et al. B7-H1-dependent sex-related differences in tumor immunity and immunotherapy responses. J Immunol. 2010;185(5):2747–53.

103. Nosrati A, Tsai KK, Goldinger SM, Tumeh P, Grimes B, Loo K, et al. Evaluation of clinicopathological factors in PD-1 response: derivation and validation of a prediction scale for response to PD-1 monotherapy. Br J Cancer. 2017;116:1141.

104. Dronca RS, Dong H. A gender factor in shaping T-cell immunity to melanoma. Front Oncol. 2015;5:8.

105. Malorni W, Campesi I, Straface E, Vella S, Franconi F. Redox features of the cell: a gender perspective. Antioxid Redox Signal. 2007;9(11):1779–801.

106. Cotter MA, Thomas J, Cassidy P, Robinette K, Jenkins N, Florell SR, et al. N-acetylcysteine protects melanocytes against oxidative stress/damage and delays onset of ultraviolet-induced melanoma in mice. Clin Cancer Res. 2007;13(19):5952–8.

107. Sander CS, Hamm F, Elsner P, Thiele JJ. Oxidative stress in malignant melanoma and non-melanoma skin cancer. Br J Dermatol. 2003;148(5):913–22.

108. Meyskens FL Jr, McNulty SE, Buckmeier JA, Tohidian NB, Spillane TJ, Kahlon RS, et al. Aberrant redox regulation in human metastatic melanoma cells compared to normal melanocytes. Free Radic Biol Med. 2001;31(6):799–808.

109. Nishikawa M. Reactive oxygen species in tumor metastasis. Cancer Lett. 2008;266(1):53–9.

110. Trouba KJ, Hamadeh HK, Amin RP, Germolec DR. Oxidative stress and its role in skin disease. Antioxid Redox Signal. 2002;4(4):665–73.

111. Thomas-Ahner JM, Wulff BC, Tober KL, Kusewitt DF, Riggenbach JA, Oberyszyn TM. Gender differences in UVB-induced skin carcinogenesis, inflammation, and DNA damage. Cancer Res. 2007;67(7):3468–74.

112. Malorni W, Straface E, Matarrese P, Ascione B, Coinu R, Canu S, et al. Redox state and gender differences in vascular smooth muscle cells. FEBS Lett. 2008;582(5):635–42.

113. Borras C, Gambini J, Lopez-Grueso R, Pallardo FV, Vina J. Direct antioxidant and protective effect of estradiol on isolated mitochondria. Biochim Biophys Acta. 2010;1802(1):205–11.

114. Berwick M, Erdei EO. Vitamin D and melanoma incidence and mortality. Pigment Cell Melanoma Res. 2013;26(1):9–15.

115. Johnson JA, Beckman MJ, Pansini-Porta A, Christakos S, Bruns ME, Beitz DC, et al. Age and gender effects on 1,25-dihydroxyvitamin D3-regulated gene expression. Exp Gerontol. 1995;30(6):631–43.

116. Evans SR, Houghton AM, Schumaker L, Brenner RV, Buras RR, Davoodi F, et al. Vitamin D receptor and growth inhibition by 1,25-dihydroxyvitamin D3 in human malignant melanoma cell lines. J Surg Res. 1996;61(1):127–33.

117. Essa S, Denzer N, Mahlknecht U, Klein R, Collnot EM, Tilgen W, et al. VDR microRNA expression and epigenetic silencing of vitamin D signaling in melanoma cells. J Steroid Biochem Mol Biol. 2010;121(1-2):110–3.

118. Seifert M, Rech M, Meineke V, Tilgen W, Reichrath J. Differential biological effects of 1,25-dihydroxyVitamin D3 on melanoma cell lines in vitro. J Steroid Biochem Mol Biol. 2004;89-90(1-5):375–9.

119. Frampton RJ, Omond SA, Eisman JA. Inhibition of human cancer cell growth by 1,25-dihydroxyvitamin D3 metabolites. Cancer Res. 1983;43(9):4443–7.

120. Frampton RJ, Suva LJ, Eisman JA, Findlay DM, Moore GE, Moseley JM, et al. Presence of 1,25-dihydroxyvitamin D3 receptors in established human cancer cell lines in culture. Cancer Res. 1982;42(3):1116–9.

121. Danielsson C, Fehsel K, Polly P, Carlberg C. Differential apoptotic response of human melanoma cells to 1 alpha,25-dihydroxyvitamin D3 and its analogues. Cell Death Differ. 1998;5(11):946–52.

122. Colston K, Colston MJ, Feldman D. 1,25-dihydroxyvitamin D3 and malignant melanoma: the presence of receptors and inhibition of cell growth in culture. Endocrinology. 1981;108(3):1083–6.

123. Yudoh K, Matsuno H, Kimura T. 1alpha,25-dihydroxyvitamin D3 inhibits in vitro invasiveness through the extracellular matrix and in vivo pulmonary metastasis of B16 mouse melanoma. J Lab Clin Med. 1999;133(2):120–8.

124. Newton-Bishop JA, Beswick S, Randerson-Moor J, Chang YM, Affleck P, Elliott F, et al. Serum 25-hydroxyvitamin D3 levels are associated with breslow thickness at presentation and survival from melanoma. J Clin Oncol. 2009;27(32):5439–44.

125. Theodoratou E, Tzoulaki I, Zgaga L, Ioannidis JP. Vitamin D and multiple health outcomes: umbrella review of systematic reviews and meta-analyses of observational studies and randomised trials. BMJ. 2014;348:g2035.

126. Yang X, Schadt EE, Wang S, Wang H, Arnold AP, Ingram-Drake L, et al. Tissue-specific expression and regulation of sexually dimorphic genes in mice. Genome Res. 2006;16(8):995–1004.

127. Gabory A, Attig L, Junien C. Sexual dimorphism in environmental epigenetic programming. Mol Cell Endocrinol. 2009;304(1-2):8–18.

128. Dorak MT, Karpuzoglu E. Gender differences in cancer susceptibility: an inadequately addressed issue. Front Genet. 2012;3:268.

129. Edgren G, Liang L, Adami HO, Chang ET. Enigmatic sex disparities in cancer incidence. Eur J Epidemiol. 2012;27(3):187–96.

130. Wu H, Luo J, Yu H, Rattner A, Mo A, Wang Y, et al. Cellular resolution maps of X chromosome inactivation: implications for neural development, function, and disease. Neuron. 2014;81(1):103–19.

131. Carrel L, Willard HF. X-inactivation profile reveals extensive variability in X-linked gene expression in females. Nature. 2005;434(7031):400–4.

132. Indsto JO, Nassif NT, Kefford RF, Mann GJ. Frequent loss of heterozygosity targeting the inactive X chromosome in melanoma. Clin Cancer Res. 2003;9(17):6476–82.

133. Elsheikh M, Dunger DB, Conway GS, Wass JA. Turner's syndrome in adulthood. Endocr Rev. 2002;23(1):120–40.

134. Schoemaker MJ, Swerdlow AJ, Higgins CD, Wright AF, Jacobs PA. Cancer incidence in women with Turner syndrome in Great Britain: a national cohort study. Lancet Oncol. 2008;9(3):239–46.

135. Guo X, Su B, Zhou Z, Sha J. Rapid evolution of mammalian X-linked testis microRNAs. BMC Genomics. 2009;10:97.

136. Sotiropoulou G, Pampalakis G, Lianidou E, Mourelatos Z. Emerging roles of microRNAs as molecular switches in the integrated circuit of the cancer cell. RNA. 2009;15(8):1443–61.

137. Brown CJ, Hendrich BD, Rupert JL, Lafreniere RG, Xing Y, Lawrence J, et al. The human XIST gene: analysis of a 17 kb inactive X-specific RNA that contains conserved repeats and is highly localized within the nucleus. Cell. 1992;71(3):527–42.

138. Yildirim E, Kirby JE, Brown DE, Mercier FE, Sadreyev RI, Scadden DT, et al. Xist RNA is a potent suppressor of hematologic cancer in mice. Cell. 2013;152(4):727–42.

139. Ruteshouser EC, Robinson SM, Huff V. Wilms tumor genetics: mutations in WT1, WTX, and CTNNB1 account for only about one-third of tumors. Genes Chromosomes Cancer. 2008;47(6):461–70.

140. Rubinfeld B, Robbins P, El-Gamil M, Albert I, Porfiri E, Polakis P. Stabilization of beta-catenin by genetic defects in melanoma cell lines. Science. 1997;275(5307):1790–2.

141. Rimm DL, Caca K, Hu G, Harrison FB, Fearon ER. Frequent nuclear/cytoplasmic localization of beta-catenin without exon 3 mutations in malignant melanoma. Am J Pathol. 1999;154(2):325–9.

142. Rivera MN, Kim WJ, Wells J, Driscoll DR, Brannigan BW, Han M, et al. An X chromosome gene, WTX, is commonly inactivated in Wilms tumor. Science. 2007;315(5812):642–5.

143. Tu Y, Wu W, Wu T, Cao Z, Wilkins R, Toh BH, et al. Antiproliferative autoantigen CDA1 transcriptionally up-regulates p21(Waf1/Cip1) by activating p53 and MEK/ERK1/2 MAPK pathways. J Biol Chem. 2007;282(16):11722–31.

144. Kandalaft LE, Zudaire E, Portal-Nunez S, Cuttitta F, Jakowlew SB. Differentially expressed nucleolar transforming growth factor-beta1 target (DENTT) exhibits an inhibitory role on tumorigenesis. Carcinogenesis. 2008;29(6):1282–9.

145. Ebert LM, Tan BS, Browning J, Svobodova S, Russell SE, Kirkpatrick N, et al. The regulatory T cell-associated transcription factor FoxP3 is expressed by tumor cells. Cancer Res. 2008;68(8):3001–9.

146. Tan B. FOXP3 over-expression inhibits melanoma tumorigenesis via effects on proliferation and apoptosis. Oncotarget. 2013;5(1):264–76.

147. Tan B. Pigment Cell Melanoma Res. 2012;25(3):398–400.

148. Kido T, Lau YF. The human Y-encoded testis-specific protein interacts functionally with eukaryotic translation elongation factor eEF1A, a putative oncoprotein. Int J Cancer. 2008;123(7):1573–85.

149. Yin YH, Li YY, Qiao H, Wang HC, Yang XA, Zhang HG, et al. TSPY is a cancer testis antigen expressed in human hepatocellular carcinoma. Br J Cancer. 2005;93(4):458–63.

150. Hodis E, Watson IR, Kryukov GV, Arold ST, Imielinski M, Theurillat JP, et al. A landscape of driver mutations in melanoma. Cell. 2012;150(2):251–63.

151. Kido T, Ou JH, Lau YF. The X-linked tumor suppressor TSPX interacts and promotes degradation of the hepatitis B viral protein HBx via the proteasome pathway. PLoS One. 2011;6(7):e22979.

152. Dreumont N, Bourgeois CF, Lejeune F, Liu Y, Ehrmann IE, Elliott DJ, et al. Human RBMY regulates germline-specific splicing events by modulating the function of the serine/arginine-rich proteins 9G8 and Tra2-{beta}. J Cell Sci. 2010;123(Pt 1):40–50.

153. Liu Y, Bourgeois CF, Pang S, Kudla M, Dreumont N, Kister L, et al. The germ cell nuclear proteins hnRNP G-T and RBMY activate a testis-specific exon. PLoS Genet. 2009;5(11):e1000707.

154. Mahadevaiah SK, Odorisio T, Elliott DJ, Rattigan A, Szot M, Laval SH, et al. Mouse homologues of the human AZF candidate gene RBM are expressed in spermatogonia and spermatids, and map to a Y chromosome deletion interval associated with a high incidence of sperm abnormalities. Hum Mol Genet. 1998;7(4):715–27.

155. Tsuei DJ, Hsu HC, Lee PH, Jeng YM, Pu YS, Chen CN, et al. RBMY, a male germ cell-specific RNA-binding protein, activated in human liver cancers and transforms rodent fibroblasts. Oncogene. 2004;23(34):5815–22.

156. Tsuei DJ, Lee PH, Peng HY, Lu HL, Su DS, Jeng YM, et al. Male germ cell-specific RNA binding protein RBMY: a new oncogene explaining male predominance in liver cancer. PLoS One. 2011;6(11):e26948.

Infantile Hemangioma

16

Shoshana Greenberger

16.1 Epidemiology and Clinical Course

Infantile hemangioma (IH), a benign vascular tumor, is the most common tumor of infancy, with an incidence of 5–10% at the end of the first year [1]. The great majority of IH are focal and solitary. Sixty percent of the tumors occur on the head and neck, 25% on the trunk, and 15% on the extremities. Epidemiological studies demonstrated an increased risk in premature neonates under the weight of 1500 g [2], in females and in Caucasians [3].

The tumor displays a distinctive life cycle that can be separated, both clinically and histologically, into three phases [4, 5]. The proliferating phase starts within few weeks from birth and ends in the first year of life, with the most growth occurring during the first 4–6 months of life [6]. At this phase, the tumor changes its presentation from mild blanching, fine telangiectasias or a red or macule to a prominent bright red papule, plaque or nodule [6]. Histologicaly, the proliferation phase is characterized by endothelial cells covered by a pericyte layer, arranged in dense, immature blood vessels. Outside the vessels reside multipotent progenitor-like cells [7, 8]. The involution phase begins on average at 12 months of age. The tumor changes color from bright red to less red and gray. Also, nodules and papules shrink and soften. Histologically, vascular channels become more mature and are lined with flattened endothelial cells. There is a prominent apoptosis of endothelial cells [9, 10] and an increase in the number of mast cells. Finally, at the involuted phase, tumor growth has stopped and the tumor regressed. Histologically, fat, fibroblasts and connective tissue had replaced the vascular tissue at this stage, with few large feeding and draining vessels evident. About half of tumors involute by age 5 years and 70% by age 7 years. In 30%, an additional 3–5 years to complete the process [11]. The regression of IH often leaves residues. These residues are correlated to the maximum size of the hemangioma. These include telangiectasias, atrophic, wrinkled skin, hyper or hypopigmentation as well as redundant fibrofatty tissue [12].

IH is a benign tumor, and in most patients no specific treatment is required. However, in 10% of cases IH is complicated, due to its location or due to excessive growth. In these circumstances, that carry the risk of irreversible disfigurement, airway obstruction or decreased vision, treatment is indicated. In recent years, beta-blockers, most specifically propranolol, became the treatment of choice for complicated IH.

S. Greenberger
The Department of Dermatology, Pediatric
Dermatology Service, Sheba Medical Center,
Ramat Gan, Israel

Sackler Faculty of Medicine, Tel Aviv University,
Tel Aviv, Israel
e-mail: Shoshana.Greenberger@sheba.health.gov.il

© Springer International Publishing AG, part of Springer Nature 2018
E. Tur, H. I. Maibach (eds.), *Gender and Dermatology*,
https://doi.org/10.1007/978-3-319-72156-9_16

16.2 Cellular Components of IH

In recent years, several cellular components of IH were isolated and characterized. These include hemangioma-derived progenitor/stem cells (HemSCs), Hemangioma endothelial cells (HemECs), perivascular cells (Hem-pericytes) and meloid cells.

16.2.1 HemSC

These cells were first isolated by Bischoff group in 2008 [7] using anti-CD133-coated magnetic beads. Itinteang et al. also demonstrated the expression of embryonic stem cell (ESC) markers, in the proliferative phase of IH with reduced expression during lesion involution [13, 14]. HemSC are rare cells, comprising 0.1–1% of the cells in proliferating phase IH have the ability to self-renew and undergo multi-lineage differentiation. Differently from Bone marrow mesenchymal progenitor cells, HemSC differentiate not only towards adipocytes, osteocytes and chondrocytes but also into endothelium, having the ability to create hemangioma like vessels de-novo.

16.2.2 Hemangioma Endothelial Cells

Endothelial cells constitute about 30% of the proliferating tumor and were shown to be clonal [15]. Morphologically the cells are plump in the proliferating tumor and spindle shape in the involuting phase [16]. The cells express typical endothelial-specific markers such as von Willebrand Factor, CD31/PECAM-1, and E-selectin KDR, TIE-2, and VE-cadherin [15, 17]. In addition, North and colleagues showed that glucose transporter-1 (GLUT1) is expressed on hemangioma endothelium, whereas no expression is noted in other types of vascular tumors and vascular malformations [18]. Consequently GLUT1 became a useful diagnostic marker.

16.2.3 Pericytes

Pericytes are contractile mural cells that are located around the EC of capillaries and venules. The cells express distinct set molecular markers including platelet-derived growth factor receptor β (PDGFRβ), CD146, aminopeptidases A and N (CD13), endoglin, neuron-glial 2 (NG2) [19–21]. Pericytes have a central role in endothelial barrier development and maintenance of integrity [22]. In addition, the microvascular tone is regulated, in large, by the pericytes [23]. In IH, pericytes are abundant in both the proliferating and the involuting phases [14], probably deriving from HemSC. Boscolo et al. demonstrated that IH pericytes differ from normal pericytes both by their phenotype and their expression profile [24]. Hemangioma pericytes have increased proliferation, increased vessel formation in vivo, and decreased ability to suppress proliferation and migration of endothelial cells. In addition, the cells secrete more VEGF-A, a critical cytokine for IH proliferation [24, 25].

16.2.4 Myeloid Cells and Macrophages

The presence of myeloid cells in IH, and more specifically macrophages, have been shown in several studies [26, 27]. Macrophages perform phagocytic clearance of dying cells and protect the host through innate immunity, both as resident tissue macrophages and as monocyte-derived recruited cells during inflammation. Classically, macrophages have been divided into two types: The M1 and M2-polarized cells [28]. Both M1 and M2 Macrophages were shown to be more prevalent in proliferating IHs than in involuting lesions [26, 29], with M1 being more prevalent. The cells are located in the interstitium, between the vessels, and were shown to increase the proliferation and significantly suppress the adipogenesis of HemSC [29].

16.3   Propranolol Treatment

Historically, systemic glucocorticoids were the mainstay therapy for complicated IH, with interferon α and vincristine used for unresponsive tumors [30, 31]. However, in recent years, beta-blockers, most specifically propranolol, have become the first line treatment. In 2008, Leaute-Labreze et al. published their serendipitous discovery of the rapid clinical effect of propranolol on IHs. In 2 children treated with propranolol for cardiopulmonary indications [32] rapid regression of the tumor was observed. Since then, many retrospective studies and case reports [33, 34] and few, placebo-controlled trials [35, 36] have supported the efficacy of this treatment. A meta-analysis of 35 studies comprising 795 patients treated with propranolol showed response rate of 97%, compared to pooled response rate of 69% to steroids after 12 months of follow-up ($p < 0.001$) [37]. The dosing is most frequently 2–3 mg per kilogram of body weight per day and there is still a lack of consensus regarding the protocols for initiation of the drug and ongoing monitoring [38, 39]. Propranolol use is not devoid of side effects. These include sleep disorders, diarrhea, bronchial hyperreactivity, cold hands and feet as well as—rarely—hypoglycemia that may be life threatening [35, 40]. In addition, propranolol is lipophilic, being able to cross of the blood–brain barrier. Evidence derived from animal studies and clinical studies on adults has shown that propranolol use is associated with central nervous system (CNS) effects such as Impairment to short- and long-term memory, changes in psychomotor functions, sleep quality, and mood [41–43]. The long term CNS effects of propranolol use for long periods, especially in the early developmental phases, is not well-studied [41]. Recently, however studies assessing psychomotor skills in infants treated with propranolol for IH have not identified a negative effect [44, 45]. Also, a parent-completed screening has found no increased developmental risk or growth impairment at age 4 years in patients with IH treated with propranolol [46].

As a result of propranolol's adverse effect and the concern over its CNS effect, the use of other β-blockers, such as atenolol become more common. Atenolol has a selective beta-blockade sparing β2 adrenergic receptors reducing the risk of bronchospasm. Furthermore, as it does not cross the blood-brain barrier it can theoretically prevent the sleep disturbances and the hypothetical CNS adverse effect associated with propranolol. An additional advantage of atenolol is its once-daily regimen, leading to better compliance. Indeed, in a number of studies atenolol showed similar efficacy with fewer adverse side-effects [47–51].

16.3.1 Beta Adrenergic Signaling and β Blocker's Mechanism of Action

The β-adrenergic signaling pathway mediates fight-or-flight stress responses through the sympathetic nervous system (SNS) [52]. The sympathetic nerve fibers innervate all tissues in the body and secrete the catecholamine neurotransmitter norepinephrine (NE) in response to environmental, psychological or physiological stimuli [53, 54]. Upon activation, catecholamine levels rises both in tissues and in circulating blood via the release of epinephrine (E) from the adrenal medulla chromaffin cells and NE overflow from vascular neuro-muscular junctions.

The biological effects of NE and E are mediated by three receptor families: α1, α2 and β-adrenergic receptors. Ligation of β-receptors by NE and E activates the Gαs guanine nucleotide-binding protein to stimulate adenylyl cyclase synthesis of cyclic 3'-5' adenosine monophosphate (cAMP). Subsequently, protein kinase A (PKA) is activated and, in turn, phosphorylates serine or threonine residues on myriad of target proteins involved in cells proliferation, differentiation, morphology and motility. Gene expression studies have demonstrated that approximately 20% of human genes are affected by PKA-induced phosphorylation [55, 56]. An additional key effector of cAMP is guanine nucleotide Exchange Protein activated by Adenylyl Cyclase (EPAC). EPAC stimulates the Ras-like guanine triphosphatase Rap1A, which then activates downstream effectors B-Raf, MEK1/2, and ERK1/2A [57]. Propranolol is an orthosteric antagonist of both β1- and β2-adrenergic receptors. In addition, it functions as central serotonin 5-HT receptor antagonist, inhibitor of noradrenaline reuptake and indirect agonist of α-adrenergic receptors [58]. The drug exists as a pair of optical isomers: S(−)propranolol and R(+)propranolol. The enantiomers bind with relatively large differences in affinity to the β-adrenoceptors [58]. Propranolol, as other pharmacological antagonists of the adrenergic receptors, counteract the agonists via the same signaling pathways.

Stress and the β-adrenergic system have been shown to have many effects on tumor biology. Though with some conflicting results, the use of β-blockers has been linked to increased survival of patients with solid cancers [59] . In addition, stressful life conditions have been shown to correlate with less favorable prognosis of cancer patients. In mouse models of tumors β-adrenergic agonists have also been found to accelerate tumor progression and metastasis [60, 61]. As expected by the high percentage of cAMP responsive genes, many cellular processes in tumors were shown to be modulated by the β-adrenergic system, including expression of pro-inflammatory cytokines, macrophages recruitment, angiogenesis, invasiveness and apoptosis [54, 62].

The mechanism of action of β blockers in hemangioma is not completely understood. Studies done on human cells isolated from IH in vitro and in vivo, on mouse models, revealed an effect on three major processes that will be detailed below: vascular tone, angiogenesis and vascuogenesis.

16.3.1.1 Vascular Tone

Following the administration of propranolol, a rapid change in the tumor consistency and color is typically noticed, especially with deep-seated IH [34, 63]. This raises the question of whether propranolol has an effect on the tumor vascular tone via vasoconstriction. Indeed, propranolol has been shown to decrease tissue blood flow to many organs following single administration [64–66]. Particularly in the skin, adrenaline-induced vasoconstriction has been shown to be increased by oral propranolol [67]. However, additional mechanisms might be involved in the slower, long-term effect of propranolol. A potential target of this mechanism of action is the pericyte. Pericytes are regulators of microvascular tone. Bosclo et al. demonstrated that pericytes from proliferating IH have lower density of the cytoskeleton component F-actin fiber compared to involuting Hemangioma pericytes and retinal pericytes. Also, these cells exhibit lower contractile capacity compared to normal pericytes [24]. In another work from the same group Lee et al. demonstrated that Epinephrine-induced relaxation of IH pericytes was prevented by propranolol. Using siRNA assay it was demonstrated that both the relaxation and its prevention by propranolol were mediated by the β2 receptor [68]. Interestingly, cultured pericytes from other sources have been shown to constrict, not relax, in response to catecholamines [69, 70]. Thus, the response of pericytes to NE and its blockers might be cell and context dependent.

In addition to direct effect of propranolol on the pericytes to induce contraction, it might exert its effect indirectly via the blocking of Nitric oxide release from HemEC. The endothelial isoform of nitric-oxide synthase (eNOS), is a key determinant of vascular tone [71, 72]. In different tissues and experimental systems, diverse adrenergic receptors subtypes have been shown to modulate eNOS expression and activity, including the β1, 2 and 3 adrenergic receptors [73, 74]. eNOS protein expression has been demonstrated to be significantly decreased in involuting versus proliferating hemangiomas [75]. In patients treated with propranolol, a significant decrease in the expression of eNOS in hemangioma tissues was noted compared with the age-matched untreated controls [75]. Also, serum concentrations of eNOS declined gradually during the first 2 months of propranolol treatment for IH [76]. On immortalized HemEC, Pan et al. has demonstrated that propranolol pretreatment robustly suppressed NO secretion and eNOS activation induced by Norepinephrine [77].

16.3.1.2 Angiogenesis

Vascular endothelial growth factor (VEGF) has been shown to play a key role in the angiogenic process in general and specifically in IH proliferation. The VEGF family consists of five ligands VEGF-A, VEGF-B, VEGF-C, VEGF-D and placental growth factor (PIGF). These ligands bind to three main subtypes of VEGF receptors: VEGFR-1 (Flt-1), VEGFR-2 (KDR/Flk-1) and VEGFR-3 [78]. Several works showed overexpression of VEGF-A in proliferating hemangioma tissue and in serum of patients with IH, compared to healthy controls [25, 79–81]. Moreover, we have shown that silencing the expression of VEGF-A in HemSC by short hairpin RNA (shRNA) was sufficient to block blood vessel formation in vivo [25]. NE enhances VEGF-A expression of both normal and tumoral cell types, [82–84]. Propranolol has been shown to reverse this effect via the blocking $\beta1$ and $\beta2$ adrenergic receptors [82–85]. Several lines of evidence suggest that propranolol acts at least in part through the blocking of VEGF. First, serum VEGF levels were shown to decrease noticeably in 91% of patients after a single month of propranolol treatment [86]. Similar results were reported by another group following the administration of relatively low doses of propranolol [76]. Second, in vitro studies have demonstrated that the NE agonist isoprenaline increased the expression of VEGF-A and the phosphorylation of VEGFR-2 in HemECs in a β-adrenergic receptor- and extracellular-signal-regulated kinase (ERK) -dependent manner. This response was blocked by β-adrenergic blockers. In HemSC, Ling Zhang et al. showed that propranolol at physiological concentrations leads to dose-dependent suppression of VEGF expression, at the mRNA and the protein level [87].

An additional major regulator of angiogenesis is Hypoxia-inducible factor (HIF)-1α. During hypoxia, HIF-1α binds the regulatory region of the VEGF gene, inducing its transcription and initiating its expression [88, 89]. HIF-1α expression has shown to be increased in the endothelium of proliferating hemangioma compared with involuting tissues [81]. Recently, it has been shown that HIF-1α was upregulated in the serum,

urine and tumor tissues of IH, and treatment of propranolol markedly inhibited its expression. In vitro, in HemEC, overexpression of HIF-1α blocked the inhibitory effects of propranolol on VEGF expression [90].

Several groups have demonstrated a direct pro-apoptotic or anti proliferative effect of propranolol on HemEC. However, a major concern is the high concentrations of propranolol required for these effects. These drug levels are unlikely to be present in the tumor's microenvironment [91]. It is possible, though, that propranolol works by opposing the growth promoting effects of catecholamines. Ji et al. showed that HemECs proliferation increased in response to isoprenaline via regulation of thee cell-cycle proteins cyclin D1 and its associated kinases, CDK-4 and CDK-6. These effects were reversed by β-adrenergic receptor antagonists. Of note, the antagonists had no effect on basal cell proliferation, but significantly decreased ISO-induced cell proliferation and cell viability [92]. An additional work has shown that hemSCs do not undergo apoptosis upon propranolol exposure, as caspase-3 levels is not upregulated. However, propranolol exposure significantly decreases HemSC proliferation via suppression of cyclin-D1 levels [93]. Also, propranolol can lower cAMP levels and activate the mitogen-activated protein kinase (MAPK) pathway downstream of βARs [94].

16.3.1.3 Vasculogenesis

Vasculogenesis, the creation of blood vessels de-novo from stem/progenitor cells, contributes the proliferation of IH. Thus, it is appealing to hypothesize that propranolol acts as an inhibitor of this process, as was shown for corticosteroids and rapamycin [95]. Against this hypothesis is the fact that late regrowth of the hemangioma seen in a subset of patients after cessation of the treatment [96]. This might mean that propranolol does not target the HemSC or even prevents their terminal differentiation or apoptosis. Effect of the adrenergic system on non-hemangioma stem/mesenchymal cells has been shown by several works. For example, NE has been shown to induce brown adipocyte differentiation of mesenchymal progenitors within white adipose tissue [97]. Also, an effect of NE on mesenchymal stem cells adipogenesis has been demonstrated in-vitro cell [98]. In work done on HemSC, Wong et al. reported that Propranolol-treated cells had a more robust response to adipogenic induction when compared to vehicle-treated HemSCs [99]. In a follow-up work the same group has shown that this adipogenic differentiation is characterized by improper adipogenic gene expression [100]. Similar results were reported by another group [101]. However, these results were achieved in very high, non-physiological concentration of propranolol.

16.3.1.4 Gender and Hemangioma

Female sex has been long recognized as a risk factor for infantile hemangiomas [102, 103]. In a questionnaire-based study on 1058 children, between 2002 and 2003, Haggstrom and collegues found that 71% were female, 29% were male [3]. In additional work, Anderson et al. identified all infants residing in Olmsted County, Minnesota, who were diagnosed with IH between 1976 and 2010. Among 999 infants, 64% were female [104]. Interestingly, female predominance was not found in a retrospective study on 973 preterm infants [2]. The etiology for female predominance is still unclear. In the following section, several hypotheses will be discussed, both sociological and biological.

16.4 Referral Bias Due to Sociological Factors

A possible explanation for the female predominance might be a referral bias. As parents perceive hemangiomas to pose a greater cosmetic concern when females are affected, they might be over-represented in dermatology clinics.

Most hemangiomas arise in exposed body areas, mainly the head and neck region (60%). Given the facts that some hemangiomas may be disfiguring, they often pose psychological stress on the caregiver. For example, in a questionnaire-based study on parents of infants with IH most parents testified to the negative commentary or stares they received from others, leading them to seek professional advice from a specialty clinic.

A quarter of parents declared that they were actually accused of child abuse because of their child's vascular lesion [105]. In additional study, disfiguring facial hemangiomas were found to be associated with parental reactions of disbelief, fear, and mourning. Reactions of strangers forced parents to confront various aspects of social stigmatization. A broad array of effects were observed regarding the effect of IH on the parent-child interaction [106]. As the social perception of the significance of physical appearance is different for boys and girls, it might be the case that parents seek more medical consultation when their daughter is affected by IH. However, a non-biased, population-based study had a similar female predominance. In 43 children with periocular infantile hemangiomas 70% were female ($p < 0.001$) [107]. Thus, a biological and not only social factors are plausible.

16.5 Pro-Angiogenic and Pro-Vasculogenic Effects of Estrogen

One might assume that differences between genders in estrogen levels or estrogen receptors lead to the female predominance. Estrogen is known to be a regulator of angiogenesis via effects on endothelial cell [108]. Many clues, both experimental and clinical suggest that estrogen has an important role in developing the vascular system and influence neovascularization. Estradiol (E2), a steroid and the primary female sex hormone is known to promote angiogenesis activity in vitro and in vivo [109, 110]. For example, E_2 stimulates VEGF expression in the utero [111]. In addition, E2 administration increases tumor extracellular levels of VEGF in estrogen-dependent animal models of breast cancer [112], whereas tamoxifen, an estrogen antagonist, suppresses it [113, 114]. Estrogen has also effects on the vascular tone. E_2 has been shown to increase the synthesis of nitric oxide (NO) in endothelial cells as well as to have anti-inflammatory and antioxidant effects [115]. In this sense, E2 might have a promoting role in the proliferation of IH.

In addition to pro-angiogenic effects, estrogen has also pro-vasculogenic effects. Circulating bone marrow–derived endothelial progenitor cells (EPCs) contribute to vasculogenesis (the de novo formation of blood vessels) by homing and incorporating into the microvascular endothelium [116]. EPC express estrogen receptor-α. Under in vitro conditions, activation of this receptor increases the proliferation of EPCs, as well as their migratory capacity and their differentiation toward mature vascular endothelial cells [117, 118]. In the setting of myocardial infarction in adult mice, estradiol has been shown to mobilize circulating EPCs from bone-marrow, resulting in incorporation into sites of neovascularization. This effect of estradiol appears to be dependent on the ability of estradiol to modulate the kinetics of bone-marrow-derived progenitor cells [119].

In infants with proliferating IH, serum levels of estrogen (estradiol 17β) have been shown to be increased compared to normal infants [120, 121]. Furthermore, estrogen receptor (ER) expression and binding activity were reported to be higher in patients with proliferating IH [81, 120]; and to later decrease following treatment with corticosteroids [120]. Plasma estradiol levels are very high at birth and later, at 8 day of life with no difference between males and females [122]. However, E2 levels in the plasma might not represent its level in the neonatal skin or the vascular tissue and it might be the case that gender differences exist as been shown for other tissues. For example, the amount of testosterone and estradiol measured in the different brain area during the perinatal period shows significant sex differences [122].

16.6 Genetic Basis

An alternative hypothesis might be that IH has a genetic basis, with dose effect of the X chromosome, meaning that two X chromosomes confer a higher risk of IH, while one X chromosome confers a lower risk of IH. Although most IHs occurs sporadically familial clustering has been reported. Grimmer et al. [123] showed a twofold increase in the risk ratio in siblings of an affected proband. Using information from the Utah Population Database, Walter et al. [124] reported 6 pedigrees with an autosomal dominant inheritance of high penetrance. By genome-wide linkage analysis of 3 unrelated families found linkage to a 38-cM interval on chromosome 5q31–q33. In a small number of patients, genetic variants were associated with germline mutations in the VEGFR2, VEGFR3, and TEM8 genes [125]; However, no genetic mutations on the X chromosome have been reported.

To sum up, the etiology of female predominance in IH, and especially the biological its basis is still obscure. Perhaps future studies will enrich our insight about the pathogenesis of hemangioma will shed a light on this enigma.

References

1. Hoornweg MJ, Smeulders MJ, Ubbink DT, van der Horst CM. The prevalence and risk factors of infantile haemangiomas: a case-control study in the Dutch population. Paediatr Perinat Epidemiol. 2012;26(2):156–62.
2. Amir J, Metzker A, Krikler R, Reisner SH. Strawberry hemangioma in preterm infants. Pediatr Dermatol. 1986;3(4):331–2.
3. Haggstrom AN, Drolet BA, Baselga E, Chamlin SL, Garzon MC, Horii KA, et al. Prospective study of infantile hemangiomas: demographic, prenatal, and perinatal characteristics. J Pediatr. 2007;150(3):291–4.
4. Enjolras O, Mulliken JB. The current management of vascular birthmarks. Pediatr Dermatol. 1993;10(4):311–3.
5. Frieden IJ, Haggstrom AN, Drolet BA, Mancini AJ, Friedlander SF, Boon L, et al. Infantile hemangiomas: current knowledge, future directions. Proceedings of a research workshop on infantile hemangiomas, April 7–9, 2005, Bethesda, MD, USA. Pediatr Dermatol. 2005;22(5):383–406.
6. Chang LC, Haggstrom AN, Drolet BA, Baselga E, Chamlin SL, Garzon MC, et al. Growth characteristics of infantile hemangiomas: implications for management. Pediatrics. 2008;122(2):360–7.
7. Khan ZA, Boscolo E, Picard A, Psutka S, Melero-Martin JM, Bartch TC, et al. Multipotential stem cells recapitulate human infantile hemangioma in immunodeficient mice. J Clin Invest. 2008;118(7):2592–9.
8. Boscolo E, Bischoff J. Vasculogenesis in infantile hemangioma. Angiogenesis. 2009;12(2):197–207.

9. Razon MJ, Kraling BM, Mulliken JB, Bischoff J. Increased apoptosis coincides with onset of involution in infantile hemangioma. Microcirculation. 1998; 5(2-3):189–95.

10. Iwata J, Sonobe H, Furihata M, Ido E, Ohtsuki Y. High frequency of apoptosis in infantile capillary haemangioma. J Pathol. 1996;179(4):403–8.

11. Bruckner AL, Frieden IJ. Hemangiomas of infancy. J Am Acad Dermatol. 2003;48(4):477–93.

12. Drolet BA, Esterly NB, Frieden IJ. Hemangiomas in children. N Engl J Med. 1999;341(3):173–81.

13. Itinteang T, Brasch HD, Tan ST, Day DJ. Expression of components of the renin-angiotensin system in proliferating infantile haemangioma may account for the propranolol-induced accelerated involution. J Plast Reconstr Aesthet Surg. 2011;64(6):759–65.

14. Spock CL, Tom LK, Canadas K, Sue GR, Sawh-Martinez R, Maier CL, et al. Infantile hemangiomas exhibit neural crest and pericyte markers. Ann Plast Surg. 2015;74(2):230–6.

15. Boye E, Yu Y, Paranya G, Mulliken JB, Olsen BR, Bischoff J. Clonality and altered behavior of endothelial cells from hemangiomas. J Clin Invest. 2001; 107(6):745–52.

16. Hopel-Kreiner I. Histogenesis of hemangiomas–an ultrastructural study on capillary and cavernous hemangiomas of the skin. Pathol Res Pract. 1980;170:70.

17. Greenberger S, Bischoff J. Pathogenesis of infantile haemangioma. Br J Dermatol. 2013;169(1):12–9.

18. North PE, Waner M, Mizeracki A, Mihm MC Jr. GLUT1: a newly discovered immunohistochemical marker for juvenile hemangiomas. Hum Pathol. 2000;31(1):11–22.

19. Crisan M, Yap S, Casteilla L, Chen CW, Corselli M, Park TS, et al. A perivascular origin for mesenchymal stem cells in multiple human organs. Cell Stem Cell. 2008;3(3):301–13.

20. Crisan M, Corselli M, Chen WC, Peault B. Perivascular cells for regenerative medicine. J Cell Mol Med. 2012;16(12):2851–60.

21. Ribatti D, Nico B, Crivellato E. The role of pericytes in angiogenesis. Int J Dev Biol. 2011;55(3):261–8.

22. van Dijk CG, Nieuweboer FE, Pei JY, YJ X, Burgisser P, van Mulligen E, et al. The complex mural cell: pericyte function in health and disease. Int J Cardiol. 2015;190:75–89.

23. Kutcher ME, Herman IM. The pericyte: cellular regulator of microvascular blood flow. Microvasc Res. 2009;77(3):235–46.

24. Boscolo E, Mulliken JB, Bischoff J. Pericytes from infantile hemangioma display proangiogenic properties and dysregulated angiopoietin-1. Arterioscler Thromb Vasc Biol. 2013;33(3):501–9.

25. Greenberger S, Boscolo E, Adini I, Mulliken JB, Bischoff J. Corticosteroid suppression of VEGF-A in infantile hemangioma-derived stem cells. N Engl J Med. 2010;362(11):1005–13.

26. Wang FQ, Chen G, Zhu JY, Zhang W, Ren JG, Liu H, et al. M2-polarised macrophages in infantile hae-

mangiomas: correlation with promoted angiogenesis. J Clin Pathol. 2013;66(12):1058–64.

27. Ritter MR, Reinisch J, Friedlander SF, Friedlander M. Myeloid cells in infantile hemangioma. Am J Pathol. 2006;168(2):621–8.

28. Mills CD. M1 and M2 macrophages: oracles of health and disease. Crit Rev Immunol. 2012; 32(6):463–88.

29. Zhang W, Chen G, Wang FQ, Ren JG, Zhu JY, Cai Y, et al. Macrophages contribute to the progression of infantile hemangioma by regulating the proliferation and differentiation of hemangioma stem cells. J Invest Dermatol. 2015;135:3163–72.

30. Zarem HA, Edgerton MT. Induced resolution of cavernous hemangiomas following prednisolone therapy. Plast Reconstr Surg. 1967;39(1):76–83.

31. Cohen SR, Wang CI. Steroid treatment of hemangioma of the head and neck in children. Ann Otol Rhinol Laryngol. 1972;81(4):584–90.

32. Leaute-Labreze C, Dumas de la Roque E, Hubiche T, Boralevi F, Thambo JB, Taieb A. Propranolol for severe hemangiomas of infancy. N Engl J Med. 2008; 358(24):2649–51.

33. Price CJ, Lattouf C, Baum B, McLeod M, Schachner LA, Duarte AM, et al. Propranolol vs corticosteroids for infantile hemangiomas: a multicenter retrospective analysis. Arch Dermatol. 2011;147(12):1371–6.

34. Sans V, de la Roque ED, Berge J, Grenier N, Boralevi F, Mazereeuw-Hautier J, et al. Propranolol for severe infantile hemangiomas: follow-up report. Pediatrics. 2009;124(3):e423–31.

35. Leaute-Labreze C, Hoeger P, Mazereeuw-Hautier J, Guibaud L, Baselga E, Posiunas G, et al. A randomized, controlled trial of oral propranolol in infantile hemangioma. N Engl J Med. 2015;372(8):735–46.

36. Hogeling M, Adams S, Wargon O. A randomized controlled trial of propranolol for infantile hemangiomas. Pediatrics. 2011;128(2):e259–66.

37. Izadpanah A, Kanevsky J, Belzile E, Schwarz K. Propranolol versus corticosteroids in the treatment of infantile hemangioma: a systematic review and meta-analysis. Plast Reconstr Surg. 2013;131(3): 601–13.

38. Biesbroeck L, Brandling-Bennett HA. Propranolol for infantile haemangiomas: review of report of a consensus conference. Arch Dis Child Educ Pract Ed. 2014;99(3):95–7.

39. Drolet BA, Frommelt PC, Chamlin SL, Haggstrom A, Bauman NM, Chiu YE, et al. Initiation and use of propranolol for infantile hemangioma: report of a consensus conference. Pediatrics. 2013; 131(1):128–40.

40. Horev A, Haim A, Zvulunov A. Propranolol induced hypoglycemia. Pediatr Endocrinol Rev. 2015;12(3): 308–10.

41. Langley A, Pope E. Propranolol and central nervous system function: potential implications for paediatric patients with infantile haemangiomas. Br J Dermatol. 2015;172(1):13–23.

42. Strange BA, Dolan RJ. Beta-adrenergic modulation of emotional memory-evoked human amygdala and hippocampal responses. Proc Natl Acad Sci U S A. 2004;101(31):11454–8.

43. Lonergan MH, Olivera-Figueroa LA, Pitman RK, Brunet A. Propranolol's effects on the consolidation and reconsolidation of long-term emotional memory in healthy participants: a meta-analysis. J Psychiatry Neurosci. 2013;38(4):222–31.

44. Moyakine AV, Spillekom-van Koulil S, van der Vleuten CJM. Propranolol treatment of infantile hemangioma is not associated with psychological problems at 7 years of age. J Am Acad Dermatol. 2017;77(1):105–8.

45. Moyakine AV, Hermans DJ, Fuijkschot J, van der Vleuten CJ. Propranolol treatment of infantile hemangiomas does not negatively affect psychomotor development. J Am Acad Dermatol. 2015;73(2):341–2.

46. Moyakine AV, Kerstjens JM, Spillekom-van Koulil S, van der Vleuten CJ. Propranolol treatment of infantile hemangioma (IH) is not associated with developmental risk or growth impairment at age 4 years. J Am Acad Dermatol. 2016;75(1):59–63.

47. Bayart CB, Tamburro JE, Vidimos AT, Wang L, Golden AB. Atenolol versus propranolol for treatment of infantile hemangiomas during the proliferative phase: a retrospective noninferiority study. Pediatr Dermatol. 2017;34(4):413–21.

48. Ji Y, Wang Q, Chen S, Xiang B, Xu Z, Li Y, et al. Oral atenolol therapy for proliferating infantile hemangioma: a prospective study. Medicine (Baltimore). 2016;95(24):e3908.

49. Abarzua-Araya A, Navarrete-Dechent CP, Heusser F, Retamal J, Zegpi-Trueba MS. Atenolol versus propranolol for the treatment of infantile hemangiomas: a randomized controlled study. J Am Acad Dermatol. 2014;70(6):1045–9.

50. Pope E, Chakkittakandiyil A, Lara-Corrales I, Maki E, Weinstein M. Expanding the therapeutic repertoire of infantile haemangiomas: cohort-blinded study of oral nadolol compared with propranolol. Br J Dermatol. 2013;168(1):222–4.

51. Tasani M, Glover M, Martinez AE, Shaw L. Atenolol treatment for infantile haemangioma. Br J Dermatol. 2017;176(5):1400–2.

52. Madamanchi A. Beta-adrenergic receptor signaling in cardiac function and heart failure. McGill J Med. 2007;10(2):99–104.

53. Daly CJ, McGrath JC. Previously unsuspected widespread cellular and tissue distribution of beta-adrenoceptors and its relevance to drug action. Trends Pharmacol Sci. 2011;32(4):219–26.

54. Cole SW, Sood AK. Molecular pathways: beta-adrenergic signaling in cancer. Clin Cancer Res. 2012;18(5):1201–6.

55. Montminy M. Transcriptional regulation by cyclic AMP. Annu Rev Biochem. 1997;66:807–22.

56. Zhang X, Odom DT, Koo SH, Conkright MD, Canettieri G, Best J, et al. Genome-wide analysis of cAMP-response element binding protein occupancy, phosphorylation, and target gene activation in human tissues. Proc Natl Acad Sci U S A. 2005;102(12):4459–64.

57. de Rooij J, Zwartkruis FJ, Verheijen MH, Cool RH, Nijman SM, Wittinghofer A, et al. Epac is a Rap1 guanine-nucleotide-exchange factor directly activated by cyclic AMP. Nature. 1998;396(6710):474–7.

58. Young R, Glennon RA. S(−)propranolol as a discriminative stimulus and its comparison to the stimulus effects of cocaine in rats. Psychopharmacology. 2009;203(2):369–82.

59. Watkins JL, Thaker PH, Nick AM, Ramondetta LM, Kumar S, Urbauer DL, et al. Clinical impact of selective and nonselective beta-blockers on survival in patients with ovarian cancer. Cancer. 2015;121(19):3444–51.

60. Sloan EK, Priceman SJ, Cox BF, Yu S, Pimentel MA, Tangkanangnukul V, et al. The sympathetic nervous system induces a metastatic switch in primary breast cancer. Cancer Res. 2010;70(18):7042–52.

61. Thaker PH, Han LY, Kamat AA, Arevalo JM, Takahashi R, Lu C, et al. Chronic stress promotes tumor growth and angiogenesis in a mouse model of ovarian carcinoma. Nat Med. 2006;12(8):939–44.

62. Tang J, Li Z, Lu L, Cho CH. Beta-adrenergic system, a backstage manipulator regulating tumour progression and drug target in cancer therapy. Semin Cancer Biol. 2013;23(6 Pt B):533–42.

63. Rosbe KW, Suh KY, Meyer AK, Maguiness SM, Frieden IJ. Propranolol in the management of airway infantile hemangiomas. Arch Otolaryngol Head Neck Surg. 2010;136(7):658–65.

64. Nies AS, Evans GH, Shand DG. Regional hemodynamic effects of beta-adrenergic blockade with propranolol in the unanesthetized primate. Am Heart J. 1973;85(1):97–102.

65. McSorley PD, Warren DJ. Effects of propranolol and metoprolol on the peripheral circulation. Br Med J. 1978;2(6152):1598–600.

66. Vandenburg MJ, Conlon C, Ledingham JM. A comparison of the effects of propranolol and oxprenolol on forearm blood flow and skin temperature. Br J Clin Pharmacol. 1981;11(5):485–90.

67. Doshi BS, Kulkarni RD, Dattani KK, Anand MP. Effect of labetalol and propranolol on human cutaneous vasoconstrictor response to adrenaline. Int J Clin Pharmacol Res. 1984;4(1):25–8.

68. Lee D, Boscolo E, Durham JT, Mulliken JB, Herman IM, Bischoff J. Propranolol targets the contractility of infantile haemangioma-derived pericytes. Br J Dermatol. 2014;171(5):1129–37.

69. Kelley C, D'Amore P, Hechtman HB, Shepro D. Vasoactive hormones and cAMP affect pericyte contraction and stress fibres in vitro. J Muscle Res Cell Motil. 1988;9(2):184–94.

70. Markhotina N, Liu GJ, Martin DK. Contractility of retinal pericytes grown on silicone elastomer substrates is through a protein kinase A-mediated

intracellular pathway in response to vasoactive peptides. IET Nanobiotechnol. 2007;1(3):44–51.

71. Balligand JL, Cannon PJ. Nitric oxide synthases and
cardiac muscle. Autocrine and paracrine influences.
Arterioscler Thromb Vasc Biol. 1997;17(10):1846–58.

72. McHugh J, Cheek DJ. Nitric oxide and regulation of
vascular tone: pharmacological and physiological
considerations. Am J Crit Care. 1998;7(2):131–40.

73. Ferro A, Coash M, Yamamoto T, Rob J, Ji Y, Queen L.
Nitric oxide-dependent beta2-adrenergic dilatation
of rat aorta is mediated through activation of both
protein kinase A and Akt. Br J Pharmacol. 2004;
143(3):397–403.

74. Dessy C, Saliez J, Ghisdal P, Daneau G, Lobysheva
II, Frerart F, et al. Endothelial beta3-adrenoreceptors
mediate nitric oxide-dependent vasorelaxation of
coronary microvessels in response to the third-
generation beta-blocker nebivolol. Circulation. 2005;
112(8):1198–205.

75. Dai Y, Hou F, Buckmiller L, Fan CY, Saad A, Suen
J, et al. Decreased eNOS protein expression in invo-
luting and propranolol-treated hemangiomas. Arch
Otolaryngol Head Neck Surg. 2012;138(2):177–82.

76. Yuan WL, Jin ZL, Wei JJ, Liu ZY, Xue L, Wang
XK. Propranolol given orally for proliferating infantile haemangiomas: analysis of efficacy and sero-
logical changes in vascular endothelial growth factor
and endothelial nitric oxide synthase in 35 patients.
Br J Oral Maxillofac Surg. 2013;51(7):656–61.

77. Pan WK, Li P, Guo ZT, Huang Q, Gao Y. Propranolol
induces regression of hemangioma cells via the
down-regulation of the PI3K/Akt/eNOS/VEGF pathway. Pediatr Blood Cancer. 2015;62(8):1414–20.

78. McMahon G. VEGF receptor signaling in tumor
angiogenesis. Oncologist. 2000;5(Suppl 1):3–10.

79. Takahashi K, Mulliken JB, Kozakewich HP, Rogers
RA, Folkman J, Ezekowitz RA. Cellular markers that
distinguish the phases of hemangioma during infancy
and childhood. J Clin Invest. 1994;93(6):2357–64.

80. Chang J, Most D, Bresnick S, Mehrara B, Steinbrech
DS, Reinisch J, et al. Proliferative hemangiomas:
analysis of cytokine gene expression and angiogenesis. Plast Reconstr Surg. 1999;103(1):1–9.

81. Kleinman ME, Greives MR, Churgin SS, Blechman
KM, Chang EI, Ceradini DJ, et al. Hypoxia-induced
mediators of stem/progenitor cell trafficking are
increased in children with hemangioma. Arterioscler
Thromb Vasc Biol. 2007;27(12):2664–70.

82. Fredriksson JM, Lindquist JM, Bronnikov GE,
Nedergaard J. Norepinephrine induces vascular
endothelial growth factor gene expression in brown
adipocytes through a beta -adrenoreceptor/cAMP/
protein kinase A pathway involving Src but independently of Erk1/2. J Biol Chem. 2000;275(18):
13802–11.

83. Lutgendorf SK, Cole S, Costanzo E, Bradley S,
Coffin J, Jabbari S, et al. Stress-related mediators
stimulate vascular endothelial growth factor secretion by two ovarian cancer cell lines. Clin Cancer
Res. 2003;9(12):4514–21.

84. Park SY, Kang JH, Jeong KJ, Lee J, Han JW, Choi
WS, et al. Norepinephrine induces VEGF expression
and angiogenesis by a hypoxia-inducible factor-
1alpha protein-dependent mechanism. Int J Cancer.
2011;128(10):2306–16.

85. Guo K, Ma Q, Wang L, Hu H, Li J, Zhang D, et al.
Norepinephrine-induced invasion by pancreatic
cancer cells is inhibited by propranolol. Oncol Rep.
2009;22(4):825–30.

86. Chen XD, Ma G, Huang JL, Chen H, Jin YB, Ye XX,
et al. Serum-level changes of vascular endothelial
growth factor in children with infantile hemangioma
after oral propranolol therapy. Pediatr Dermatol.
2013;30(5):549–53.

87. Zhang L, Mai HM, Zheng J, Zheng JW, Wang YA,
Qin ZP, et al. Propranolol inhibits angiogenesis via
down-regulating the expression of vascular endothelial growth factor in hemangioma derived stem cell.
Int J Clin Exp Pathol. 2014;7(1):48–55.

88. Ziello JE, Jovin IS, Huang Y. Hypoxia-inducible
factor (HIF)-1 regulatory pathway and its potential
for therapeutic intervention in malignancy and ischemia. Yale J Biol Med. 2007;80(2):51–60.

89. Dery MA, Michaud MD, Richard DE. Hypoxia-
inducible factor 1: regulation by hypoxic and non-
hypoxic activators. Int J Biochem Cell Biol. 2005;
37(3):535–40.

90. Li P, Guo Z, Gao Y, Pan W. Propranolol represses
infantile hemangioma cell growth through the beta2-
adrenergic receptor in a HIF-1alpha-dependent manner. Oncol Rep. 2015;33(6):3099–107.

91. Wong L, Nation RL, Chiou WL, Mehta PK. Plasma
concentrations of propranolol and 4-hydroxypro-
pranolol during chronic oral propranolol therapy. Br
J Clin Pharmacol. 1979;8(2):163–7.

92. Ji Y, Chen S, Li K, Xiao X, Zheng S, Xu T. The role
of beta-adrenergic receptor signaling in the proliferation of hemangioma-derived endothelial cells. Cell
Div. 2013;8(1):1.

93. Kum JJ, Khan ZA. Propranolol inhibits growth of
hemangioma-initiating cells but does not induce
apoptosis. Pediatr Res. 2014;75(3):381–8.

94. Munabi NC, England RW, Edwards AK, Kitajewski
AA, Tan QK, Weinstein A, et al. Propranolol targets
hemangioma stem cells via cAMP and mitogen-activated protein kinase regulation. Stem Cells Transl Med.
2016;5(1):45–55.

95. Greenberger S, Yuan S, Walsh LA, Boscolo E,
Kang KT, Matthews B, et al. Rapamycin suppresses
self-renewal and vasculogenic potential of stem
cells isolated from infantile hemangioma. J Invest
Dermatol. 2011;131(12):2467–76.

96. Bagazgoitia L, Hernandez-Martin A, Torrelo A.
Recurrence of infantile hemangiomas treated with
propranolol. Pediatr Dermatol. 2011;28(6):658–62.

97. Vegiopoulos A, Muller-Decker K, Strzoda D,
Schmitt I, Chichelnitskiy E, Ostertag A, et al.
Cyclooxygenase-2 controls energy homeostasis in
mice by de novo recruitment of brown adipocytes.
Science. 2010;328(5982):1158–61.

98. Li H, Fong C, Chen Y, Cai G, Yang M. Beta2- and beta3-, but not beta1-adrenergic receptors are involved in osteogenesis of mouse mesenchymal stem cells via cAMP/PKA signaling. Arch Biochem Biophys. 2010; 496(2):77–83.

99. Wong A, Hardy KL, Kitajewski AM, Shawber CJ, Kitajewski JK, Wu JK. Propranolol accelerates adipogenesis in hemangioma stem cells and causes apoptosis of hemangioma endothelial cells. Plast Reconstr Surg. 2012;130(5):1012–21.

100. England RW, Hardy KL, Kitajewski AM, Wong A, Kitajewski JK, Shawber CJ, et al. Propranolol promotes accelerated and dysregulated adipogenesis in hemangioma stem cells. Ann Plast Surg. 2014;73(Suppl 1):S119–24.

101. Ma X, Zhao T, Ouyang T, Xin S, Ma Y, Chang M. Propranolol enhanced adipogenesis instead of induction of apoptosis of hemangiomas stem cells. Int J Clin Exp Pathol. 2014;7(7):3809–17.

102. Finn MC, Glowacki J, Mulliken JB. Congenital vascular lesions: clinical application of a new classification. J Pediatr Surg. 1983;18(6):894–900.

103. Bree AF, Siegfried E, Sotelo-Avila C, Nahass G. Infantile hemangiomas: speculation on placental trophoblastic origin. Arch Dermatol. 2001;137(5):573–7.

104. Anderson KR, Schoch JJ, Lohse CM, Hand JL, Davis DM, Tollefson MM. Increasing incidence of infantile hemangiomas (IH) over the past 35 years: correlation with decreasing gestational age at birth and birth weight. J Am Acad Dermatol. 2016;74(1):120–6.

105. Williams EF, Iii HM, Rodgers BJ, Brockbank D, Shannon L, et al. A psychological profile of children with hemangiomas and their families. Arch Facial Plast Surg. 2003;5(3):229–34.

106. Tanner JL, Dechert MP, Frieden IJ. Growing up with a facial hemangioma: parent and child coping and adaptation. Pediatrics. 1998;101(3):446–52.

107. Alniemi ST, Griepentrog GJ, Diehl N, Mohney BG. Incidence and clinical characteristics of periocular infantile hemangiomas. Arch Ophthalmol. 2012;130(7):889–93.

108. Losordo DW, Isner JM. Estrogen and angiogenesis: a review. Arterioscler Thromb Vasc Biol. 2001;21(1): 6–12.

109. Johns A, Freay AD, Fraser W, Korach KS, Rubanyi GM. Disruption of estrogen receptor gene prevents 17 beta estradiol-induced angiogenesis in transgenic mice. Endocrinology. 1996;137(10):4511–3.

110. Morales DE, McGowan KA, Grant DS, Maheshwari S, Bhartiya D, Cid MC, et al. Estrogen promotes angiogenic activity in human umbilical vein endothelial cells in vitro and in a murine model. Circulation. 1995;91(3):755–63.

111. Bausero P, Cavaille F, Meduri G, Freitas S, Perrot-Applanat M. Paracrine action of vascular endothelial growth factor in the human endometrium: production and target sites, and hormonal regulation. Angiogenesis. 1998;2(2):167–82.

112. Dabrosin C, Margetts PJ, Gauldie J. Estradiol increases extracellular levels of vascular endothelial growth factor in vivo in murine mammary cancer. Int J Cancer. 2003;107(4):535–40.

113. Takei H, Lee ES, Jordan VC. In vitro regulation of vascular endothelial growth factor by estrogens and antiestrogens in estrogen-receptor positive breast cancer. Breast Cancer. 2002;9(1):39–42.

114. Garvin S, Dabrosin C. Tamoxifen inhibits secretion of vascular endothelial growth factor in breast cancer in vivo. Cancer Res. 2003;63(24):8742–8.

115. Resanovic I, Rizzo M, Zafirovic S, Bjelogrlic P, Perovic M, Savic K, et al. Anti-atherogenic effects of 17β-estradiol. Horm Metab Res. 2013;45(10): 701–8.

116. Nolan DJ, Ciarrocchi A, Mellick AS, Jaggi JS, Bambino K, Gupta S, et al. Bone marrow-derived endothelial progenitor cells are a major determinant of nascent tumor neovascularization. Genes Dev. 2007;21(12):1546–58.

117. Suriano R, Chaudhuri D, Johnson RS, Lambers E, Ashok BT, Kishore R, et al. 17β-estradiol mobilizes bone marrow–derived endothelial progenitor cells to tumors. Cancer Res. 2008;68(15):6038–42.

118. Baruscotti I, Barchiesi F, Jackson EK, Imthurn B, Stiller R, Kim J-H, et al. Estradiol stimulates capillary formation by human endothelial progenitor cells: role of ER-α/β, heme oxygenase-1 and tyrosine kinase. Hypertension. 2010;56(3):397–404.

119. Iwakura A, Shastry S, Luedemann C, Hamada H, Kawamoto A, Kishore R, et al. Estradiol enhances recovery after myocardial infarction by augmenting incorporation of bone marrow–derived endothelial progenitor cells into sites of ischemia-induced neovascularization via endothelial nitric oxide synthase–mediated activation of matrix metalloproteinase-. Circulation. 2006;113(12): 1605–14.

120. Sasaki GH, Pang CY, Wittliff JL. Pathogenesis and treatment of infant skin strawberry hemangiomas: clinical and in vitro studies of hormonal effects. Plast Reconstr Surg. 1984;73(3):359–70.

121. Liu W, Zhang S, Hu T, Jiang X, Hu X, Feng J. Sex hormone receptor of hemangioma and vascular malformation in children. Zhonghua Wai Ke Za Zhi. 1999;37(5):295–7.

122. Konkle AT, McCarthy MM. Developmental time course of estradiol, testosterone, and dihydrotestosterone levels in discrete regions of male and female rat brain. Endocrinology. 2011;152(1):223–35.

123. Grimmer JF, Williams MS, Pimentel R, Mineau G, Wood GM, Bayrak-Toydemir P, et al. Familial clustering of hemangiomas. Arch Otolaryngol Head Neck Surg. 2011;137(8):757–60.

124. Walter JW, Blei F, Anderson JL, Orlow SJ, Speer MC, Marchuk DA. Genetic mapping of a novel familial form of infantile hemangioma. Am J Med Genet. 1999;82(1):77–83.

125. Walter JW, North PE, Waner M, Mizeracki A, Blei F, Walker JW, et al. Somatic mutation of vascular endothelial growth factor receptors in juvenile hemangioma. Genes Chromosomes Cancer. 2002;33(3):295–303.

Cutaneous Leishmaniasis

17

Michal Solomon and Eli Schwartz

17.1 Introduction

Leishmaniasis is a group of chronic cutaneous, mucocutaneous, and visceral diseases caused by infection with one of several species of the protozoan parasite, Leishmania [1]. Members of the genus Leishmania are obligate intracellular parasitic protozoa in the family Trypanosomatidae. They exist as elongate, 10–15 μm, flagellated forms called promastigotes in their sand fly vectors. When an infected sand fly bites a mammalian host, it injects the promastigotes into the skin. Tissue macrophages phagocytize the organisms, which then transform into round or oval, 2–3 μm non-flagellated forms called amastigotes. The amastigotes undergo successive asexual division until the macrophage ruptures releasing the amastigotes, which enter other macrophages to continue the cycle. When a sand fly bites an infected mammalian host, it ingests amastigote-laden macrophages along with its blood-meal. The amastigotes transform into promastigotes and reproduce in the gut of the fly before migrating to the proboscis of the fly to complete the cycle with the next fly bite.

The sand-fly female in the genera Phlebotomus in the Old World, and Lutzomyia and Psychodopygus in the New World transmit the Leishmania organisms via their bite. Several non-human mammals serve as reservoirs for leishmaniasis including domestic and wild canines and various rodents depending on the geographic distribution and the species of Leishmania involved.

17.2 Clinical Manifestations

There are three major clinical manifestations:

1. Cutaneous Leishmaniasis (CL)
2. Mucocutaneous Leishmaniasis (MCL)
3. Visceral Leishmaniasis (VL) (Beyond the scope of this chapter)

M. Solomon (✉)
Department of Dermatology,
Chaim Sheba Medical Center,
Tel Hashomer, Israel

The Sackler School of Medicine,
Tel Aviv University, Tel Aviv, Israel

E. Schwartz
The Sackler School of Medicine,
Tel Aviv University, Tel Aviv, Israel

Center for Geographic Medicine and Tropical
Diseases, Chaim Sheba Medical Center,
Tel Hashomer, Israel

© Springer International Publishing AG, part of Springer Nature 2018
E. Tur, H. I. Maibach (eds.), *Gender and Dermatology*,
https://doi.org/10.1007/978-3-319-72156-9_17

17.3 Cutaneous Leishmaniasis

Based on its geographical distribution, cutaneous leishmaniasis can be divided into [2]:

1. *Old World* (including, the Middle East, Southern Europe, parts of South-West Asia and Africa)
2. *New World leishmaniasis* (from Southern USA through Latin America to the highlands of Argentina)

Old World species cause mostly benign and often self-limiting cutaneous disease, while New World species cause a broad spectrum of manifestations, from benign to severe, including mucosal involvement.

17.3.1 Old World Cutaneous Leishmaniasis (OWCL)

Common names include Oriental sore, Rose of Jericho, Delhi boil, and Aleppo boil.

17.3.2 Etiology and Epidemiology

Four species: *L. major, L. tropica, L. aethiopica,* and *L. infantum* cause OWCL.

L. major is characterized by being rural, wet, and zoonotic cutaneous leishmaniasis. The animal reservoirs are desert rodents. It is endemic in desert areas of northern Africa, Central Asia, the Sudan, and the Middle East.

L. tropica is characterized by being urban, dry, and more often anthroponotic cutaneous leishmaniasis. In a recent outbreak in Israel, Rock hyraxes were found to be the reservoir. Endemic areas include urban areas of the Mediterranean basin, Central Asia, and the Middle East. Although in Israel it is widespread in villages communities.

L. aethiopica occurs mainly in Ethiopia and Kenya in rural mountain areas. Hyraxes, are the animal reservoir.

L. infantum occurs in the Mediterranean basin, China, Central Asia, and the Middle East. Adults

infected with this species tend to develop a mild self-limited cutaneous disease, whereas infants tend to develop visceral disease. Animal reservoirs include domesticated and wild canines.

17.3.3 Clinical Features

Following inoculation by the sand fly, characteristic skin lesions generally appear within 6 weeks, but may be delayed for prolonged periods depending on the size of the inoculum. The lesion begins as a small, pruritic, erythematous papule that slowly enlarges and breaks down to form a small ulcer or is sometimes a nodular lesion. Lesions may be single or multiple and occur on exposed skin surfaces. Ulcers persist for a variable time and heal slowly with scarring.

L. major often causes multiple lesions with an exudative base. The lesions may be healed spontaneously in 6–12 months. Spread to regional lymph nodes is rare [3].

L. tropica usually causes a single/multiple, more severe ulcer that may require 1–3 years for spontaneous healing.

L. aethiopica produces an even more severe ulcer that may persist for several years. Diffuse cutaneous leishmaniasis, an anergic state with extensive skin infiltration by organisms resembling lepromatous leprosy, occurs in approximately 20% of endemic *L. aethiopica* infections.

17.3.4 New World Cutaneous Leishmaniasis (NWCL)

Common names include: American cutaneous leishmaniasis, Chiclero's ulcer, espundia, bush yaws, uta, and picatura de pito (Fig. 17.1).

17.3.5 Etiology and Epidemiology

NWCL is a disease of rural forest and jungle areas of most of Central and South America. Forest workers, agricultural workers, and others travelling in rural, forested areas are primarily at risk, as

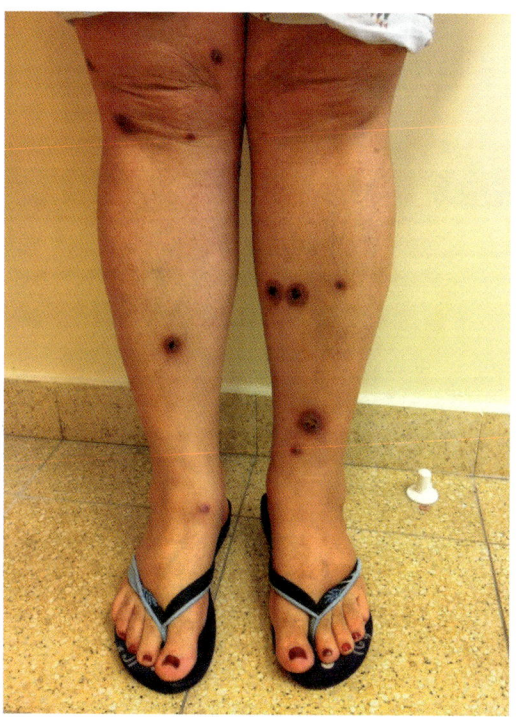

Fig. 17.1 Multiple lesions on the legs of a patient with *L. major* infection

Table 17.1 New World cutaneous leishmaniasis

Subgenus	Common species
L. Viannia	*L. (V.) brasiliensis*
	L. (V.) guyanensis
	L. (V.) panamensis
	L. (V.) peruviana
L. Mexicana	*L. mexicana*
	L. amazonensis
	L. venezuelensis

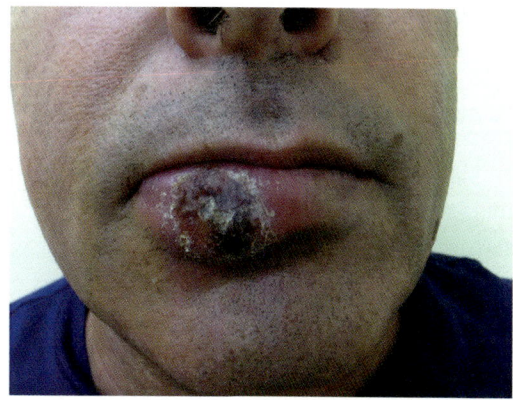

Fig. 17.2 Skin ulcer on the lower lip of a patient with *L. tropica*

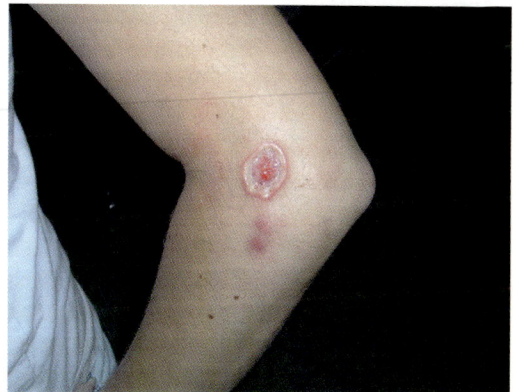

Fig. 17.3 Lesion in a traveller with *L. braziliensis*. Note the subcutaneous nodules distal to the ulcer

the sand fly vectors do not readily bite humans. Several species belonging to the *L. viannia* and *L. mexicana* complexes cause NWCL (Table 17.1). Species from either complex may be principal causes of leishmaniasis in each area. Both complexes are pathogenic throughout the range of the regions in the New World, with the exceptions of southern Texas and the Dominican Republic, where *L. mexicana* is the sole identified species. Animal reservoirs include foxes, sloths and forest rodents depending on the species (Fig. 17.2).

17.3.6 Clinical Features

Cutaneous lesions may resemble those of OWCL with a few distinctive differences. Lesions tend to be larger, up to 7 cm in diameter, with an elevated, indurated border which is mostly ulcerative. In addition, subcutaneous nodules with sporotrichoid distribution, and regional lymphadenopathy may be present (Fig. 17.3). The cutaneous lesions heal very slowly, and they may spread to the oropharyngeal mucosa causing mucocutaneous leishmaniasis.

Chiclero's ulcer refers to cutaneous disease found in the Yucatan, Belize, and Guatemala caused primarily by *L. mexicana*. Lesions tend to be solitary and occur most frequently on the ear. Ear ulcers may persist for many years before healing and may result in destruction of the ear. Lesions in other skin areas often heal within 6 months. Mucosal spread is rare.

Mucocutaneous leishmaniasis results primarily from infections caused by *L. (Viannia) braziliensis.* The cutaneous lesions spread along lymphatics, resembling sporotrichosis, and mucosal disease occurs in 10% of cases. Mucosal involvement occurs by metastatic spread of infection from the skin and presents months to years after the initial cutaneous lesions. It begins as erythema, edema, and ulceration of the nasal septum, with gradual extension to the palate, pharynx, and larynx. Occasionally, the anus and other mucosal sites may be involved. This destructive, granulomatous process of the soft tissue can involve cartilage but not bone. Perforation of the nasal septum and collapse of the nasal bridge is typical, giving the so-called tapir nose. Mucosal disease is progressive and mutilating and may be fatal. The severe form of mucosal disease is called espundia. OWCL leishmaniasis may be seen in travelers to endemic areas [4, 5].

17.3.7 Diagnosis of Cutaneous Leishmaniasis

Diagnosis requires demonstrating the organism in a sample from the lesion. Variable numbers of amastigotes, also called Leishman–Donovan (LD) bodies, are present in lesions, and they may be seen in smears or biopsies or culture.

17.3.8 Smear

Parasite isolation is performed on material obtained from scratches from the lesion margins, using a sterile surgical blade (scalpel). In case of non-ulcerated lesions (nodular, sporotrichoid, lupoid), aspirated punctures are performed using disposable syringes containing 0.3–0.5 ml of sterile saline solution.

Smears are bleached using *May-Grünwald-Giemsa* stain to identify amastigotes forms by means of optical microscopy with sensitivity rate ranging from 64% [6] to 80% [7] depending on technique quality. The specificity of the dermal smear is excellent (100%) (Fig. 17.4).

17.3.9 Culture

The parasite can be isolated in NNN/Schneider medium (incubation at 28°C) from a tissue fragment removed from the border of an active lesion. Culture usually requires 3–10 days to grow and sometimes more with some leishmania New World species. Specimen should not

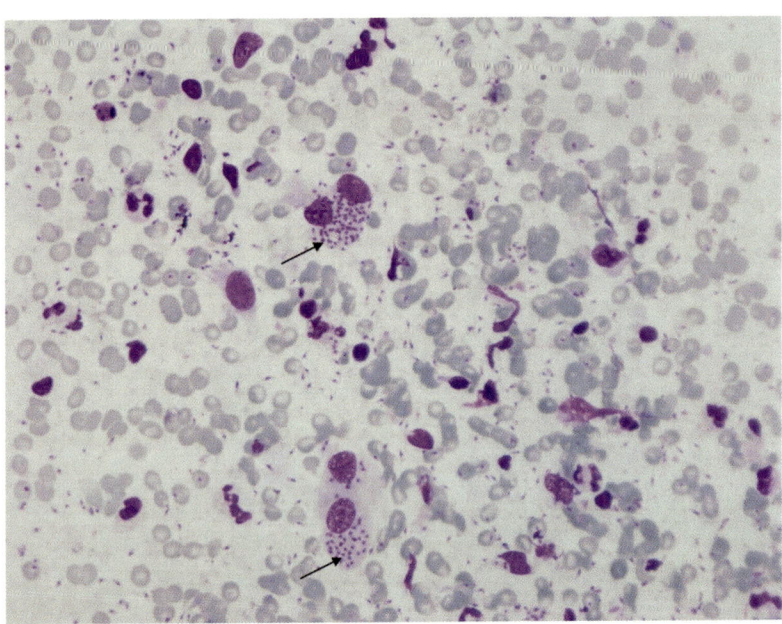

Fig. 17.4 Smear of skin lesion of leishmanial- note the LD bodies in the macrophages

be discarded unless they are negative for 4 weeks. Positivity of the culture varies depending on presence of amastigotes in the smear. Specificity is about 100%, but sensitivity rate is in challenge [6].

17.3.10 Biopsy

Skin biopsies should be taken from the margin of the lesion. Histopathologic analysis of infected tissues stained with hematoxylin-eosin allows a diagnostic confirmation of the disease in most cases. The histopathological presentation of CL shows a great variability, but a predominant pattern characterized by the presence of unorganized granuloma without necrosis. The leishmania organisms are typically intensely blue with Giemsa stain. The Leishman-Donovan bodies, that are 2–4 μm in diameter and round or oval are usually seen in macrophages, but mat be also present in the extracellular areas [8].

17.3.11 PCR

The above-mentioned tests are genus-specific tests, identifying whether the person is infected with leishmania. However, since the clinical spectrum of the disease and its response to treatment vary according to the species, a species-specific diagnosis is often warranted. The polymerase chain reaction (PCR) is now considered to be the method of choice [9, 10]. It is a rapid tool with a high specificity to differentiate between Old and New World leishmaniasis. It is highly sensitive and requires minute amounts of DNA from dermal scrapings of cutaneous lesions, and its sensitivity ranges from 89% to 100% [11].

17.3.12 Treatment of Cutaneous Leishmaniasis

Risk-benefit considerations should be made in treating cutaneous leishmaniasis. On one hand, the infection can be mild and self-limited, and the benefits of treatment need to be weighed against potential toxicity. On the other hand, the infection can manifest as a significant skin lesion with the potential of spreading, or with an actual mucosal lesion.

Uncomplicated versus complicated infection—The approach to management of cutaneous leishmaniasis (CL) begins with establishing the clinical severity of infection [2].

Features of uncomplicated CL include:

1. Infection with species not likely to be associated with mucosal leishmaniasis (e.g. OWCL)
2. No mucosal involvement
3. Single lesion or a few lesions
4. Small lesion size (eg, <1 cm)
5. Immunocompetent host

Features of complicated CL include:

1. Infection with species associated with mucosal leishmaniasis (ML; primarily *Viannia* subgenus, especially in the "mucosal belt" of Bolivia, Peru, and Brazil)
2. More than four lesions of significant size (e.g., >1 cm)
3. Individual lesions ≥5 cm
4. Subcutaneous nodules
5. Regional adenopathy >1 cm size (somewhat controversial)
6. Size or location of lesions for which local treatment is not feasible
7. Lesions on face, fingers, toes, or genitalia
8. Immunosuppressed host
9. Clinical failure of local therapy after 2–3 months posttreatment

Forms of CL that should be managed as complicated infection with expert consultation include:

1. Leishmaniasis recidivans (due to *L.L. tropica*)
2. Disseminated/diffuse CL (due to *L.V. braziliensis, L.L. mexicana* or *L.L. amazonensis*)
3. Infections due to *L.L. aethiopica*

Numerous forms of treatment, both systemic and local, have been advocated, including systemic treatment by pentavalent antimonials, amphotericin B (liposomal), pentamidine, and recently oral Miltefosine. Local treatment by cryotherapy, Thermotherapy and many others [12]. Many of them never been investigated systematically. Treatment options are summarized in Table 17.2.

The main treatment options for OWCL are topical treatment with paromomycin ointment (Leshcutan, Teva) [13], liquid nitrogen, or intralesional injectable sodium stibogluconate (pentostam^R) [14, 15]. Occasionally, there are cases of OWCL that require systemic therapy, such as in cases that lack response to local treatment, cases

of multiple lesions or if affected areas of the body are such that local treatment cannot be applied. Individuals with multiple lesions (sometimes as many as 30–40 lesions) cannot feasibly be treated with topical therapy. In these cases, we recommend using systemic treatment (intravenous sodium stibogluconate with a 10-day course [16].

L. Tropica seems to be more resistant to treatment and has less of a response to paromomycin ointment. In these cases, therefore, our practice is to treat with sodium stibogluconate, either intralesional or intravenous. Another treatment option is using intravenous liposomal Amphothericin B for 6 days with good response [17].

The most common systemic treatment is intravenous sodium stibogluconate (pentostam^R). This treatment may cause serious side effects, therefore in recent years we use intravenous liposomal Amphotericin B (AmBisome^R) as the first line treatment, with a high success rate.

Treatment with oral miltefosine is another option although there are no enough data about its efficacy [18].

Standard treatment for NWCL especially for *L. braziliensis* is intravenous therapy in order to prevent its spread to the nasopharynx which can cause permanent destruction of the cartilage in these areas. The drug of choice is intravenous liposomal amphotericin B, and in cases of treatment failure, intravenous sodium stibogluconate (pentostam) can be used [19, 20]. Another treatment option is oral Miltefosine tablets. It is contra indicated during pregnancy and nursing.

Table 17.2 Treatment of cutaneous leishmanisis

Local therapy		
Pentavalent antimonials	Sodium stibogluconate	0.5–2 mL of 100 mg/mL pentavalent antimony (Sb^{5+}) intralesionally every 3 weeks until healed
Paromomycin	Paromomycin ointment	Apply topically to lesions twice daily for 10 days, rest for 10 days, then reapply for 10 days
Physical therapy	Cryotherapy	
	Thermotherapy	
	Photodynamic therapy	
Oral systemic therapy		
Miltefosine	Miltefosine	2.5 mg/kg (maximum 150 mg) orally in 3 divided doses for 28 days
Parenteral systemic therapy		
Pentavalent antimonials	Sodium stibogluconate	20 mg Sb^V/kg/day intravenously or intramuscularly for 10–20 days
	Meglumine antimoniate	20 mg Sb^V/kg/day intravenously or intramuscularly for 10–20 days
Amphotericin	Liposomal amphotericin B (AmBisome)	3–5 mg/kg intravenously daily for 5–7 doses, such as days 1–5, 10

17.4 Gender and Leishmaniasis

Most studies of CL and MCL provide scarce information regarding gender and leishmania infection. It is estimated that leishmaniasis is more common in males. Differences between the sexes in the incidence and severity of infection might be attributed to genetic and physiological constitutions [21] including attractiveness to vectors, processing of pathogens and cellular responses to the pathogen [usually refers to 'Sex' difference], but also to differences in exposures, to participation in high-risk activities, and use of preventive strategies [22]. [refers to behavioral difference or 'Gender' differences] [22].

In a recent study in Israel, we sought to evaluate the sex and gender differences across CL and MCL among Israeli patients. Among 145 cases of imported MWCL in returning Israeli travelers 121 (83%) were males. This high percentage of males is high above the known distribution of Israeli travelers to the tropics, which is about 50% of each gender. All these infections were acquired in in the Amazon region of Bolivia, a known *Leishmania (V.) braziliensis* endemic areas. Thus, we cannot exclude the option that female travelers are less likely to travel specifically to this region or that they are keeping more strict precautions.

CL is also endemic in Israel and all cases should be reported to the Ministry of Health (MOH). In their data base, males are also more likely to be infected by leishmania with incidence of 5/100,000 in males vs. 3.5 in females (*Ministry of Health website, Jerusalem, Israel*). Because of the known fact, that there is a significant under-reporting of the diseases, we decided to conduct a demographic survey in several locations where CL is highly endemic. One region was in Southern Israel (Negev) where *L. major* is the common species. Another region was in Central part of Israel where *L. tropica* is the common species. Altogether 612 people were screened. Results showed that In the *L. major* endemic region, 49% were males. In the *L. tropica* endemic region, 41% were males and 59% were females [23].

These data clearly show that when population-based screening is done, avoiding referral bias and or risky travel to endemic regions, the rate of infection is similar between males and females.

An additional interesting observation we have made by assessing the rate of mucosal leishmania among those who contracted the disease in Bolivia. Among the cohort mention above of 145 travelers with NWCL there were 17 cases in whom MCL was developed. The rate of transformation from CL to MCL among males was slightly higher 14 vs. 4% in females (but non-significant difference) [24].

Our study is, to our knowledge, the first to explore the spectrum of CL in terms of sex and gender, and with the use of standard analyses, we found significant differences in the spectrum of NWCL illness in male travelers compared to women but not in population-based study of OWCL. It may be postulated that leishmania infection is more common in men because of more risk-taking behaviors and travel to more remote destinations, where the chance of acquiring tropical diseases is higher. Additionally, men may be less likely to adhere to preventive measures and therefore, are at an increased risk of contracting disease [25].

References

1. Herwaldt BL. Leishmaniasis. Lancet. 1999;354: 1191–9.
2. Aronson N, Herwaldt BL, Libman M, et al. Diagnosis and treatment of leishmaniasis: clinical practice guidelines by the Infectious Diseases Society of America (IDSA) and the American Society of Tropical Medicine and Hygiene (ASTMH). Clin Infect Dis. 2016;63:1539–57.
3. Solomon M, Greenberger S, Baum S, Pavlotsky F, Barzilai A, Schwartz E. Unusual forms of cutaneous leishmaniasis due to Leishmania major. J Eur Acad Dermatol Venereol. 2016;30:1171–5.
4. Herwaldt BL, Stokes SL, Juranek DD. American cutaneous leishmaniasis in U.S. travelers. Ann Intern Med. 1993;118:779–84.
5. Schwartz E, Hatz C, Blum J. New world cutaneous leishmaniasis in travellers. Lancet Infect Dis. 2006;6:342–9.
6. Faber WR, Oskam L, van Gool T, et al. Value of diagnostic techniques for cutaneous leishmaniasis. J Am Acad Dermatol. 2003;49:70–4.
7. Chargui N, Bastien P, Kallel K, et al. Usefulness of PCR in the diagnosis of cutaneous leishmaniasis in Tunisia. Trans R Soc Trop Med Hyg. 2005;99: 762–8.
8. Andrade-Narvaez FJ, Medina-Peralta S, Vargas-Gonzalez A, Canto-Lara SB, Estrada-Parra S. The histopathology of cutaneous leishmaniasis due to Leishmania (Leishmania) mexicana in the Yucatan peninsula, Mexico. Rev Inst Med Trop Sao Paulo. 2005;47(4):191.
9. Marfurt J, Niederwieser I, Makia ND, Beck HP, Felger I. Diagnostic genotyping of old and new world leishmania species by PCR-RFLP. Diagn Microbiol Infect Dis. 2003;46:115–24.
10. Van der Auwera G, Maes I, De Doncker S, et al. Heat-shock protein 70 gene sequencing for Leishmania species typing in European tropical infectious disease clinics. Euro Surveill. 2013;18:20543.
11. Bensoussan E, Nasereddin A, Jonas F, Schnur LF, Jaffe CL. Comparison of PCR assays for diagno-

sis of cutaneous leishmaniasis. J Clin Microbiol. 2006;44:1435–9.

12. Blum J, Desjeux P, Schwartz E, Beck B, Hatz C. Treatment of cutaneous leishmaniasis among travellers. J Antimicrob Chemother. 2004;53:158–66.

13. el-On J, Halevy S, Grunwald MH, Weinrauch L. Topical treatment of old world cutaneous leishmaniasis caused by leishmania major: a double-blind control study. J Am Acad Dermatol. 1992;27:227–31.

14. Solomon M, Baum S, Barzilai A, Pavlotsky F, Trau H, Schwartz E. Treatment of cutaneous leishmaniasis with intralesional sodium stibogluconate. J Eur Acad Dermatol Venereol. 2009;23:1189–92.

15. Faris RM, Jarallah JS, Khoja TA, al-Yamani MJ. Intralesional treatment of cutaneous leishmaniasis with sodium stibogluconate antimony. Int J Dermatol. 1993;32:610–2.

16. Herwaldt BL, Berman JD. Recommendations for treating leishmaniasis with sodium stibogluconate (Pentostam) and review of pertinent clinical studies. Am J Trop Med Hyg. 1992;46:296–306.

17. Solomon M, Pavlotsky F, Leshem E, Ephros M, Trau H, Schwartz E. Liposomal amphotericin B treatment of cutaneous leishmaniasis due to Leishmania tropica. J Eur Acad Dermatol Venereol. 2011;25:973–7.

18. van Thiel PP, Leenstra T, Kager PA, et al. Miltefosine treatment of leishmania major infection: an observational study involving Dutch military personnel returning from northern Afghanistan. Clin Infect Dis. 2010;50:80–3.

19. Solomon M, Pavlotzky F, Barzilai A, Schwartz E. Liposomal amphotericin B in comparison to sodium stibogluconate for Leishmania braziliensis cutaneous leishmaniasis in travelers. J Am Acad Dermatol. 2013;68:284–9.

20. Wortmann G, Miller RS, Oster C, Jackson J, Aronson N. A randomized, double-blind study of the efficacy of a 10- or 20-day course of sodium stibogluconate for treatment of cutaneous leishmaniasis in United States military personnel. Clin Infect Dis. 2002;35:261–7.

21. Jansen A, Stark K, Schneider T, Schoneberg I. Sex differences in clinical leptospirosis in Germany: 1997–2005. Clin Infect Dis. 2007;44:e69–72.

22. Schlagenhauf P, Chen LH, Wilson ME, et al. Sex and gender differences in travel-associated disease. Clin Infect Dis. 2010;50:826–32.

23. Solomon M, Fucs I, Glazer I, Schwartz E. Gender and Cutaneous Leishmaniasis. Submitted for publication. 2017.

24. Solomon M, Sachar N, Pavlotzky F, et al. Mucosal leishmaniasis in travelers. In: Poster presentation at world leish 6, 2017 May 16–20; Toledo, Spain.

25. Solomon M, Benenson S, Baum S, Schwartz E. Tropical skin infections among Israeli travelers. Am J Trop Med Hyg. 2011;85:868–72.

Fungal Infections (Onychomycosis, Tinea Pedis, Tinea Cruris, Tinea Capitis, Tinea Manuum, Tinea Corporis, different *Candida* Infections, and Pityriasis Versicolor) and Mycological Laboratory Analyses

18

Avner Shemer and Meir Babaev

18.1 Onychomycosis

Onychomycosis is a fungal infection of the nail and it represents 50% of nail diseases [1]. Pathogens that cause onychomycosis include dermatophyte—with *Trichophyton rubrum* being the most common (in 60% of cases)—and non-dermatophyte molds and yeasts. *Candida spp.* is responsible for up to 30% of fingernail onychomycosis, which was found to be more frequent in females, probably due to more frequent immersion of the hands in water [2]. Onychomycosis is more common in the elderly, having increased in prevalence recently because the habit of wearing tight shoes, using lockers, and neglecting proper foot care. Tinea pedis frequently appears first, and after the fungal infection extends to the nail bed, onychomycosis appears. Nail trauma, occlusive footwear, genetic predispositions, and humidity are well-known risk factors for onychomycosis [3, 4]. Clinical findings frequently seen in onychomycosis include thick and discolored nails, though thick nails can be also seen in the elderly, after nail trauma, and in psoriasis, eczema and metabolic disorders, such as hypothyroidism.

Onychomycosis can occur in both sexes, but most studies found onychomycosis to be more frequent in males [5]. Because onychomycosis and nail trauma are more frequent in men, thick nails are observed more frequently in men than in women. In addition, women usually nurture and cut their nails more often than men, and women have a greater awareness of the appearance of their nails [6]. However, because women tend to wear tight shoes more often than men, a deformation of the fifth toenail is frequent in women, caused by constant retrograde pressure applied from the sides of the shoes through the nail plate toward the nail matrix [7].

Treatment options for onychomycosis include topical and systemic therapies. The advantage of topical therapy is the safety and lack of drug interactions, but major disadvantages include its low efficacy and longer treatment periods. Topical therapy is usually indicated for onychomycosis with distal nail involvement, as well as when there is a contraindication for systemic treatment or a risk of drug–drug interactions.

A. Shemer (✉)
Sackler Faculty of Medicine, Tel-Aviv University, Tel Aviv, Israel

Department of Dermatology, Sheba Medical Center, Tel-Hashomer, Ramat Gan, Israel

M. Babaev
Division of Medicine, Faculty of Health Sciences, Ben-Gurion University of the Negev, Beer-Sheva, Israel

© Springer International Publishing AG, part of Springer Nature 2018
E. Tur, H. I. Maibach (eds.), *Gender and Dermatology*,
https://doi.org/10.1007/978-3-319-72156-9_18

Possible topical treatments for mild to moderate onychomycosis include efinaconazole, amorolfine, tavaborole, and ciclopirox. Topical treatment for onychomycosis is usually not effective enough because of its limited penetration of the nail bed. Systemic treatment is usually advised when onychomycosis involves the nail matrix. The causative organism found in the culture will help the clinician to decide on the most suitable systemic treatment. Adverse effects and drug interactions should also be considered when selecting an appropriate treatment.

Terbinafine is a first-line systemic agent for dermatophyte onychomycosis, and the recommended treatment regimen for fingernail onychomycosis is 250 mg of terbinafine for 6 weeks. For toenail onychomycosis, a course of 12–16 treatments is advised. A meta-analysis found a mycological cure rate of 76% using terbinafine [8]. Some studies show a higher prevalence of *candida* onychomycosis among women, but there are no significant effects of gender on differences in other onychomycosis pathogens [2, 9].

Itraconazole and fluconazole belong to the azoles group—all are fungistatic. Itraconazole is an alternative systemic treatment for patients who fail to respond or have an adverse reaction to terbinafine. A pulse dose of 400 mg daily for 1 week per month for 3 months was proven equally effective as a dose of 200 mg daily for 3 months in the case of toenail onychomycosis. Pulsed itraconazole showed mycologic cure rates of 63% and for continuous itraconazole dosing showed cure rates of 59% [8]. The potential for drug–drug interactions is higher with itraconazole than with terbinafine. Itraconazole is considered the treatment of choice for *candida* and non-dermatophyte mold onychomycosis [10, 11]. Fluconazole is another systemic agent that can be used in onychomycosis treatment with a weekly dose of 150–300 mg for three to 12 months [12].

Systemic treatment for onychomycosis should not be administered during periods of pregnancy and lactation. Regarding safety in pregnancy, terbinafine is a category B drug and considered the safest. Itraconazole and fluconazole are categorized as C and D, respectively, and treatment with those agents should be avoided during pregnancy. Pregnancy category B implies that animal reproduction studies did not show any risk to a fetus, while pregnancy category C means that adverse effects have been shown in animal reproduction studies, and there are not enough data about safety in humans. Finally, category D implies positive evidence of human fetal risk [13].

In women, treatment outcomes can appear less favorable than they really are because of an oxidation process due to nail polish products that give the nails a darker coloring. Some clinicians advise their female patients to avoid wearing nail polish during topical treatment for onychomycosis, but there are not enough data on the impact of toenail polish application on drug penetration [14]. One study demonstrated better results of topical efinaconazole in women [15].

18.2   Tinea Pedis

Tinea pedis, also known as athlete's foot, is dermatophytosis of the feet, the most common fungal infection [16]. The prevalence of tinea pedis increases with age [17], and it is higher in males than females [18]. Males are infected at approximately three times the rate of females [19]. This is probably due to habitual and occupational differences between genders. Women participate less often in sporting activities and they wear open shoes more often than males. Moreover, women devote more time to foot hygiene than men [6]. Common causes of tinea pedis include *T. rubrum*, *Trichophyton interdigitale*, and *Epidermophyton floccosum*. Direct contact with the causative organism is the usual method of infection, which may occur through barefoot contact between the feet and an infected surface in locker rooms and swimming pools. In the winter, the use of occlusive footwear is more common, and this leads to increased incidences of tinea pedis. Tinea pedis is more frequent in athletes and blue-collar workers, which can be explained by the habit of wearing occlusive footwear. Multiple risk factors for tinea pedis have been identified, including working in damp areas, visits to swimming pools, the use of communal showers, obesity, and diabetes.

Tinea pedis can present in three different variants: interdigital (most common variant), moccasin (hyperkeratotic variant), and vesiculobullous (inflammatory variant). Mild cases respond well to topical treatment, such as topical terbinafine, ciclopirox, and econazole. Severe cases and cases in which topical treatment has failed require systemic treatment, as one third of tinea pedis cases fail to respond to topical therapy [20]. Systemic treatment must be administered for 2–4 weeks and in stubborn cases, 12 weeks of treatment may be required. Systemic terbinafine treatment for 1 week has a cure rate above 80% due to fungicidal action.

18.3   Tinea Cruris

Tinea cruris, sometimes called jock itch, is a superficial dermatophyte infection that involves the proximal medial thighs. It has a worldwide distribution, affecting adolescents and adults predominantly. Different studies report a varied prevalence of tinea cruris between 2.5 and 52% [21, 22]. Fungal infections occur due to the inoculation of fungi from a reservoir of dermatophytes in the feet, hands, or nails. *T. rubrum* is the most common cause of tinea cruris [23], which is an almost exclusively male disease because of the humid environment created from contact between the scrotum and groin skin [24, 25]. However, tinea cruris has also been reported in female sex workers [26]. Risk factors for tinea cruris include obesity, hot climates, excessive sweating, humidity, occlusive undergarments, and the immunocompetence of the host [23, 26]. Tinea cruris is rare in children. The typical presentation is itchy and burning circinate plaque with an active inflammatory border. The groin area is usually involved, sparing the scrotal skin. A central clearing can be noted sometimes due to the centrifugal spread of the fungus. The treatment for tinea cruris usually involves 2–4 weeks of topical allylamines or azoles, which will provide a cure rate of 80%.

18.4   Tinea Capitis

Tinea capitis is a common dermatophyte infection of the scalp, most commonly seen in children between the ages of three and 14 years. The most common pathogens causing tinea capitis are *Trichophyton tonsurans* and *Microsporum canis*. In cases of a *Trichophyton* infection, there are no gender differences, as males are affected at a similar rate as females. In cases of *M. canis*, males are more likely to be infected then females [27]. There are variations in the pathogens of tinea capitis in different geographic areas for which several factors are responsible, including population migrations, differences in habits, and the availability of medical supplies. The sebum of adults is rich in triglycerides, and this imposes fungistatic features on the sebum of the scalp. This explains the low incidence of tinea capitis after puberty [28].

Tinea capitis is traditionally classified into several types. Wood's lamp can help the clinician to differentiate endothrix from ectothrix infections. In the former, the spores are located inside the hair shaft and there is no fluorescence, but in the latter, the spores are inside and outside the hair shaft and there is fluorescence. In black dot tinea capitis, round areas of broken and short hair stubs can be observed. This is caused by the zoophilic pathogens *Trichphyton violaceum* and *T. tonsurans*. In black dot tinea capitis, there is no fluorescence under Wood's lamp, while the grey patch form of tinea capitis presents with scaly patches with grey discoloration, and it is usually caused by zoophilic fungi; as well, there is fluorescence under Wood's lamp. Diffuse scale tinea capitis resembles seborrheic dermatitis, and it presents as diffuse plaque with pustules. Kerion celsi is a combination of an inflammatory reaction and fungal infection, and it usually presents as a boggy lump with pus. Kerion is caused by *M. canis*, *T. tonsurans*, *Trichophyton mentagrophytes*, and *Trichophyton verrucosum*. Favus is another type of tinea capitis caused by *Trichophyton schoenleinii*, and it may appear in children and adults. Both males and females are affected equally.

The carrier stage of tinea capitis is characterized by minimal or no clinical findings and a positive fungal culture. The carrier stage is observed more frequently in adults who have had close contact with infected children. Shorter scalp hair is more contagious, making the carrier stage and infection more frequent in males than in females. Asymptomatic carriers are common and serve as a reservoir for the disease, making tinea capitis difficult to eradicate. A fungal culture from asymptomatic carriers will most often yield anthropophilic rather than zoophilic pathogens.

Systemic antifungal treatment is mandatory in tinea capitis, as topical agents fail to penetrate the hair follicle. Topical therapy is only used as an adjuvant therapy to systemic antifungals. The first step in the diagnosis of tinea capitis is the performance of a fungal culture. Treatment should be tailored to the pathogen found in the culture. Griseofulvin has been the gold standard treatment for tinea capitis since 1959, and a pediatric dose of 20–25 mg/kg/day was found safe and effective. The recommended treatment duration is 8–12 weeks, and treatment should be continued for 2 weeks after a clinical cure has been observed [27]. The disadvantage of griseofulvin is its long treatment duration. Systemic itraconazole, fluconazole, and terbinafine appear safe and effective. In a comparison of griseofulvin and itraconazole, neither was found superior, and the same efficacy was found against M. canis [29]. In an efficacy meta-analysis of griseofulvin versus terbinafine and azole antifungals, data from 21 studies and 1813 patients demonstrated a similar efficacy. Terbinafine and azoles may be preferred because of their shorter treatment durations and better treatment adherence [30]. Another meta-analysis that included 25 studies and 4449 patients concluded that terbinafine is more effective for T. tonsurans and griseofulvin for M. canis infections [31]. Some authors recommend the addition of oral glucocorticoids to the antifungal treatment of kerion to reduce the risk of scarring. Other authors doubt this approach and recommend antifungal therapy without corticosteroids [32].

A fungal culture should be taken from the scalp of people living in close contact with the infected individuals. If the culture is positive, treatment should be given to reduce re-infection, and infected animals should be treated as well.

18.5   Tinea Manuum

Tinea manuum is a fungal infection of the hands or palms. The prevalence of tinea manuum is rare, and it occurs slightly more often in males than in females. This difference between genders can be explained by occupational differences. Tinea manuum is observed in occupations associated with extensive use of the palms, and these occupations are usually held by males. Other risk factors for tinea manuum include the picking of infected nails, repetitive occupational trauma, hyperhidrosis, and the use of alkaline soaps [33]. When both feet and one hand are infected with dermatophytes, it is referred to as one hand to feet syndrome. The most frequently identified pathogen involved is T. rubrum [33].

Tinea manuum tends to be unilateral and it usually involves the right hand. In many cases, there is evidence of concomitant tinea pedis and tinea unguium. Clinical forms include a dyshidrotic form and a hyperkeratotic form that presents with dryness and peeling of the palmar skin. Systemic treatment for 1–2 months is indicated to treat tinea manuum, although mild cases can be treated with topical agents.

18.6   Tinea Corporis

Tinea corporis is defined as dermatophytosis of all skin areas except the soles, palms, scalp, beard, and groin. After tinea pedis and onychomycosis, tinea corporis is the third most prevalent form of cutaneous mycosis. Factors that predispose individuals to tinea corporis include warm and humid climates, tight occlusive clothing, diabetes mellitus, atopic dermatitis, and immunosuppressive states. Tinea corporis is more common in athletes and people that participate in combat sports. Among judo fighters and wrestlers, the term tinea corporis gladiatorum was coined, and the prevalence of tinea corporis in such a population was reported to be 11–14% [34]. The deep follicular invasion of the hyphae presents as red plaque with follicular papules, and this clinical entity is called Majocchi granuloma [35].

The classic presentation of tinea corporis is annular plaque with a circular, scaly, raised red border, and a typical lesion has a central clearing and scales. Topical treatment with terbinafine, azoles, ciclopirox olamine, and amorolfine is usually recommended. In large lesions and in cases of topical treatment failure, systemic treatment should be administered.

18.7 Cutaneous Candidiasis

Candida is a genus of yeast-like fungi, and it is the leading cause of fungal infections worldwide. *Candida* can present in the form of true hyphae and pseudohyphae. *Candida spp.* is a leading cause of fungal infections in immunocompromised individuals. The most common mycosis of the oral cavity is oral candidiasis, as *candida spp.* is a common commensal organism in the oral cavity. Renal failure, pregnancy, immunosuppression, malignancy, xerostomia, and diabetes mellitus are also factors that predispose people to oral candidiasis. The most common form of acute oral candidiasis is pseudomembranous candidiasis. The clinical presentation is soft white plaque on the buccal mucosa and tongue. The plaque can be wiped away with gauze, exposing a red mucosa. The most common form of oral chronic candidiasis is hyperplastic candidiasis, and it presents as firm white plaque on the lips, tongue, and cheeks. Denture-related stomatitis is another type of chronic oral candidiasis, characterized by diffuse redness and swelling of the denture-bearing area. Some studies have found that women are more affected with denture stomatitis than men. A *candida* infection is very common in flexural areas and is often associated with intertrigo, which appears in moist and warm areas of the skin. Clinical findings of intertrigo candidiasis include red plaque with pustules, maceration,

and fissures. The borders of lesions sometimes have a characteristic white rim and satellite lesions located outside the borders of the main lesion. Erosio interdigitalis blastomycetica is candidiasis of the fingers or toe webs that have been subjected to friction, a wet environment, and occlusion. Characteristic web spaces that are involved include the third web space on the hands and the fourth web space on the feet. Other forms of cutaneous candidiasis include folliculitis, paronychia, and onychomycosis. Candida folliculitis is an infection of hair follicles of the beard and moustache area in men. Frequent contact of hands with water is associated with paronychia and candida onychomycosis, which is more common in females.

The second most common cause of vaginitis is candida vulvovaginitis, a common condition that will affect 75% of women at least once in their lifetime, while 10% of women will experience recurrent events. Candida vulvovaginitis is associated with increased estrogen levels, such as oral contraceptive use and pregnancy. The clinical presentation includes itch, vaginal discharge, dyspareunia, and dysuria. Physical findings include erythematous plaque on the labia, vaginal redness, and vaginal discharge, but the cervix has a normal appearance.

Candida balanitis is characterized by an itch, white patches, vesicles, and exudate on the penis or adjacent thighs, scrotum, and gluteal area. Balanitis is thought to be acquired through sexual contact with a partner that has candida vulvovaginitis. Uncircumcised males have a higher frequency of balanitis [36].

18.8 Pityriasis Versicolor

Pityriasis versicolor (PV) is a chronic superficial mycosis that affects young people in their twenties and thirties, though cases of PV are reported in children [37, 38] and infants [39, 40]. PV is more common in hot and humid climates and during the summer. The *Malassezia* genus is the main pathogen involved in PV. The most common *Malassezia* spp. cultured from PV lesions include globosa, sympodialis, and furfur [41].

Clinical findings in PV include round scaly patches distributed on the upper trunk and arms. Lesions may vary in color from white to tan brown. Usually the patches are asymptomatic, but sometimes an itch can be an associated complaint [41]. Factors that predispose individuals to PV include hyperhidrosis and the use of moisturizers and drugs (mainly systemic steroids and anticoagulants). Systemic corticosteroids elevate the chances of contracting PV by changing the lipid composition of the sebaceous glands and because of the immunosuppressive effect on the skin [42, 43]. A genetic predisposition can also play a role in PV, as it is more common among first, second, and even third degree family members [44]. Topical agents are the first choice of treatment for PV, where 2.5% selenium sulfide shampoo acts by physically peeling the stratum corneum, and it is an effective PV treatment. Topical antifungal agents are another option for treating PV, including azoles, ciclopirox olamine, allylamines, benzylamines, and tacrolimus [41]. Rilopirox, a new antifungal agent, and adapalene gel, originally used for acne, have a demonstrated efficacy in PV treatment. Probable mechanisms of action include the inhibition of sebaceous gland secretion, peeling of the stratum corneum, and anti-inflammatory properties [45, 46]. The recommended treatment regimen for shampoos is daily application for several weeks. The patient should be instructed to leave the shampoo on the skin for five minutes and then rinse. Creams are applied once or twice a day for 1 month. For recurrent cases, prophylactic treatment is advised once a week. Different systemic antifungal regimens exist for the treatment of PV, including itraconazole at a dose of 200 mg per day for 5 or 7 days and fluconazole at a dose of 300 mg per week for 2 weeks. Fluconazole is considered the safest systemic agent for treating PV [47].

18.9   Mycological Laboratory Analysis

A diagnostic laboratory confirmation should be obtained before starting long-term systemic antifungal treatment, usually in cases of onychomycosis. For appropriate treatment, it is advisable to obtain a laboratory confirmation of other types of superficial mycoses. A direct microscopy of the Kalium Hydroxide (KOH) preparation provides an immediate result of the fungal hyphae. A fungal culture is the most specific test for diagnosing a fungal infection, as it identifies the specific organism, enabling an appropriate treatment plan. Sometimes the culture can provide false negative results, but these can be minimized by repeating the sample collection. If the diagnosis is uncertain, a histopathological examination with Periodic Acid Schiff (PAS) can help in a diagnosis. A histological examination will demonstrate the depth of the penetration of the fungal infection, and it can distinguish invasive pathogens that require eradication. Recent studies have utilized the newest molecular method to detect fungal DNA or RNA, where a polymerase chain reaction (PCR) technique is used. Specific molecular probes include common organisms, such as *T. rubrum*, whereas panfungal probes include a panel of multiple possible pathogens.

References

1. Gupta AK, Jain HC, Lynde CW, Macdonald P, Cooper EA, Summerbell RC. Prevalence and epidemiology of onychomycosis in patients visiting physicians' offices: a multicenter canadian survey of 15,000 patients. J Am Acad Dermatol. 2000;43(2 Pt 1):244–8.
2. Ellabib MS, Agaj M, Khalifa Z, Kavanagh K. Yeasts of the genus Candida are the dominant cause of onychomycosis in Libyan women but not men: results of a 2-year surveillance study. Br J Dermatol. 2002;146(6):1038–41.
3. Elewski BE. Onychomycosis: pathogenesis, diagnosis, and management. Clin Microbiol Rev. 1998;11(3):415–29.
4. Elewski BE, Charif MA. Prevalence of onychomycosis in patients attending a dermatology clinic in northeastern Ohio for other conditions. Arch Dermatol. 1997;133(9):1172–3.
5. Sigurgeirsson B, Baran R. The prevalence of onychomycosis in the global population: a literature study. J Eur Acad Dermatol Venereol. 2014;28(11):1480–91.
6. Rossaneis MA, Haddad Mdo C, Mathias TA, Marcon SS. Differences in foot self-care and lifestyle between men and women with diabetes mellitus. Rev Lat Am Enfermagem. 2016;24:e2761.

7. Avner S, Nir N, Henri T. Fifth toenail clinical response to systemic antifungal therapy is not a marker of successful therapy for other toenails with onychomycosis. J Eur Acad Dermatol Venereol. 2006;20(10):1194–6.

8. Gupta AK, Ryder JE, Johnson AM. Cumulative meta-analysis of systemic antifungal agents for the treatment of onychomycosis. Br J Dermatol. 2004;150(3):537–44.

9. Segal R, Shemer A, Hochberg M, Keness Y, Shvarzman R, Mandelblat M, Frenkel M, Segal E. Onychomycosis in Israel: epidemiological aspects. Mycoses. 2015;58(3):133–9.

10. Gupta AK, De Doncker P, Haneke E. Itraconazole pulse therapy for the treatment of Candida onychomycosis. J Eur Acad Dermatol Venereol. 2001;15(2):112–5.

11. Gupta AK, Gregurek-Novak T, Konnikov N, Lynde CW, Hofstader S, Summerbell RC. Itraconazole and terbinafine treatment of some nondermatophyte molds causing onychomycosis of the toes and a review of the literature. J Cutan Med Surg. 2001;5(3):206–10.

12. Scher RK, Breneman D, Rich P, Savin RC, Feingold DS, Konnikov N, Shupack JL, Pinnell S, Levine N, Lowe NJ, Aly R, Odom RB, Greer DL, Morman MR, Bucko AD, Tschen EH, Elewski BE, Smith EB. Once-weekly fluconazole (150, 300, or 450 mg) in the treatment of distal subungual onychomycosis of the toenail. J Am Acad Dermatol. 1998;38(6 Pt 2):S77–86.

13. Food, Drug Administration HHS. Content and format of labeling for human prescription drug and biological products; requirements for pregnancy and lactation labeling. Final Rule Fed Regist. 2014;79(233):72063–103.

14. Del Rosso JQ. Application of nail polish during topical management of onychomycosis: are data available to guide the clinician about what to tell their patients? J Clin Aesthet Dermatol. 2016;9(8):29–36.

15. Rosen T. Evaluation of gender as a clinically relevant outcome variable in the treatment of onychomycosis with efinaconazole topical solution 10. Cutis. 2015;96(3):197–201.

16. Ilkit M, Tanir F, Hazar S, Gumusay T, Akbab M. Epidemiology of tinea pedis and toenail tinea unguium in worshippers in the mosques in Adana. Turkey J Dermatol. 2005;32(9):698–704.

17. Cheng S, Chong L. A prospective epidemiological study on tinea pedis and onychomycosis in Hong Kong. Chin Med J. 2002;115(6):860–5.

18. Kamihama T, Kimura T, Hosokawa JI, Ueji M, Takase T, Tagami K. Tinea pedis outbreak in swimming pools in Japan. Public Health. 1997;111(4):249–53.

19. Aste N, Pau M, Aste N, Biggio P. Tinea pedis observed in Cagliari, Italy, between 1996 and 2000. Mycoses. 2003;46(1-2):38–41.

20. Vella Zahra L, Gatt P, Boffa MJ, Borg E, Mifsud E, Scerri L, Vella Briffa D, Pace JL. Characteristics of superficial mycoses in Malta. Int J Dermatol. 2003;42(4):265–71.

21. al-Sogair SM, Moawad MK, al-Humaidan YM. Fungal infection as a cause of skin disease in the eastern province of Saudi Arabia: tinea corporis and tinea cruris. Mycoses. 1991;34(9-10):423–7.

22. Imwidthaya S, Thianprasit M. A study of dermatophytoses in Bangkok (Thailand). Mycopathologia. 1988;102(1):13–6.

23. Odom R. Pathophysiology of dermatophyte infections. J Am Acad Dermatol. 1993;28(5 Pt 1):S2–7.

24. Blank F, Mann SJ. Trichophyton rubrum infections according to age, anatomical distribution and sex. Br J Dermatol. 1975;92(2):171–4.

25. Blank F, Mann SJ, Reale RA. Distribution of dermatophytosis according to age, ethnic group and sex. Sabouraudia. 1974;12(3):352–61.

26. Otero L, Palacio V, Vazquez F. Tinea cruris in female prostitutes. Mycopathologia. 2002;153(1):29–31.

27. Shemer A, Plotnik IB, Davidovici B, Grunwald MH, Magun R, Amichai B. Treatment of tinea capitis - griseofulvin versus fluconazole - a comparative study. J Dtsch Dermatol Ges. 2013;11(8):737–41. 737-42

28. Aste N, Pau M, Biggio P. Tinea capitis in adults. Mycoses. 1996;39(7-8):299–301.

29. Lopez-Gomez S, Del Palacio A, Van Cutsem J, Soledad Cuetara M, Iglesias L, Rodriguez-Noriega A. Itraconazole versus griseofulvin in the treatment of tinea capitis: a double-blind randomized study in children. Int J Dermatol. 1994;33(10):743–7.

30. Gonzalez U, Seaton T, Bergus G, Jacobson J, Martinez-Monzon C. Systemic antifungal therapy for tinea capitis in children. Cochrane Database Syst Rev. 2007;4:CD004685.

31. Chen X, Jiang X, Yang M, Bennett C, Gonzalez U, Lin X, Hua X, Xue S, Zhang M. Systemic antifungal therapy for tinea capitis in children: an abridged Cochrane review. J Am Acad Dermatol. 2017;76(2):368–74.

32. Proudfoot LE, Higgins EM, Morris-Jones R. A retrospective study of the management of pediatric kerion in Trichophyton tonsurans infection. Pediatr Dermatol. 2011;28(6):655–7.

33. Daniel CR 3rd, Gupta AK, Daniel MP, Daniel CM. Two feet-one hand syndrome: a retrospective multicenter survey. Int J Dermatol. 1997;36(9):658–60.

34. Ohno S, Tanabe H, Kawasaki M, Horiguchi Y. Tinea corporis with acute inflammation caused by Trichophyton tonsurans. J Dermatol. 2008;35(9):590–3.

35. Elgart ML. Tinea incognito: an update on Majocchi granuloma. Dermatol Clin. 1996;14(1):51–5.

36. Sneppen I, Thorup J. Foreskin morbidity in uncircumcised males. Pediatrics. 2016;137(5):e20154340. https://doi.org/10.1542/peds.2015-4340.

37. Terragni L, Lasagni A, Oriani A, Gelmetti C. Pityriasis versicolor in the pediatric age. Pediatr Dermatol. 1991;8(1):9–12.

38. Sunenshine PJ, Schwartz RA, Janniger CK. Tinea versicolor. Int J Dermatol. 1998;37(9):648–55.

39. Wyre HW Jr, Johnson WT. Neonatal pityriasis versicolor. Arch Dermatol. 1981;117(11):752–3.

40. Jubert E, Martin-Santiago A, Bernardino M, Bauza A. Neonatal pityriasis versicolor. Pediatr Infect Dis J. 2015;34(3):329–30.

41. Gupta AK, Batra R, Bluhm R, Boekhout T, Dawson TL Jr. Skin diseases associated with Malassezia species. J Am Acad Dermatol. 2004;51(5):785–98.

42. Gaitanis G, Magiatis P, Hantschke M, Bassukas ID, Velegraki A. The Malassezia genus in skin and systemic diseases. Clin Microbiol Rev. 2012;25(1):106–41.

43. Mendez-Tovar LJ. Pathogenesis of dermatophytosis and tinea versicolor. Clin Dermatol. 2010;28(2):185–9.

44. He SM, Du WD, Yang S, Zhou SM, Li W, Wang J, Xiao FL, Xu SX, Zhang XJ. The genetic epidemiology of tinea versicolor in China. Mycoses. 2008;51(1):55–62.

45. Shi TW, Ren XK, Yu HX, Tang YB. Roles of adapalene in the treatment of pityriasis versicolor. Dermatology. 2012;224(2):184–8.

46. Shi TW, Zhang JA, Tang YB, Yu HX, Li ZG, Yu JB. A randomized controlled trial of combination treatment with ketoconazole 2% cream and adapalene 0.1% gel in pityriasis versicolor. J Dermatolog Treat. 2015;26(2):143–6.

47. Rivard SC. Pityriasis versicolor: avoiding pitfalls in disease diagnosis and therapy. Mil Med. 2013; 178(8):904–6.

Vered Atar-Snir

Atopic Dermatitis (AD) is a chronic pruritic inflammatory disease that occurs most frequently in children, buy also affects substantial number of adults.

It is often associated with elevated level of immunoglobulin E, as other IgE dependent diseases as bronchial asthma, allergic rhinitis and food allergy [1, 2].

The terms "Eczema" and "dermatitis" used interchangeably. It often refers to atopic eczema. The term "eczematous" describes some blister formation and serous oozing. The disease significantly reduces the quality of life of patients and their families which leads to serious socioeconomic consequences [3, 4].

19.1   Epidemiology

AD affects 5–20% of children worldwide and 0.9–5% adults [5]. It is leveled off or even decreased in western countries, while in the developing countries it is still in rise [5].

Immigrants from developing countries living in developed countries have a higher incidence of AD than the regular population.

AD affects persons of all races.

V. Atar-Snir
Clalit Health Care Services, Tel Aviv, Israel

Schneider Children's Medical Center,
Petah Tikva, Israel
e-mail: mrveredat@clalit.org.il

AD most often begins in early childhood. It is believed that 60% of all cases begin in the first year of life and 90% before age of 5 years.

The disease tends to regress before 5 years of age in 40–80% of patients and in 60–90% it subsides before 15 years of age [1, 6].

The remaining (10–40%) continue to have eczema into adolescent or experience relapse of symptoms after some symptom free years.

Many with adult onset AD or relapsing AD develop hand eczema as the main manifestation.

19.2   Gender Variations

Female to male ratio for atopic dermatitis is 1.14:1.

In a multicenter study on 10,464 Italian patients age 20–44 years, the authors found that eczema and hay fever are highly prevalent (3.4–8.1%) in Italian young adults, especially in women [7].

Another study done in Israel [8] in adolescents (ages 17–18 years) found that atopic dermatitis rose three-fold for both genders during the study period (1998–2008). The increase was higher in females (0.5–1.2%) than males (0.3–0.9%).

Mild and moderate disease was higher in females than males.

Ziyab et al. [9] conducted a study in both genders 1–18 years of age and showed that up to 10 years of age, gender did not influence prevalence. From 10–18 years, eczema became more

© Springer International Publishing AG, part of Springer Nature 2018
E. Tur, H. I. Maibach (eds.), *Gender and Dermatology*,
https://doi.org/10.1007/978-3-319-72156-9_19

prevalent among girls (16.3% for girls vs 8.3% for boys), which might suggest a role for gender specific pubertal factors.

A Danish study [10] among ages 1–17 years showed that the frequency of positive patch test reactions and allergic contact dermatitis was significantly higher among girls.

In Taiwan [11], they found that the prevalence of atopic dermatitis in females was lower than in males before age of 8 years, but became higher after that.

In the Singapore study [12] there were slightly more boys with atopic dermatitis among 6–12 years age group, but more girls were affected among the age 16 years and older (1.57:1).

Same tendency was shown in England [13] where girls 13–14 years of age had higher prevalence rates of asthma, rhinitis and eczema symptoms than boys.

19.3 Risk Factors

Approximately 70% of patients have a positive family history of atopic diseases (eczema, asthma, allergic rhinitis). Child with one atopic parent has two to threefold increased risk to develop AD. The risk increases to three to fivefolds if both parents are atopic [14].

A genetic basis for AD is suggested by twin studies that found rates of 80% AD in monozygotic twins compared to 20% in dizygotic twins [15].

Another study [16] showed strong association between atopic and mutations in the filaggrin gene, positioned on chromosome 1. This gene is the strongest known genetic risk factor for AD.

Ten percent of people in western countries carry mutations in this gene, whereas around 50% of AD patients carry this mutation.

This gene mutation gives rise to functional impairment in the filaggrin protein and thereby disrupt the skin barrier. The clinical manifestation in these patients is dry skin with fissures and higher risk of eczema.

Environmental risk factors were also considered as causative factor for AD: for example; children who grew up in a farming environment with exposure to variety of microflora from unpasteurized cow milk, live stocks etc' were protected to some extent against developing allergic diseases [17, 18].

19.4 Pathophysiology

Two main hypothesis were suggested to explain the inflammatory lesions in AD:

19.4.1 The Skin Barrier Hypothesis

It is based on the observation that patients with filaggrin gene mutation have increased risk of developing AD [16].

The filaggrin gene encodes structural proteins in the stratum corneum and stratum granulosum that help bind the keratinocytes together which maintain the intact skin barrier and the hydrated stratum corneum. Filaggrin gene impairment leads to dry and fissured skin which increases penetration of allergens into the skin resulting in allergic sensitization, asthma and hay fever [19, 20].

19.4.2 The Immunological Hypothesis

Suggests that AD results from imbalance of T cells particularly T helper cells type 1, 2, 17, 22 [21]. In the allergic state (acute eczema), The TH2 differentiation of CD4+ T cells predominates, which increases production of interleukins (IL 4,5,13) that leads to increase level of IgE and the TH1 differentiation is correspondingly inhibited [22].

19.5 Clinical Manifestation

Dry skin and severe pruritus as the cardinal signs of AD. However, the manifestations can vary depending upon age and disease activity.

Age 0–2 years: AD presents with pruritic, red scaly and crusted lesions of the extensor surfaces, cheeks or scalp. Usually there is sparing of the diaper areas [23, 24]. The lesions are characterized by erythema, papules, vesicles, excoriations, oozing and formation of crusts.

Age 2–16 years: the lesions are often confined to the flexures of the elbows and knees as well as wrists and ankles. The eczema becomes drier and lichenified with excoriations, papules and nodules.

Adults: the lesions frequently localize to the face and neck. Thirty percent develop atopic hand eczema.

There are several exposures that may aggravate the eczema: hot water, infection with staphylococcus, woolen clothing and certain foods that the patient is allergic to.

19.6 Diagnosis

The diagnosis of AD is clinical. Based upon history, morphology and distribution of skin lesions [14].

The UK working group on AD published criteria for diagnosing AD that include one mandatory and five major criteria [25, 26]:

- Evidence of pruritic skin including the report by a parent of a child rubbing or scratching. In addition to itchy skin, 3 or more of the following are needed to make the diagnosis:

1. History of skin creases being involved: antecubital fossae, popliteal fossae, neck areas around the eyes and fronts of ankles.
2. History of asthma or hay fever or history of atopic disease in a first degree relative for children under 4 years of age.
3. The presence of generally dry skin within the past year.
4. Symptoms beginning in a child before the age of 2 years.
5. Visible dermatitis involving flexural surfaces, for children under 4 years of age, This criteria is met by dermatitis affecting the cheeks or forehead and outer aspects of the extremities.

Skin biopsy and laboratory testing including IgE levels are not routinely used and not recommended.

19.7 Differential Diagnosis

1. Allergic dermatitis: the localization of dermatitis, history of exposure to irritations and patch test can help to differentiate.
2. Seborrheic dermatitis: the most common in infants. The two conditions may coexist. Involvement of the scalp, little or no pruritus, Support diagnosis of seborrheic dermatitis.
3. Psoriasis: often involve the diaper area with well demarcated erythematous patches.
4. Scabies: involvement of skin folds (in infants—diaper area), presence of vesicopostules on the palms and soles, all these suggest scabies. Demonstration of mites or eggs confirm the diagnosis.

19.8 Treatment

AD is not curable. Patients experience a chronic course of the disease [27]. The goals of treatment are to reduce symptoms (pruritus and dermatitis), prevent exacerbations and minimize therapeutic risk.

Standard treatment modalities are the use of topical anti-inflammatory preparations and mositurization of the skin, but patients with severe disease may require phototherapy or systemic treatment [28, 29].

The first aim is prevention: this is best achieved by reducing the dryness of the skin by daily use of skin moisturizing creams or emollients and avoidance of irritants as allergens, noncotton clothing, hot baths.

The emollient should be applied several times a day. This has been shown to reduce the need for steroid creams [30, 31]. The emollients act as an occlusive layer on the top of the skin minimizing the evaporation. Also itching is reduced.

There are several emollients, the choice depends on the individual patient. Thick layer of cream is used for the driest skin while creams and lotions with higher water content are used for mild eczema. Emollient with perfume should be avoided since they may provoke secondary allergic sensitization.

19.8.1 Topical Steroids

Used for the treatment of moderate to severe atopic dermatitis in children and adults. Mild to moderate steroid creams are reserved for children while adults can be treated with stronger preparations. The amount applied on the skin should fit a fingertip.

Many studies showed large therapeutic efficacy of topical corticosteroids compared with placebo. No clear benefit has been demonstrated with more than once daily application [32, 33].

Long term use of topical steroids on large body area may lead to adrenal suppression. Other adverse effects include skin thinning, telangiectasia, folliculitis and contact dermatitis.

19.8.2 Topical Calcineurin Inhibitors

Pimecrolimus cream and tacrolimus ointment (topical calcineurin inhibitors) used both for treatment of acute flares and for maintenance therapy of atopic dermatitis [34]. They are non-steroidal immunomodulating agents that unlike topical steroids, do not cause skin atrophy or other steroid adverse effects. They can be used as an alternative to topical steroids for the treatment of mild to moderate atopic dermatitis involving the face (including eyelids) and skin folds [35].

19.8.3 Phototherapy

In children—phototherapy is not suitable for infants and young children. In older children and adolescents with AD not controlled with topical therapies, narrow band UVB phototherapy may be an option.

In adults with moderate to severe AD that is not controlled with topical therapy, narrow band UVB phototherapy is recommended usually 3 times a week. Emollients may be necessary since phototherapy may increase skin dryness.

Prolonged treatment may lead to an increased risk of melanoma and non-melanoma skin cancer [36, 37].

19.8.4 Systemic Immunosuppressant Treatments

In adults: oral cyclosporine is a short term treatment option in cases of moderate to severe AD that is not adequately controlled with topical therapy, when phototherapy is not available or contraindicated [38].

In children: oral cyclosporine is not indicated in infants and in young children with AD. In older children and adolescents, it should be reserved to the most severe cases that failed to respond to topical treatment.

19.8.5 Other Medications

Dupilumab is an interleukin (IL)–4 receptor alpha antagonist that was recently approved for treatment of adult patients with moderate to severe AD not controlled with topical therapy [39]. It inhibits IL-3,4, cytokines TH2 that are believed to play a key role in atopic diseases as asthma and AD.

19.8.6 Immunotherapy

Allergens specific immunotherapy (SIT) with dust mite extract in sensitized patients with AD has been studied using subcutaneous or sublingual administration with conflicting results [40].

19.8.7 New Agents

Tofacitinib—is an oral molecule of JAK inhibitor that blocks multiple interleukins (IL-3,4,5). The efficacy of topical Tofacitinib for the treatment of AD has been evaluated in the phase IIB randomized trial with promising results [41]. More studies are needed to evaluate long term efficacy and safety.

Nemolizumab—is a humanized monoclonal antibody against receptor A of IL–31. A randomized trial evaluated its efficacy in the treatment of AD in adults with moderate to severe AD not controlled by topical steroids or calcineurin inhibitors with promising results [42].

Again, longer studies are needed to evaluate long term efficacy and safety.

References

1. Sprengel JM. From atopic dermatitis to asthma: the atopic march. Am Allergy Asthma Immunol. 2010;105:99.
2. Schlapbach C, Simon D. Update on skin allergy. Allergy. 2014;69:1571–81.
3. Brown MM, Chamlin SL. Quality of life in pediatric dermatology. Dermatol Clin. 2013;31:211–21.
4. Carroll CL, Balkrishnan R, Feldman SR, et al. The burden of atopic dermatitis: impact on the patent, family and society. Pediatr Dermatol. 2005;22:192–9.
5. Asher MI, Montfort S, et al. Worldwide time trends in the prevalence of symptoms of asthma, allergic rhinoconjunctivitis and eczema in childhood. Lancet. 2006;368(9537):733–43.
6. William HC. Atopic dermatitis. N Engl J Med. 2005;352(22):2314–66.
7. Pesce G, Harcon A, Carosso A, et al. Adult eczema in Italy: prevalence and associations with environmental factors. J Eur Acad Dermatol Venerol. 2015;29(6):1180–7.
8. Wohly Y, Wainstein J, Bar-Dayan Y. Atopic dermatitis in Israeli adolescents—a large retrospective cohort study. Acta Derm Venereol. 2014;94(6):695–8.
9. Ziyab HA, Raza A, Karmaus W, et al. Trends in eczema in the first 18 years of life. Results from the isle of Wight birth cohort study. Clin Exp Allerg. 2010;40(12):1776–84.
10. Simonsen AB, Deleuran M, et al. Allergic contact dermatitis in Danish children referred from patch testing—a nationwide multicenter study. Contact Dermatitis. 2014;70(2):104–11.
11. Hwang CY, Chen YJ, Lin MW, et al. Prevalence of atopic dermatitis, allergic rhinitis and asthma in Taiwan. A national study 2000–2007. Acta Derm Venereol. 2010;96(6):589–94.
12. Tay YK, Khool L, Cl G, Giam YC. The prevalence and descriptive epidemiology of atopic dermatitis in Singapore school children. Br J Dermatol. 2002;146(1):101–6.
13. Shamssain MH, Shamsian N. Prevalence and severity of asthma, rhinitis and atopic eczema in 13–14 years old school children from northeast of England. Ann Allergy Asthma Immunol. 2001;86(4):428–32.
14. Eichenfield LF, Tom WL, Chamlin SL, et al. Guidelines of care for the management of atopic dermatitis. Section 1: diagnosis and assessment of atopic dermtitis. J Am Acad Dermatol. 2014;70:338.
15. Schultz LF. Atopic dermatitis: a genetic epidemiologic study in a population based twin sample. J Am Acad Dermatol. 1993;28:719.
16. Palmer CNA, Irvine AD, et al. Common loss of function variants of the epidermal barrier protein filaggrin are a major predisposing factor for atopic dermatitis. Nat Genet. 2006;38(4):441–6.
17. Strachan DP. Hay fever, hygiene and household size. Br Med J. 1989;299(6710):1259–60.
18. Von Mutius E. Maternal farm exposure ingestion of unpasteurized cow milk and allergic disease. Curr Opin Gastroenterol. 2012;28:570–6.
19. De Bendetto A, Kubo A, Beck LA. Skin barrier disruption: a requirement for allergen sensitization. J Invest Dermatol. 2012;132(3):949–63.
20. Thomsen SF. Atopic dermatitis: natural history diagnosis and treatment. ISRN Allergy. 2014;2014:354250.
21. Eyerich K, Novak N. Immunology of atopic eczema overcoming the Th1/Th2 paradigm. Allergy. 2013;68:974–82.
22. Leung DYM, Guttmn-Yassky E. Diciphering the complexties of atopic dermatitis shifting paradigms in treatment approaches. J Allergy Clin Immunol. 2014;134:769.
23. Radikoff D, Lebwohl M. Atopic dermatitis. Lancet. 1998;351:1715.
24. William L Weston, William Howe. Atopic dermatitis (eczema), pathogenesis, clinical manifestation and diagnosis. Uptodate 10/2017.
25. Williams HC. Clinical practice. Atopic dermatitis. N Engl J Med. 2005;352:2314.
26. Williams HC, et al. The UK working party's diagnostic criteria for atopic dermatitis. BR J Dermat. 1994;131:406.
27. Ring J, Alomar A, Bieber T, et al. Guidelines for treatment of atopic eczema. J Eur Acad Dermatol Venereol. 2012;26:1045–60.
28. Eichenfield LF, Tom WL, Berger TG, et al. Guidelines of care for the management of atopic dermatitis section 2: management and treatment of atopic dermatitis with topical therapies. J Am Acad Dermatol. 2014;71:116.
29. Sibbury R, Davis DM, Cogen DE, et al. Guidelines of care for the management of atopic dermatitis section 3: management and treatment with phototherpy and systemic agents. J Am Acad Dermatol. 2014;71:327.
30. Simpson EL. Atopic dermatitis: a review of topical treatment options. Curr Med Res Opin. 2010;26(3):633–40.
31. Ricci G, Dondi A, Patrizi A. Useful tools for the management of atopic dermatitis. Am J Clin Dermatol. 2009;10(5):287–300.
32. Hoare C, Li Wan Po A, Williams H. Systematic review of treatments for atopic eczema. Health Technol Assess. 2000;4:1.
33. Green C, Colquitt JL, Kirby J, et al. Clinical and cost effectiveness of once daily versus more frequent use of same potency topical corticosteroids for atopic eczema. A systematic review and economic evaluation. Health Technol Assess. 2004;8(47):1–120.
34. El-Batawy MMY, Bassrila MA, Mashaly HM. Topical calcineurin inhibitors in atopic dermatitis: a systemic review and meta-analysis. J Dermatol Sci. 2009;54(2):76–87.

35. Ascroft DM, Dimmock P, Garside R, et al. Efficacy and tolerability of topical pimecrolimus and tacrolimus in the treatment of atopic dermatitis; meta-analysis of randomized controlled trials. Br Med J. 2005;330:516.

36. Garristen FM, Brouner MW. Photo (chemo) therpy in the management of atopic dermatitis: and updated systematic review with implications for practice and research. Br J Dermatol. 2014;170:501.

37. Stern RS, Nicholsky KT. Malignant melanoma in patients treated for psoriasis with methoxsalen (psoralen) and ultraviolet radiation (PUVA) the PUVA follow up study. N Engl J Med. 1997;336:1041.

38. Ring J, Alomar A, Bieber T, et al. Guidelines for treatment of atopic eczema (atopic dermatitis) part II. J Eur Acad Dermatol Venereol. 2012;26:1176.

39. Beck LA, Thaci D, Hamilton JD, et al. Dupilumab treatment in adults with moderate to severe atopic dermatitis inadequately controlled by topical treatment: a randomized, placebo controlled dose ranging phase IIB trial. Lancet. 2016;387:40.

40. Pajno GB, Caminitil L, Vita D, et al. Sublingual immunotherapy in mite sensitized children with atopic dermatitis; a randomized, double blind, placebo controlled study. J Allergy Clin Immunol. 2007;120:164.

41. Bissonnette R, Papp KA, Poulin Y, et al. Topical tofacitinib for atopic dermatitis a phase IIa randomized trial. Br J Dermatol. 2016;175:902.

42. Ruzicka T, Hanifin JM, Furue M, et al. Anti interleukin-31 receptor A antibody for atopic dermatitis. N Engl J Med. 2017;376:826.

Occupational Dermatitis in Nail Salon Workers

20

Liran Horev

20.1 Introduction

The number and popularity of beauty salons and nail salons has grown dramatically, as they provide generalized services related to skin health, facial aesthetic, foot and hand care, hair removal, etc. as well as an enjoyable experience. Professional manicure work has only been recognized as a profession since the 1980s, but has recently become one of the fastest growing industries in the United States. Within the last 20 years there has been a 345% increase in the number of registered manicurists, with over 400,000 licensed professionals in the country in 2011 [1].

Nail salons are an important work arena for women, with 97% of nail technicians being women [1]. In California, Manicurists are predominately Asian women, with Vietnamese comprising 62.1% and Non-Hispanic White women comprising 23.2% of the group, while 31.2% of the general female population [2].

There are limited published studies investigating work-related ill-health in nail salon technicians [3–5]. Available literature cites individuals suffering from occupational asthma, allergic contact dermatitis and musculoskeletal disorders as a result of maintaining awkward postures of the upper body and limbs while performing highly repetitive tasks. Dermatological disorders are among the most common work-related diseases and injuries, with contact dermatitis accounting for 90% of occupational skin disease. Occupational skin disease has a guarded prognosis. Despite proper treatment, only 27% of patients have clearance of the dermatitis, even with a change in jobs [6]. The negative impact results in lost worker productivity, medical care and disability payments. Skin hazards to nail salon workers, is the subject of this chapter.

20.2 Services Available at a Nail Salon

As techniques for nail building and color have been improved and became very popular, new parlors dedicated for nail industry only, have been opened. Nail salons usually offer the following services: Manicure and pedicure treatments, acrylic, UV gel and silk/fiberglass coatings and extensions, acrylic and UV gel sculpted extensions, nail art, etc.

Fingernail coatings encompass two types [7]:

1. Coatings that harden upon evaporation
2. Coatings that polymerize

L. Horev
Department of Dermatology, Hadassah and Hebrew University Medical Center, Jerusalem, Israel

Yitzhak Shamir Medical Center, Zerifin, Israel
e-mail: rlirano@hadassah.org.il

© Springer International Publishing AG, part of Springer Nature 2018
E. Tur, H. I. Maibach (eds.), *Gender and Dermatology*,
https://doi.org/10.1007/978-3-319-72156-9_20

The types of evaporating nail coat are the nail enamel (nail polish, nail varnish), base coat and top coat. Nail enamel consists of a film-former, such as nitrocellulose, and film modifiers, the most common of which is toluene sulfonamide/formaldehyde resin (TSFR). In addition, it contains plasticizers (e.g. dibutyl phthalate and camphor), solvents, diluents, viscosity modifiers and color additives. Base coat and top coat have similar basic formulations to the nail polish, with base coats containing more resin for better adherence and top coats more nitrocellulose and plasticizers and often ultraviolet (UV) absorbing material. The allergen in nail enamel is usually the thermoplastic resin (TSFR) [8], while the non-resin components of nail enamel rarely sensitize. Also in use in regular manicure are nail hardeners [9], which are nail polishes used to strengthen the nails that may be either based on formaldehyde, or resins, and nail polish removers. Nail polish removers are liquid solvents, such as acetone, alcohol, ethyl acetate, or butyl acetate. There are used to strip the nail polish from the nail plate.

Coatings that polymerize include sculptured nails, preformed artificial nails, nail mending and wrapping and light-curing gels:

20.2.1 Sculptured Nails

Sculptured nail kits typically contain the following items: Metallized paper nail forms that are placed on the nail surface to shape the nail; A glue based on an acrylic monomer such as ethyl methacrylate or isobutyl methacrylate, which also might contain hydroquinone; A powdered polymethyl methacrylate or polyethyl methacrylate polymer, containing, as an initiator, benzoyl peroxide, and, as a stabilizer, resorcinol, eugenol, thymol, or hydroquinone/methyl ethyl hydroquinone. The polymer may also contain monomers such as methyl methacrylate and ethyl methacrylate; A catalyst, typically *N,N*-dimethyl *p*-toluidine (DMPT), to trigger the production of free radicals of benzoyl peroxide in the polymer powder; Plasticizers, such as tricresyl or phthalate phosphate; Solvents and dyes.

In the typical application procedure the nail is soaped, brushed and cleaned with antiseptic and antifungal agents, and dried with a nail dehydrator based on diethyl ether. A metallized paper form is then applied to the nail, which is primed with a methacrylic acid solvent acting as a double-sided bond that adheres to both the natural nail and the acrylate. The DMPT catalyst is mixed with the acrylic polymer in powder form and this product is molded to the nail [10].

20.2.2 Preformed Artificial Nails

Preformed artificial nails or "Tips" are made of lightweight plastic plates, "nail"-shaped, that are glued on the natural nail. The whole nail is then covered by Methacrylate. The tips are attached by a cyanoacrylate instant glue, that may cause local and distant allergic reactions, and very often contains also hydroquinone. This technique is less in use nowadays.

20.2.3 Nail Mending and Wrapping

Nail wraps are used to repair nail plates that are split or cracked along their entire length. The wrap, which is made of paper, silk, linen, plastic, or fiberglass, is cut and shaped to fit the natural nail, and is then glued to the nail surface. Several layers of a polish are then applied. The glue used for the wrap is again, cyanoacrylate-based.

20.2.4 Light Curing Gels

Gel system products are either acrylic-based (14% of the market) or cyanoacrylate-based (1% or less of the market). The long lasting cover of the gels that may last for up to 2 weeks and the lack of odor gained much popularity. The application process of gel-based manicures includes serial applications to the nail plate with a base primer, followed by a color coat and a top coat, like a nail polish. It is then cured with either UV or visible light, or with a brush-on, dropper-applied or spray catalyst. Removal of gel manicures requires soaking the nail plate with 100% acetone for 10–15 min. The gel polish system is a relatively new form of acrylic-containing manicure, and may be responsible to the growing frequency of ACD in nail technicians in recent years.

20.3 Occupational Dermatological Disorders in Nail Technicians

Products handled regularly by nail salon employees include solvents, glues, polishes, hardeners, disinfectants and artificial nails. A partial list of the chemicals ingredients includes formaldehyde, toluene, dibutyl phthalate, methyl ethyl ketone, ethyl acetate, acetone, acetonitrile etc. [11]. As mentioned earlier, the increased use of gel and artificial nails constitute a main source of exposure to (meth)acrylates.

Allergic contact dermatitis (ACD) to artificial nail acrylic components was first reported in 1956 [12]. The case report described a manicurist whose thumb and middle fingers of the left hand were constantly exposed to a mixture of acrylic materials, while she held customers' fingers. Soon after first exposure, the patient developed dermatitis of the involved skin. Skin patch tests were positive to the mixture and to the self- curing monomer, but not to the polymer powder. The dermatitis was cleared when she refrained from exposure. At that time, allergic contact dermatitis to (meth)acrylates was already well known among dental personal, dentists, dental nurses and technicians and among employees in the print industry. Use of similar materials by nail technicians has made them similarly affected by skin symptoms.

Still, (meth)acrylates allergy among beauticians and nail technicians was infrequently reported, until recent years.

Kwok et al., in a study published at 2014 [13], used the Health and Occupation Research (THOR) database of 1996–2011 to identify occupational disease in beauticians. In total, 257 cases of contact dermatitis in beauticians were identified, which were associated with 502 suspected agents. Of these, 84 cases (32.7%) were attributed to acrylates. Trend analysis showed a small average annual percentage increase in work-related contact dermatitis in beauticians for all agents, including acrylates. Other common sources of allergic contact dermatitis in this population were fragrance substances and rubber chemicals.

Nail technicians are not only prone to allergic contact dermatitis. Technicians' hands are also exposed to contact irritation due to wet work from hand-washing between clients and due to dust of nail filing. Some of the chemicals in use, such as nail enamel removers (acetone, butyl acetate, ethyl acetate, methyl ethyl acetone) and nail cuticle removers (Sodium hydroxide and potassium hydroxide) have a significant irritant potential. Methacrylic acid, the initiator of the polymerization process of artificial nails, has a strong irritant potential and may produce third-degree burns [14]. Contact irritation and atopic tendency probably add their share to the problem.

20.4 Incidence of (Metha)Crylate Allergy

It is believed that the increasing use of gel nails and sculptured nails has led to a rise in incidence of (metha)crylate allergy among beauticians and nail technicians. Lack of regulation, insufficient training and lack of awareness of risk, probably contribute to the growing number of cases. While the general incidence of (meth)acrylates allergy is unknown, but is estimated to be ~1% of all patients patch tested, it is much higher in nail technicians [15]. As opposed to clients, nail technicians are at particularly increased risk of developing (meth)acrylate contact sensitization, as they are exposed to the monomers, before they are polymerized, on a daily basis. Some of the technicians wear sculptured nails and/or gel nails themselves, thus increasing their risk.

In a study by Ramos et al. [16], among 122 who went through extended (meth)acrylate series, 37 allergic individuals were found. Twenty-five cases (67.6%) were occupational and 28 were related to artificial nails. Beauty technicians working with artificial nails were the most affected group, and constituted 80% of the occupational cases. Dermatitis developed during the first year of their activity as a nail beautician in 60%, in some cases while they were still apprentices.

20.5 Symptoms of (Meth) Acrylates Allergy in Nail Technicians

The hands are the most common site at which allergic contact dermatitis develops. Symptoms of sensitization consist of subacute or chronic eczema located on the pads of the fingers that come into direct contact with the acrylic resin, typically the finger pads of the first, second, and third finger of both hands are affected. The non-dominant hand may be involved from holding the client's nail and the dominant hand from holding the brush. Lesions also frequently occur on the sides of the hands where they come in contact with work surfaces that are likely to carry monomer residues. Periungual dermatitis, onycholysis and nail shedding that may be permanent may also appear, as are eczematous lesions away from the site of contact, for example of the face and neck, probably as a result of transportation of residues. Finger numbness and decreased dexterity, and respiratory symptoms, rhinoconjunctivitis and angioedema were also described, the last three, probably due to airborne spread of the chemicals [17].

Other reactions have also been described. Thickening of the keratin layer of the nail bed, with or without onycholysis, due to an irritant reaction to the monomer, as well as a mechanical or traumatic dermatitis, may also develop [18]. TSFR, the main allergen in nail polish, produces dermatitis that typically involves the eyelids, lips and neck, and not the hands [19]. Nail hardeners may be either based on formaldehyde, or resins. The prevalence of nail hardener reactions caused by formaldehyde is considered low, but may result in a nail damage that simulates psoriasis [20].

20.6 Diagnosis

(Meth)acrylates are tricky molecules to test, because the concentration that will reveal allergic sensitization is close to the irritancy threshold [18]. There is significant cross-reaction among (meth)acrylates, as demonstrated in both animal studies and case reports. The pattern of acrylate cross-reactivity among the most frequently positive acrylates suggests that a functional group, probably a carboxyethyl side group, may be a requisite for allergic contact dermatitis to acrylates. Chemical analyses have shown that many acrylate-based industrial products contain numerous acrylates as impurities, so some cross reactions could in fact be concomitant reactions [21].

Several authors tried to conclude which tests should be held in the detection of allergic contact dermatitis to acrylates among beauticians. Kanerva [22] reported that 6 out of 23 patients who were acrylate-sensitive were sensitive to ethyl methacrylate, which was consequently defined as a significant allergen.

In a series of 11 patients, Koppula [23] used 0.1% ethyl acrylate in petrolatum to detect 91% of the acrylate-allergic, artificial nail users and proposed the following five chemicals to be used as screens: ethyl acrylate, 2-hydroxyethyl acrylate, ethylene glycol dimethacrylate, ethyl cyanoacrylate and triethylene glycol diacrylate. In a study performed by Spencer [15], four individual (meth)acrylates (2-hydroxyethyl acrylate, 2-hydroxypropyl methacrylate, bisphenol A glycerolate dimethacrylate, and ethylacrylate), used as a screening tool, have identified 90.4% of the positive tests, and were proposed for potential screening. Among beauticians that worked with long lasting nail polish only (light curing gels), 2 hydroxy propyl methacrylate, 2 hydroxy ethyl methacrylate and tetra hydrofurfuryl methacrylate were sufficient to detect all allergies [24] (Fig. 20.1).

In two other studies from Portugal, 2 Hydroxyethyl methacrylate alone, detected 85.3% of the cases of allergic contact dermatitis to (meth)acrylates among beauticians. It was concluded that it may serve as a good yet not perfect screening tool for this population [16, 25].

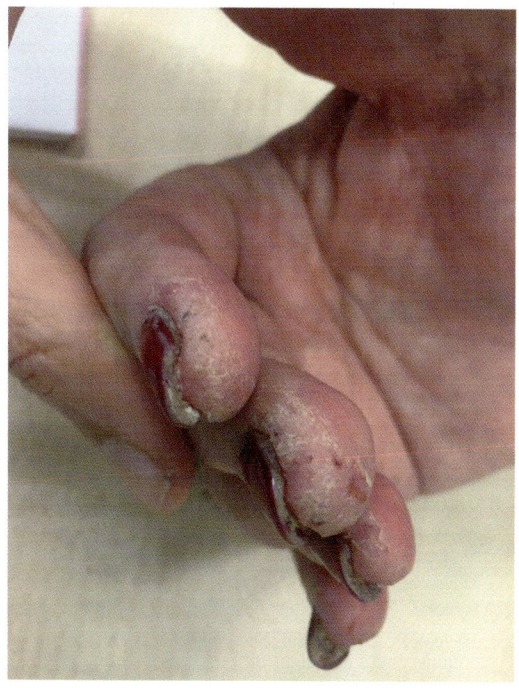

Fig. 20.1 Contact dermatitis due to (meth)acrylates exposure in a nail technician. Patch tests were reactive to 2 Hydroxyethyl methacrylate (HEMA) and 2 hydroxy propyl methacrylate (HPMA)

20.7 Protective Measures

Primary prevention is recommended as the best approach [10]. The most effective approach would be to replace current products with non-toxic alternatives as protective measures against (meth)acrylates allergy are difficult to apply. Improved ventilation in the work surrounding by engineering control is mandatory. For contact sensitivity protection, the commonly used nitril gloves, offer some benefit over latex or vinil gloves, but they are also permeated by the (meth) acrylates with prolonged exposure, so should be replaced very often. Double-gloving with nitrile gloves and changing these gloves frequently is recommended [18]. Double gloving with nitrile gloves, or polyethylene gloves under nitrile gloves, affords adequate protection for tasks that do not exceed 30–60 min. Gloves that have better resistance to (meth)acrylates, such as 4H® (Honeywell Safety Products, Smithfield, Rhode Island, USA), impair manual dexterity and are

not suitable for work. A suggested solution is to wear fingers cut from the 4H gloves under more flexible gloves. Protection using face masks and suitable clothing is also recommended. Surgical masks, many times used by technicians, do not protect from chemical vapors and dust.

Education among nail technicians regarding safer use of nail products is important. They should avoid skin contact with uncured (meth) acrylates by careful work techniques and ensure that monomers are cured with well-maintained ultraviolet lamps for the full time recommended [15]. Patients who have positive reactions to one or more (meth)acrylates should be advised to avoid all (meth)acrylates, because of significant co-sensitization between the various molecules.

20.8 Summary

Nail salons are a working area for women, where skin and airways exposure to many different chemicals may be prevalent. In particularly, demand for long-lasting cosmetic nails has led to widespread use of gel nails and acrylic nails. As a result, a rise in incidence of (Meth)acrylate induced contact dermatitis among nail technicians using these products has been observed. Education among nail technicians regarding safer use of nail products is mandatory, as is production of nontoxic alternatives to replace current products.

References

1. Nails Big Book 2015–2016. Nails magazine. Available at: http://files.nailsmag.com/Feature-Articles-in-PDF/NABB2015-16stats.pdf.
2. Quach T, Gunier R, Tran A, Von Behren J, Doan-Billings PA, Nguyen KD, Okahara L, Lui BY, Nguyen M, Huynh J, Reynolds P. Characterizing workplace exposures in Vietnamese women working in California nail salons. Am J Public Health. 2011;101(Suppl 1):S271–6.
3. Park SA, Gwak S, Choi S. Assessment of occupational symptoms and chemical exposures or nail salon technicians in Daegu City, Korea. J Prev Med Public Health. 2014;47:169–76.
4. Harris-Roberts J, Bowen J, Sumner J, Stocks-Greaves M, Bradshaw L, Fishwick D, Barber CM. Work-

related symptoms in nail salon technicians. Occup Med (Lond). 2011;61:335–40.

5. Reutman SR, Rohs AM, Clark JC, Johnson BC, Sammons DL, Toennis CA, Robertson SA, MacKenzie BA, Lockey JE. A pilot respiratory health assessment of nail technicians: symptoms, lung function, and airway inflammation. Am J Ind Med. 2009;52:868–75.

6. Mälkönen T, Jolanki R, Alanko K, Luukkonen R, Aalto-Korte K, Lauerma A, Susitaival P. A 6-month follow-up study of 1048 patients diagnosed with an occupational skin disease. Contact Dermatitis. 2009;61:261–8.

7. Baran R. Nail cosmetics allergies and irritations. Am J Clin Dermatol. 2002;3:547–55.

8. Hausen BM, Milbrodt M, Koenig WA. The allergens of nail polish. Allergenic constituents of common nail polish and toluenesulfonamide-formaldehyde resin (TS-F-R). Contact Dermatitis. 1995;33:157–64.

9. Scientific Committee on Consumer Safety (SCCS), Bernauer U, Coenraads PJ, Degen GH, Dusinska M, Lilienblum W, Luch A, Nielsen E, Platzek T, Rastogi S, Rousselle C, van Benthem J, Bernard A, Giménez-Arnau AM, Vanhaecke T. Opinion of the Scientific Committee on Consumer Safety (SCCS)–The safety of the use of formaldehyde in nail hardeners. Regul Toxicol Pharmacol. 2015;72:658–9.

10. Roche E, de la Cuadra J, Alegre V. Sensitization to acrylates caused by artificial acrylic nails: review of 15 cases. Actas Dermosifiliogr. 2008;99:788–94.

11. Sainio EL, Engstrom K, Henriks-Eckerman ML, Kanerva L. Allergenic ingredients in nail polishes. Contact Dermatitis. 1997;37:155–62.

12. Canizares O. Contact dermatitis due to acrylic materials used in artificial nails. Arch Dermatol. 1956;74:141–3.

13. Kwok C, Money A, Carder M, Turner S, Agius R, Orton D, Wilkinson M. Cases of occupational dermatitis and asthma in beauticians that were reported to The Health and Occupation Research (THOR) network from 1996 to 2011. Clin Exp Dermatol. 2014;39:590–5.

14. Cosmetic Ingredient Review Expert Panel. Final report of the safety assessment of methacrylic acid. Int J Toxicol. 2005;24:33–51.

15. Spencer A, Gazzani P, Thompson DA. Acrylate and methacrylate contact allergy and allergic contact disease: a 13-year review. Contact Dermatitis. 2016;75:157–64.

16. Ramos L, Cabral R, Gonçalo M. Allergic contact dermatitis caused by acrylates and methacrylates–a 7-year study. Contact Dermatitis. 2014;71:102–7.

17. Henriks-Eckerman ML, Korva M. Exposure to airborne methacrylates in nail salons. J Occup Environ Hyg. 2012;9:D146–50.

18. Sasseville D. Acrylates in contact dermatitis. Dermatitis. 2012;23:6–16.

19. Engasser PG, Tylor JS, Maibach HI. Cosmetologists. In: Kanerva L, editor. Handbook of occupational dermatology. Berlin: Springer; 2000. p. 893–8.

20. Mestach L, Goossens A. Allergic contact dermatitis and nail damage mimicking psoriasis caused by nail hardeners. Contact Dermatitis. 2015;74:110–27.

21. Henriks-Eckerman ML, Kanerva L. Product analysis of acrylic resins compared to information given in material safety data sheets. Contact Dermatitis. 1997;36:164–5.

22. Kanerva L, Estlander T, Jolanki R. Statistics on allergic patch test reactions caused by acrylate compounds, including data on ethyl methacrylate. Am J Contact Dermat. 1995;6:75–7.

23. Koppula SV, Fellman JH, Storrs FJ. Screening allergens for acrylate dermatitis associated with artificial nails. Am J Contact Dermatitis. 1995;6:78–85.

24. Gatica-Ortega ME, Pastor-Nieto MA, Mercader-García P, Silvestre-Salvador JF. Allergic contact dermatitis caused by (meth)acrylates in long-lasting nail polish–are we facing a new epidemic in the beauty industry? Contact Dermatitis. 2017;77(6):360–6.

25. Raposo I, Lobo I, Amaro C, Lobo ML, Melo H, Parente J, Pereira T, Rocha J, Cunha AP, Baptista A, Serrano P, Correia T, Travassos AR, Dias M, Pereira F, Gonçalo M. Allergic contact dermatitis caused by (meth)acrylates in nail cosmetic products in users and nail technicians–a 5-year study. Contact Dermatitis. 2017;77(6):356–9.

Universal Concepts of Beauty and Their Implications on Clinical Approach to Female Cosmetic Patient

Marina Landau

21.1 Introduction

While beauty in general has been explored by artists, poets and philosophers along the existence of humanity, scientific study of facial attractiveness has developed mainly in the past 30 years. Almost all of the research has been conducted in disciplines outside of dermatology. This chapter presents scientifically based information on facial attractiveness and discusses its relevance and implications while working with female cosmetic patient.

21.2 What is Beauty and Why Beauty is Important?

Human view on beauty is contradictory. Aphorisms such as "Beauty is only skin deep" and "Do not judge a book by its cover", allegedly reflect the belief that beauty is a trivial quality and should be ignored. In practice, the pursuit of beauty has always been an integral part of every human culture. It has been scientifically proven that physically attractive people have advantages that unattractive peers do not. Attractive people receive more attention in most facets of life. In fact, research suggests that physical appearance may be the single most important element of first impressions [1]. People are attracted to beauty because their brain refers to attractive people good qualities. The more attractive the face is judged, there is tendency to refer to its "owner" characteristics such as success, content, intelligence, creativity and honesty [2–4]. It seems that pretty faces "prime" the minds to make an association between beauty and positive emotions. Physical attractiveness of females, as reflected in Facebook profile photograph, is more important than the owner's personal information (likes and interests) [5]. Perceived attractiveness of an unfamiliar face activates dopaminergic regions in the brain that are strongly linked to reward prediction [6, 7].

21.2.1 Beauty Canons

The classic Greek canons of proportions were formulated by the Renaissance artists, such as Leonardo da Vinci and others. Being based on the anatomical analysis performed by the artists, these canons have been also accepted by the medical profession. These neoclassical canons include various concepts, such as: the head can be divided into equal halves at a horizontal line through the eyes; the face can be divided into equal thirds; the length of the ear is equal to the length of the nose; the distance between the eyes is equal to the width of the nose; the distance between the eyes is equal

M. Landau
Dermatology Unit, Wolfson Medical Center,
Holon, Israel

© Springer International Publishing AG, part of Springer Nature 2018
E. Tur, H. I. Maibach (eds.), *Gender and Dermatology*,
https://doi.org/10.1007/978-3-319-72156-9_21

to the width of each eye, etc. When these canons were tested experimentally, they were not found to represent adequately the ideal facial proportions. They did not differentiate between "average," "attractive" and "most attractive" faces in Caucasians and Asians [8, 9].

21.2.2 Golden Ratio

Used since the time of Egyptians in art and architecture, the ratio of 1:1.618 is known as the divine proportion. This mathematical relationship has been consistently reported to be present in beautiful things, both living and men-made [10]. Golden mask, derived from the golden ratio was created by Marquardt to support the claim that our perception of facial beauty is based on how closely one's features reflect phi in their proportions [11].

21.3   Evolutionary Esthetics

Long-held view was that standards of beauty are arbitrary cultural conventions [12, 13]. However, some observations opposed this view. It has been shown that people from different cultures generally agree on the attractiveness of human faces [14]. Beauty preferences emerge early in the development, before cultural standards of beauty are assimilated [15, 16].

Because beauty preferences affect mate choice, they may have evolved through biological, rather than cultural selection in order to enhance reproductive success [17]. This is a central pillar of evolutionary psychology. Evolutionary psychologists believe that morphologic characteristics, such as attractiveness are honest indicators of fitness, health, and reproductive value. This branch of science rests on Darwin's theories of natural and sexual selection, that claim that because of sexual selection, any characteristics that are attractive to the opposite sex enhance the reproductive success of their owner [18].

Facial attractiveness in humans has evolved as an important marker for both phenotypic and genetic quality. The ability of the human brain to subconsciously judge facial attractiveness in only 150 ms, is based on highly efficient assessment of three basic traits: averageness, symmetry, sexual dimorphism and youthfulness. All of these cues are used simultaneously [19–21].

21.3.1 Averageness

Contradicting the "romantic" view of beauty as an extraordinary trait, the appeal of computer-generated averaged composites of faces has been demonstrated more than 20 years ago [22]. The artificially composite faces have been judged as more attractive than the real component ones.

An average face has mathematically average trait values for a population. Faces with high averageness are low in distinctiveness. Typical faces, which are closer to the population average, are consistently rated as more attractive than distinctive faces [23, 24]. Furthermore, the attractiveness of individual faces can be increased or reduced by moving their configuration toward or away from an average configuration for that sex [25, 26].

Trying to explain these counterintuitive results, the evolutionary psychologists hypothesize that average traits reflect developmental stability, i.e. the ability to withstand stress and increase disease resistance [27–29]. Average trait may also be functionally optimal (e.g. average nose for optimal breathing). Therefore, averageness signals mate quality, such as good condition and heritable resistance to diseases.

21.3.2 Symmetry

Facial asymmetries negatively affect judgement of attractiveness. Manipulated perfectly symmetric faces were found to be more attractive than the original, slightly asymmetric, and their appeal could not be explained by any associated increase in averageness [30].

Reviews of numerous studies across multiple species have shown that increased asymmetry is associated with losses in fitness components [31–

35] In humans, men with lower asymmetry have more sexual partners, have better sperm quality and more offsprings, and are more often the choice of women for extra-pair copulations [36–38], Perfectly symmetric faces, are judged as more attractive than the asymmetric ones since they signal for better health [30, 39, 40].

21.4 Sexual Dimorphism

The third trait of evolutionary esthetics is preference for sexual dimorphism, i.e., for feminine traits in female faces and masculine traits in male faces. Male and female faces do not differ at birth, but the difference becomes much more marked with the onset of puberty. During the puberty in males, testosterone stimulates the growth of the jaw, brow ridges, center of the face and facial hair, creating the characteristic male traits (Table 21.1, Fig. 21.1). Men who had developed broader chins are perceived as more dominant, as they probably have had higher levels of the male hormone. Women seem to choose sexual partners based on a male's ability to protect and provide the mate and her offspring [41]. Dominancy is associated with higher resource providing potential, therefore women are more attracted to dominant males.

In females, growth of these traits is inhibited by estrogen, which is also responsible for fuller lips, higher cheekbones, wider and bigger eyes and raised thin eyebrows [42]. (Table 21.2, Fig. 21.2). Lip fullness parallels the estrogen-dependent fat deposits on the hips and breasts and reaches its maximum value between 14 and 15 years of age. Full lips are a hormone marker indicating high estrogen exposure during this developmental phase [43].

Overall, femininity is highly attractive, whether "normal" or "manipulated" images were used for the analysis. Most studies combine data from male and female raters, so the rater sex could not affect the results. The preference generalizes across faces from different races. Therefore, it has been suggested that female attractiveness is virtually synonymous with femininity. Femininity is attractive in female faces and preferred to averageness [44–47]. In both sexes, dimorphic traits signal sexual maturity, reproductive potential and mate quality [48, 49].

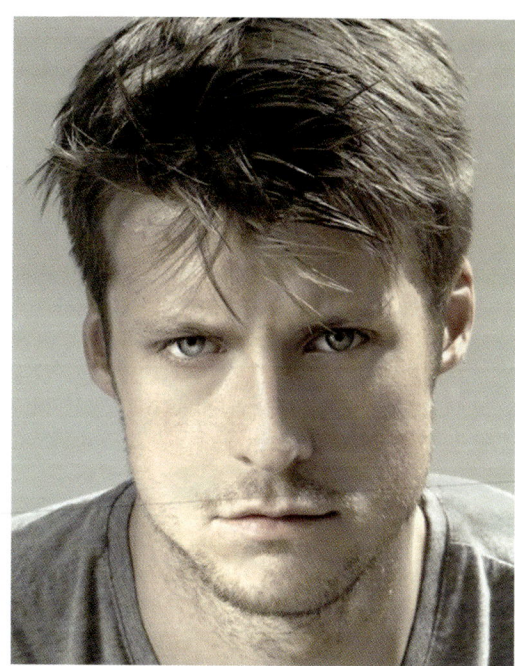

Fig. 21.1 Attractive male face presenting characteristic dimorphic features: such as prominent brow ridges, square jaw line and chin, low set eyebrows and thin lips. Photo credit: Shutterstock

Table 21.1 Male traits

Pronounced brow ridges
Prominent nose
Full low set eyebrows
Sunken narrow eyes
Wider face, nose and mouth
Wider and more prominent lower jaw
Thinner lips

Table 21.2 Female traits

Smooth round forehead
Small nose
Wider set bigger eyes
Higher and arched eyebrows
Higher cheekbones
Shorter and narrower lower jaw
Full lips

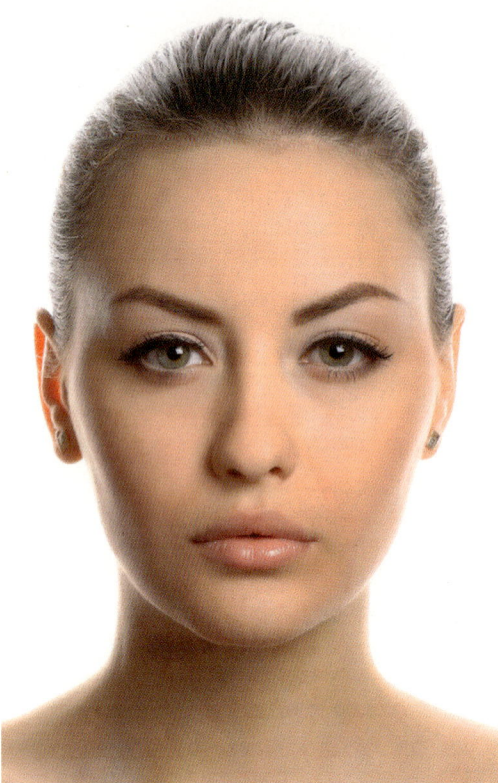

Fig. 21.2 Attractive female face presenting characteristic dimorphic female traits: smooth and round forehead, high arched eyebrows, high cheekbones and full lips. Photo credit: Shutterstock

It is felt and experimentally supported, that extremes of secondary sexual characteristics are more attractive. These differences occur because of sex hormones, which are "handicapping" and suppress the immune system. Thus, to manifest highly sexually dimorphic traits, signals to have high quality, and robust immune system.

21.4.1 Youthfulness

Many studies have confirmed that youthful faces are more attractive than older ones [50]. Childlike facial features increase female's attractiveness [51, 52]. Neoteny or babyness refer to features characteristic of newborns: among them are large eyes, small nose, round cheeks, smooth skin, glossy hair and lighter coloration. Interestingly, that these neonate features are shared by a wide range of mammalian species

[53]. Adults with neonate features elicit attraction and care providing "reflexes", evolved originally with young children. This was supported in studies showing that individuals from both genders with bigger eyes and smaller noses are found to be more attractive [54, 55]. Female faces that were digitally manipulated to have larger eyes were found to be appearing women as mating partners since they have a long period of fertility ahead of them.

21.4.2 The Magnificent Seven

A list of seven features influencing our perception of facial beauty has been recently suggested by Swift and Remington [56]. It includes facial shape, forehead height, eyebrow shape, eye size and inter-eye distance, nose shape, lips length and height, and skin clarity, texture and color. Four out of the list are features amenable to injection therapy with fillers and neuromodulators (Botulinum toxin), while skin clarity and texture can be improved by topical agents or energy based devices. Interestingly, the authors argue the importance of perfect symmetry as a beautifying trait. According to their opinion facial symmetry is not an absolute value. Both sides of the face should be similar, but not identical, while the two halves of the lips must carry perfect symmetry.

21.5   Beauty and Ethnicity

Every ethnic group presents its esthetically unique aspects, but the most beautiful and attractive people of each race tend to look similar in terms of face shape, and harmony of facial features. As faces display more distinct ethnic features, they become less attractive. Possible speculation for preference of "mixed-race" faces can be that owners of theses face are more likely to have heterozygous mixture of genes enhancing disease resistance [57].

Nevertheless, every ethnic group has its esthetically strong and weak points. For example, while Caucasian faces are generally narrower with greater vertical height and pronounced three dimensionality, Asians tend to have a wider and flatter faces with shorter vertical height. On the other hand, they possess greater infraorbital volume, fuller lips, and better skin quality [58]. Mindful of this concept of universal beauty, physicians in Asia seek to enhance "deficient" features and improve esthetic balance. In Asians, attractiveness is achieved by aiming to create an oval facial shape, by narrowing the lower face and increasing vertical height of the face. The anterior projection of the brow, medial cheek, nose, and chin is increased to improve the three-dimensionality of the face, and the appearance of the eyes is enlarged [59–61]. In addition, the ideal ratio between the lower and upper lip in Asians is closer to 1:1, and not 1:1.6 as in Caucasians [59].

21.5.1 Why All This is Important?

When planning facial cosmetic procedure, the physician should consider all the scientific data. Principally, the aim should be to produce a face close to the ideal ethnic prototype, respecting bilateral symmetry, and enhancing sexual dimorphic features. It is pertinent to recognize that the approach to male and female cosmetic patients is not identical. Masculinity depends on the dominancy of the lower face: the jaw and the chin. Flatter and low set eyebrows, prominent supraorbital ridges, sturdier muscles of midface, less projected cheeks, longer nose and less detailed upper lip- all have to be respected in male patient to avoid feminization [62]. (Fig. 21.3). On the contrary, procedures, such as lip enhancement, cheek augmentation and eyebrow lift, are appropriate to enhance feminine beauty. Restoration of youthfulness is another basic tenet of increased female attractiveness and is achieved by procedures that enhance skin quality. Aging process changes the 3D topography of the underlying facial structures, resulting in deflation and ptosis of the midface. Volumization of midface by injectable products restores the triangle of youth and provides support to sagging soft tissues.

Herein we present basic principles of injection of dermal fillers, as employed by dermatologists,

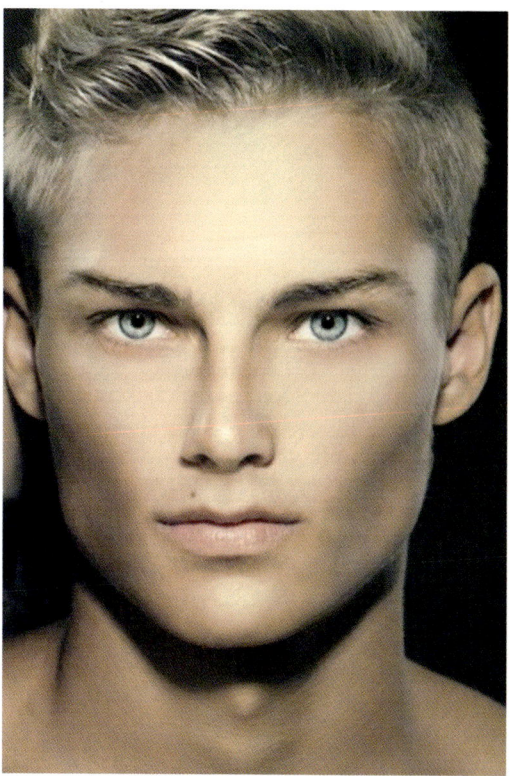

Fig. 21.3 High cheekbones, fuller lips and arched eyebrows cause feminization of male face. Photo credit: Shutterstock

to enhance female facial attractiveness. The discussion on characteristics and choice of the specific products is beyond the scope of this chapter.

21.5.2 Lips Enhancement

Lips are one of the major elements of the lower third of the face and serve as a focus of attention during communication. Female lips are considered to be the only legitimately visible sexual organ. Lips and the perioral area are of outstanding importance in youthful appearance, attractiveness, and beauty. Lip fullness is the estrogen-dependent trait and reaches its pick at puberty. Full lips are sexually dimorphic for women, signal for maturity and fertility, therefore increase facial attractiveness.

Genetics, intrinsic aging, sun exposure, smoking, and repetitive pursing of the orbicularis oris

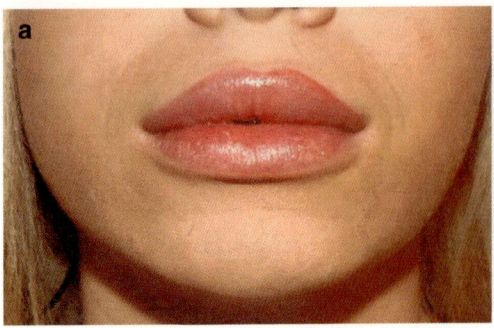 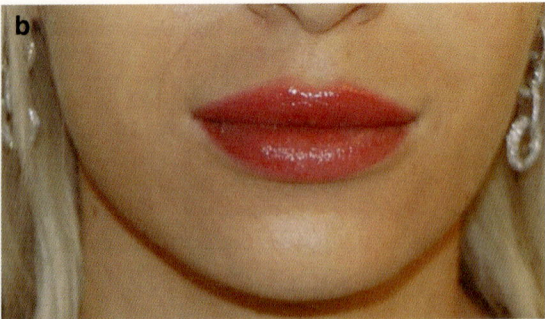

Fig. 21.4 Overfilled and disproportioned lips stigmatize the aesthetic procedures world-wide. (**a**) A patient being refused to be treated on her lips after multiple lip injec- tions elsewhere, (**b**) The same patient presents attractive and harmonious lips 7 years after avoiding any lip injec- tions. Photo credit: Shutterstock

muscle produce angular, radial, and vertical wrinkles [63]. Gravity, osteoporosis, dental changes, maxillomandibular bony resorption, and soft tissue volume loss cause the oral com- missures to turn downward in a perpetual frown. The lip margin itself becomes blunted with loss of sharp vermilion-cutaneous junction demarca- tion, philtral columns become flattened and lip volume decreases and projection of the Cupid's bow is lost.

Lip augmentation has become a very popular trend in the last years. Nevertheless, the stigma of the overinflated, disproportioned lip has perme- ated the media worldwide (Fig. 21.4a, b). The art of injecting lips, whether the goal is to restore aging lips or to beautify younger ones, revolves around subtle enhancement and not volumiza- tion. When properly carried out, lip enhancement rejuvenates, feminizes and increases facial attractiveness.

To perform this task successfully, the injecting physician should be familiar with the basic prin- ciples of ideal lip esthetics. In Caucasian lips, the height ratio of the upper lip to the lower lip is 1:1.6 to 1:2, while in Asians the ratio is closer to 1:1 (Fig. 21.5) [64]. On the lateral view, if a straight line is drawn from the sub-nasion to the tip of the chin (pogonion), the upper lip projects 3.5 mm and the lower lip 2.2 mm anterior to the line. Developmentally, the upper lip is composed of two, while the lower lip of three parts, appear- ing as lip tubercles.

"Six steps to the perfect lip" have been pub- lished and they include: sculpting of the philtral

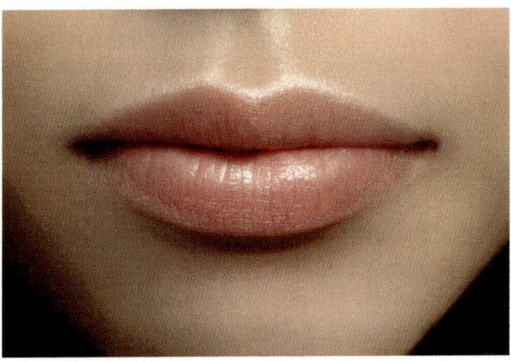

Fig. 21.5 For harmonious female Caucasian lips ratio of 1:1.6 between the upper and lower lips should be pre- served. Photo credit: Shutterstock

columns, enhancement of the Cupid's bow, re- definition of the vermilion-cutaneous junction, volumization of the lips by restoration of the tubercles, enhancing the support of the oral com- missures, and filling the upper lip wrinkles [65]. The procedure is always carried out using hyal- uronic acid based filler, as the only safe material to be used in the perioral area.

The philtrum tends to flatten with aging. Reshaping of the philtrum is achieved by super- ficial injection along the philtrum while pinch- ing the columns to control the flow of the filler. Inverted V-shape of the philtrum should be pre- served [66]. By enhancing the philtral columns, illusion of shortening of the distance between the subnasal area to the upper lip can be created (Fig. 21.6). To restore the lip border including the Cupid's bow, the needle is positioned at the vermilion border near lateral edge of the mouth

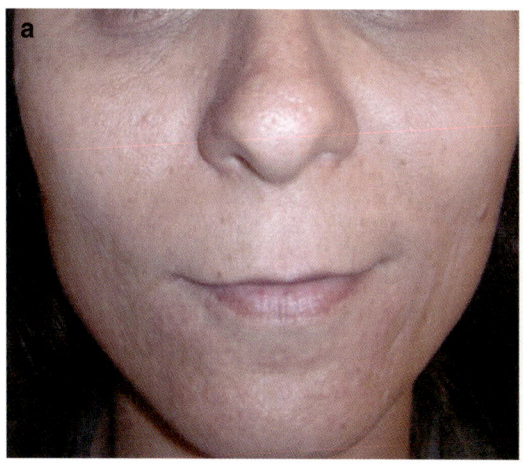
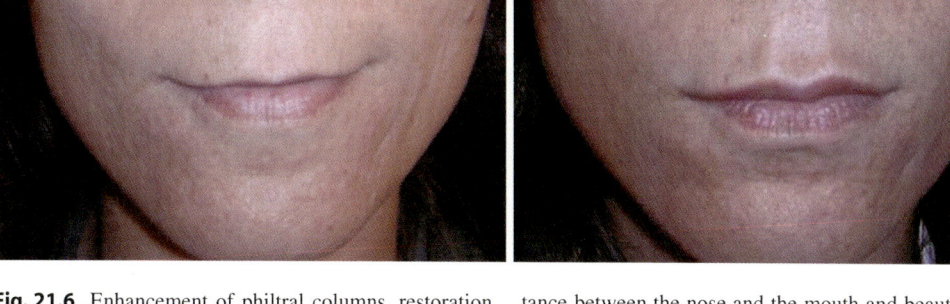

Fig. 21.6 Enhancement of philtral columns, restoration of the Cupid's bow and mild volumization of the upper lip—all together create illusion of shortening of the dis- tance between the nose and the mouth and beautification of the lips: (**a**) before, (**b**) after. Photo credit: Shutterstock

below the mucocutaneous junction. Slow injection is performed with deposition of a linear thread as the needle is advanced. Administration of strictly equal volumes of the product is performed into the Cupid's bow unless gross asymmetry was noted before the treatment [66]. To correct perioral lines is possible only when the lines are stretchable. For non- stretchable lines, resurfacing procedure by laser or deep chemical peel, provides better cosmetic outcome. For stretchable lines, perpendicular to the wrinkle injection of soft hyaluronic acid based filler is recommended. While stretching the skin a minimal amount of the product is delivered intradermally, as evidenced by skin blanching [66, 67].

Procedures on lips are usually not performed on male patients, unless some extent of feminization is intentionally required.

21.5.3 Cheek Enhancement

High cheekbones are among symbols of female attractiveness; thus, enhancement of malar area increases femininity. In addition, malar augmentation creates the illusion of tissues lifting, therefore rejuvenates the appearance. The female cheek is ovoid and does not extend higher than the lower limbus of the eyelid. The cheek axis is angled from the mouth commissure to the ear tragus. Each malar prominence has a defined apex. Depending on the injector's preference, the procedure can be performed using hyaluronic acid based product or calcium hydroxyapatite.

Several schemes exist to augment malar mound harmoniously and attractively. The simplified approach suggests three potential injection sites: lateral cheek, anterior cheek, and medial cheek. In the lateral cheek a volumizing filler is administered by supraperiosteal two small-bolus injections. In the medial and anterior cheek a filler is injected below the orbital rim supraperiosteally or deep subcutaneously [68]. According to Swift and Remington, a line is drawn from the mouth commissure to the canthus of the ipsilateral eye [55]. A second line is drawn from the same commissure to the inferior tragus of the ipsilateral ear. The highpoint of the cheek is marked by a horizontal line at a level of the limbus of the lower eyelid. Lastly a line is drawn from the lateral canthus to the base of the triangle. The cheek oval is drawn within these boundaries and with the apex located one third of a way along the last line. Since some parts of the marking are dependent on injector's esthetic vision and no specifications are made regarding the injection methodology, a modification to this scheme has been suggested. According to it, a

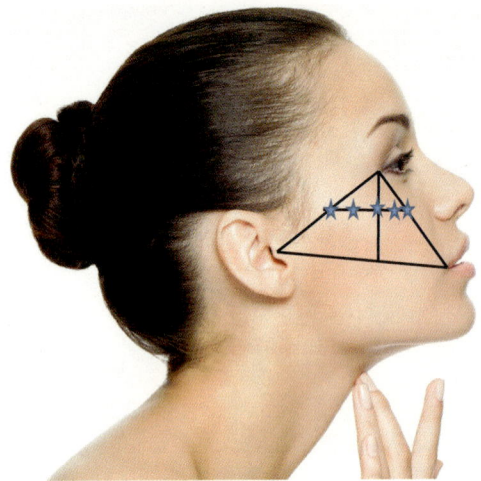

Fig. 21.7 The scheme for "5 stars technique for malar enhancement": Line 1 is drawn between the lateral canthus to the ipsilateral tragus; line 2 is drawn between the lateral canthus to the ipsilateral mouth corner; line 3 is drawn between the tragus to mouth corner; line 4 is drawn horizontally to the triangle base starting laterally at the tear trough; line 5 is drawn perpendicularly to the triangle base. Intersection between lines 4 and 5 creates a point of maximal projection. Injection technique and amount of the product are specified in the text. Photo credit: Shutterstock

triangle is drawn between lateral canthus, ipsilateral mouth commissure and ear tragus. The resultant equilateral triangle is now divided to upper third and lower two thirds by a line, which runs parallel to the triangle base and meets tear trough medially. This line denotes the augmentation plane along which the filler is injected. The last line runs vertically form the triangle apex to its base. The intersection between the vertical and horizontal lines creates a point of maximal projection. Here the maximal amount of the filler is injected. The product is either viscous hyaluronic acid or calcium hydroxyapatite, both to be delivered supraperiosteally by single boluses in 5 locations ("star") along the augmentation plane. While central "star" gets maximal amount of the filler, adjacent "stars" get half the volume and the most lateral ones–one fourth of the initial volume. The procedure is accomplished by gentle massaging of the area (Fig. 21.7). This method is used by the author for the last 10 years and is called internationally "Five stars technique for malar enhancement" (Fig. 21.8).

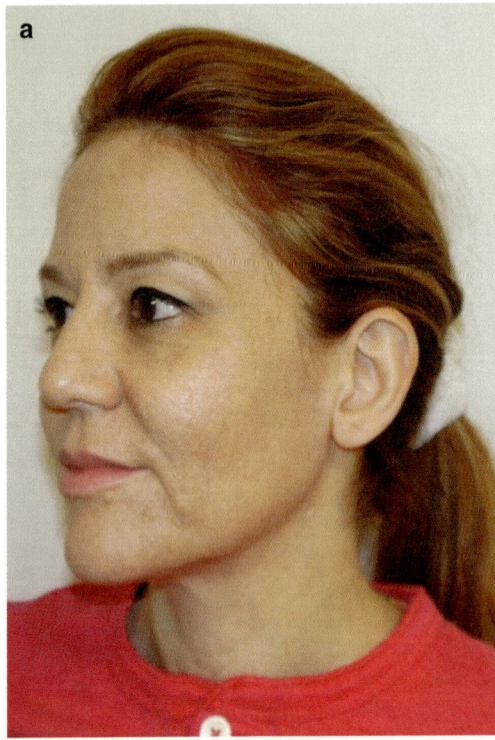

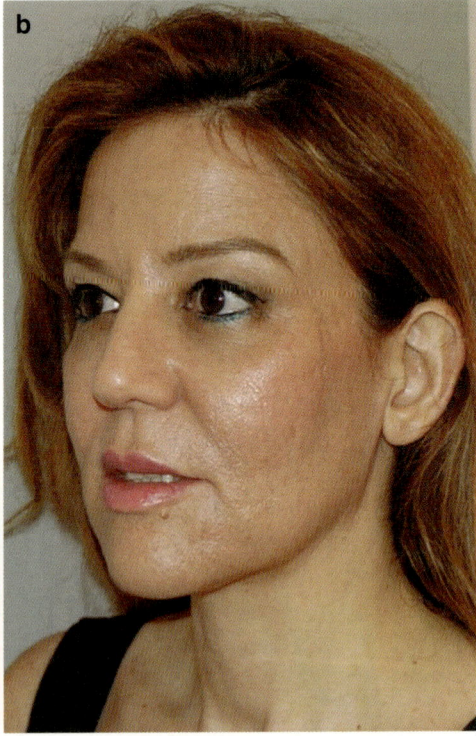

Fig. 21.8 Patient treated for enhancement of the cheekbones using "5 stars technique". (**a**) Before the injection sagging of the midface with accentuation of marionette lines are visible. (**b**) After the injection illusion of midface lifting with partial correction of marionette lines is seen. Photo credit: Shutterstock

21.5.4 Eyebrow Shaping

The medial eyebrow begins in line with medial canthus. It's length is 1.68 (phi number) of the intercanthal distance laterally. An appealing female eyebrow climbs 10–20° from medial to lateral and arches after two thirds of the way. The lateral tip should always be higher than the medial tip of the brow and there should be soft tissue fullness below the brow [66]. The position and shape of the eyebrow change with aging. Hyaluronic acid based fillers are used to improve the elevation if the brow tail alone or in combination with Botulinum toxin. After identification by palpation of the orbital rim, the filler is delivered at two adjacent points, while a finger is protecting to avoid migration of the filler into the upper eyelid. The first injection is performed at the lateral end of the brow and the second immediately medial to it. Small boluses are delivered deep supraperiosteally [69].

21.6   Summary

Human attractiveness has biological reasons. Inter-gender sexual attraction is inspired by characteristic dimorphic features in both sexes. Most of these characteristics can be restored or enhanced by injectable dermal fillers. While performing cosmetic procedures, dermatologist has to be recognizant with the universal concepts of beauty and respect them strictly to avoid masculinization or feminization of the opposite sex.

References

1. Hatfield E, Sprecher S. Mirror, mirror: the importance of looks in everyday life. New York: SUNY Press; 1986.
2. Dion K, Berscheid E, Walster E. What is beautiful is good. J Pers Soc Psychol. 1972;24:285–90.
3. Eagly AH, Ashmore RD, Makhijani MG, Longo LC. What is beautiful is good: a meta-analytic reviewof research on the physical attractiveness stereotype. Psychol Bull. 1991;110:109–28.
4. Langlois JH, Kalakanis L, Rubenstein AJ, Larson A, Hallam M, Smoot M. Maxims or myth of beauty? A meta-analytic and theoretical review. Psychol Bull. 2000;126:390–423.
5. Seidman G, Miller OS. Effects of gender and physical attractiveness on visual attention to Facebook profiles. Cyberpsychol Behav Soc Netw. 2013;16(1):20–4.
6. Schultz W, Dayan P, Montague PR. A natural substance of prediction and reward. Science. 1997;275:1593–9.
7. Kampe KW, Frith CD, Dolan RJ, Frith U. Reward value of attractiveness and gaze. Nature. 2001;413:589.
8. Farkas LG, Kolar JC. Anthropometrics and art in the aesthetics of women's faces. Clin Plast Surg. 1987;14:599–616.
9. Wang D, Qian G, Zhang M, Farkas LG. Differences in horizontal, neoclassical facial canons in Chinese (Han) and North American Caucasian populations. Aesthet Plast Surg. 1997;21:265–9.
10. Livio M. The golden ratio: the story of phi: the world's most astonishing number. New York: Broadway Books; 2002.
11. Available at: www.beautyanalysis.com. Accessed Sept 2017.
12. Berry DS. Attractiveness, attraction, and sexual selection: evolutionary perspectives on the form and function of physical attractiveness. In: Zanna MP, editor. Advances in experimental social psychology, vol. 32. San Diego: Academic; 2000. p. 373–42.
13. Etcoff N. Survival of the prettiest: the science od beauty, vol. 325. New York: Anchor-Doubleday; 1999.
14. Cunningham MR, Roberts AR, Barbee AP, Druen PB, Wu C-H. Their ideas of beauty are, on whole, the same as ours: consistence and variability in the cross-cultural perception of female attractiveness. J Pers Soc Psychol. 1995;68:261–79.
15. Langlois JH, Roggman LA, Casey RJ, Ritter JM, Reiser-Danner LA, Jenkins VY. Infent preferences for attractive faces: rudiments of stereotype? Dev Psychol. 1987;23:363–9.
16. Langlois JH, Ritter JM, Roggman LA, Vaughn LS. Facial diversity and infant preferences for attractive faces. Dev Psychol. 1991;27:79–84.
17. Rhodes G, Simmons L, Peters M. Attractiveness and sexual behavior: does attractiveness enhance mating success? Evol Hum Behav. 2005;26:186–201.
18. Prum RO. Aesthetic evolution by mate choice: Darwin's really dangerous ides. Philos Trans R Soc Lond B Biol Sci. 2012;367:2253–65.
19. Rhodes G, Zebrowitz LA. Facial attractiveness: evolutionary, cognitive and social perspectives. Westport: Ablex; 2002. p. 311.
20. Thornhill R, Gangestad SW. Facial attractiveness. Trends Cogn Sci. 1999;3:452–60.
21. Rubenstein AJ, Langlois JH, Roggman LA. What makes a face attractive and why: the role of averageness in defining facial beauty. In: Rhodes G, Zebrowitz LA, editors. Facial attractiveness: evolutionary, cognitive, and social perspectives, Advances in visual cognition, vol. 1. Westport: Ablex; 2002. p. 1–33.
22. Langlois JH, Roggman LA. Attractive faces are only average. Psychol Sci. 1990;1:115–21.
23. Light LL, Hollander S, Kayra-Stuart F. Why attractive people are harder to remember. Personal Soc Psychol Bull. 1981;7:269–76.
24. Morris PR, Wickham LHV. Typicality and face recognition a critical re-evaluation of the two factor theory. Q J Exp Psychol A. 2001;54:863–77.

25. O'Toole AJ, Price T, Vetter T, Barlett JC, Blanz V. 3D shape and 2D shape surface textures of human faces: the role of "averages" in attractiveness and age. Image Vis Comput. 1999;18:9–19.

26. Rhodes G, Tremewan T. Averageness, exaggeration, and facial attractiveness. Psychol Sci. 1996;7:105–10.

27. Thornhill R, Gangestad SW. Human facial beauty: averageness, symmetry, and parasite resistance. Hum Nat. 1993;4:237–69.

28. Thornhill A, Moller AP. Developmental stability, disease and medicine. Biol Rev Camb Philos Soc. 1997;72:497–548.

29. Gangestad SW, Buss DM. Pathogen prevalence and human mate preferences. Ethol Sociobiol. 1993;14:89–96.

30. Perret DI, Burt DM, Penton-Voak IS, Lee KJ, Rowland DA, Edwards R. Symmetry and human facial attractiveness. Evol Hum Behav. 1999;20:295–307.

31. Moller AP, Swaddle JP. Developmental stability and evolution. New York: Oxford University Press; 1997.

32. Leung B, Forbes MR. Fluctuating asymmetry in relation to stress and fitness: effect of trait type as revealed by meta-analysis. Ecoscience. 1996;3:400–13.

33. Moller AP. Developmental stability and fitness: a review. Am Nat. 1997;149:916–32.

34. Moller AP, Thornhill R. A meta-analysis of the heritability of developmental stability. J Evol Biol. 1997;10(1):16.

35. Moller AP, Thornhill R. Bilateral symmetry and sexual selection: a meta-analysis. Am Nat. 1998;151:174–92.

36. Thornhill R, Gangestad SW. Human fluctuating asymmetry and sexual behavior. Psychol Sci. 1994;5:297–302.

37. Manning JT, Scutt D, Lewis-Jones DI. Developmental stability, ejaculate size, and sperm quality in men. Evol Hum Behav. 1998;19:273–82.

38. Waynforth DC. Male mating strategies among the Mayas of Belize (men). Ph.D. thesis, Albuquerque: University of New Mexico; 1999.

39. Rhodes G, Proffitt F, Grady JM, Sumich A. Facial symmetry and the perception of beauty. Psychonom Bull Rev. 1998;5:659–69.

40. Rhodes G, Roberts J, Simmons L. Reflections on symmetry and attractiveness. Psychol Evol Gend. 1999;1:279–95.

41. Little AC, Hancock PJ. The role of masculinity and distinctiveness in judgments of human male facial attractiveness. Br J Psychol. 2002;9:451–64.

42. Bashour M. History and current concepts in the analysis of facial attractiveness. Plast Reconstr Surg. 2006;118:741–56.

43. Farkas LG. Anthropometric facial proportions in medicine. Springfield: Charles C Thomas; 1981.

44. Perret DI, Lee KJ, Penton-Voak I, Rowland D, Yoshkawa S, et al. Effects of sexual dimorphism on facial attractiveness. Nature. 1998;394:884–7.

45. Penton-Voak IS, Jacobson A, Trivers R. Population differences in attractiveness judgments of male and female faces: comparing British and Jamaican samples. Evol Hum Behav. 2004;25:355–70.

46. Rhodes G, Hickford C, Jeffery L. Sex typicality and attractiveness: are supermale and superfemale faces super-attractive? Br J Psychol. 2000;191:125–40.

47. O'Toole AJ, Deffenbacher KA, Valentin D, McKee K, Huff D, Abdi H. The perception of face gender: the role of stimulus structure in recognition and classification. Mem Cogn. 1998;26:146–60.

48. Johnston VS, Franklin M. Is beauty in the eye of the beholder? Ethol Sociobiol. 1993;14:183–99.

49. Penton-Vaok IS, Perret DI. Consistency and individual differences in facial attractiveness judgements: an evolutionary perspective. Soc Res. 2000;67:219–44.

50. Henns R. Perceiving age and attractiveness in facial photographs. J Appl Soc Psychol. 1991;21:933–46.

51. Mathes EW, Brennan SM, Haugen PM. Ratingsof physical attractiveness as a function of age. J Soc Psychol. 1985;125:157–68.

52. Zebrowitz LA, Olson K, Hoffman K. Stability of babyfaceness and attractiveness across the life span. J Pers Soc Psychol. 1993;64:453–66.

53. Eibl-Ebesfeldt I. Human ethology. New York: Aldine De-Gruyter; 1989.

54. Cunningham MR, Barbee AP, Pike CL. What do women want? Facialmetric assessment of multiple motives in the perception of male physical attractiveness. J Pers Soc Psychol. 1990;59:61–72.

55. Cunningham MR. Measuring the physical and physical attractiveness: Quasi-experiments on the sociobiology of female facial beauty. J Pers Soc Psychol. 1986;50:925–35.

56. Swift A, Remington K. BeautiPHIcation™: a global approach to facial beauty. Clin Plast Surg. 2011;38:347–77.

57. Rhodes G, Lee K, Palermo R, Weiss M, Yoshikawa M, McLean I. Attractiveness of own-race, other-race and mixed-race faces. Perception. 2005;34:319–40.

58. Liew S, Wu WT, Chan HH, Ho WWS, Kim H-J, Goodman GJ, Peng PHL, Rogers JD. Consensus on changing trends, attitudes, and concepts of Asian beauty. Aesthetic Plast Surg. 2016;40:193–201.

59. Wu WT. Botox facial slimming/facial sculpting: the role of botulinum toxin-A in the treatment of hypertrophic masseteric muscle and parotid enlargement to narrow the lower facial width. Facial Plast Surg Clin North Am. 2001;18:133–40.

60. Jayaratne YS, Deutsch CK, McGrath CP, Zwahlen RA. Are neoclassical canons valid for southern Chinese faces? PLoS One. 2012;7(12):e52593.

61. Rho NK, Chang YY, Chao YY, Furuyama N, Huang PY, Kerscher M, Kim HJ, Park JY, Peng HL, Rummaneethorn P, Rzany B, Sundaram H, Wong CH, Yang Y, Prasetyo AD. Consensus recommendations for optimal augmentation of the Asian face with hyaluronic acid and calcium hydroxylapatite fillers. Plast Reconstr Surg. 2015;136:940–56.

62. de Maio M. Ethnic and gender consideration in the use of facial injectables: male patient. Plast Reconstr Surg. 2015;136:40s–3s.
63. Wollina U. Perioral rejuvenation: restoration of attractiveness in aging females by minimally invasive procedures. Clin Interv Aging. 2013;8:1149–55.
64. Popenko NA, Tripathi PB, Devcic Z, Karimi K, Osann K, Wong BJF. A quantitative approach to determining the ideal female lip aesthetic and its effect on facial attractiveness. JAMA Facial Plast Surg. 2017;19:261–7.
65. Sarnoff DS, Gotkin RH. Six steps to the "perfect" lip. J Drugs Dermatol. 2012;11:1081–8.
66. de Maio M, Wu WTL, Goodman GJ, Monheit G. Facial assessment and injection guide for botulinum toxin and injectable hyaluronic acid fillers: focus on the lower face. Plast Reconstr Surg. 2017;140:393e–404e.
67. Sudaram H, Cassuto D. Biophysical characteristics of hyaluronic acid soft-tissue fillers and their relevance to aesthetic applications. Plast Reconstr Surg. 2013;132:5s–21s.
68. de Maio M, BeBulle K, Braz A, Rohrich RJ. Facial assessment and injection guide for botulinum toxin and injectable hyaluronic acid fillers: focus on the midface. Plast Reconstr Surg. 2017;140:540e–50e.
69. de Maio M, Swift A, Signorini M, Fagien S. Facial assessment and injection guide for botulinum toxin and injectable hyaluronic acid fillers: focus on the upper face. Plast Reconstr Surg. 2017;140:265e–76e.

Gender Differences in Mohs Micrographic Surgery

Yoav C. Metzger

22.1 Introduction

Mohs micrographic surgery (MMS) is a specialized type of margin controlled surgery that yields higher cure rates than other options in the treatment of skin cancers. The technique, in which 100% of the surgical margin is examined prior to reconstruction of the surgical defect, was developed by Dr. Frederic E. Mohs in 1938. The technique originally required in situ tissue fixation before excision, and nowadays most Mohs micrographic surgeons use the fresh tissue technique. Horizontal frozen histologic sections of the excised tumor enable complete microscopic examination of the surgical margin as opposed to the traditional bread loaf vertical sections method. Residual tumor is graphically mapped and the positive margins are pursued with staged re-excisions until the entire tumor is removed. Maximum sparing of tumor-free adjacent tissue is achieved with histologic mapping of the tumor boundaries, thus optimizing subsequent wound reconstruction [1].

The defect size after MMS has been used as a precise measure of morbidity and can be influenced by delay in treatment, initial misdiagnosis, failure to obtain a biopsy before treatment, or multiple surgical removals [2].

22.2 Indications for MMS

MMS is the treatment of choice for skin tumors in critical sites, large or recurrent tumors, tumors in sites of radiation therapy, and tumors with aggressive histologic features [3].

MMS is used mainly for the treatment of non-melanoma skin cancer (NMSC). The utilization of MMS has increased over the years from 3% in 1995 to 17% in 2010 [4].

MMS has the best long-term cure rate of any basal cell carcinoma (BCC) treatment and is indicated for the removal of all BCCs on the central face, eyelids, eyebrows, nose, lips, and chin (area H). With the exception of primary superficial BCCs less than or equal to 0.5 cm in healthy individuals, MMS is also appropriate for all BCCs of the cheeks, forehead, scalp, neck, jawline, and pretibial surface (area M). MMS is also appropriate for primary aggressive and recurrent aggressive squamous cell carcinoma (SCC) in all areas. In areas H and M for any size tumor and for all lesions greater than 2 cm, MMS is suitable for primary SCC without aggressive histologic features.

Utility of MMS in the treatment of Lentigo Maligna is somewhat of a controversy and is best performed in dedicated facilities or by "Slow MMS"—in which the histologic specimen is processed properly in paraffin and stained with relevant stainings if necessary.

Y. C. Metzger
The Tel Aviv Sourasky Medical Center,
Tel Aviv, Israel

© Springer International Publishing AG, part of Springer Nature 2018
E. Tur, H. I. Maibach (eds.), *Gender and Dermatology*,
https://doi.org/10.1007/978-3-319-72156-9_22

With time, more nontraditional indications for MMS are being studied. Recently it has been suggested that MMS is beneficial for treating Lentigo maligna of the trunk [5].

The American Academy of Dermatology (AAD), in collaboration with the American College of Mohs Surgery (ACMS), the American Society for Mohs Surgery (ASMS) and the American Society for Dermatologic Surgery Association (ASDS) has developed appropriate use criteria (AUC) for MMS. This is available on line (https://www.aad.org/practicecenter/quality/appropriate-use-criteria/mohs-surgery-auc) and also as an application for any smartphone (https://www.aad.org/members/aad-apps/mohs-auc).

22.3 Gender Considerations in MMS

Gender differences in MMS stem from three main origins:

- *The patient's tumor*—the tumor location, size and subtype are influenced by biological along with gender-specific lifestyle, psychosocial and behavior differences.
- *The patient's preference*—which differs due to gender-specific considerations and aesthetic concerns.
- *The physician*—the referring dermatologist and the Mohs surgeon may treat the same tumor differently in different patients due to the patients' gender.

22.4 Tumor Prevalence and Subtype

Lee et al. [6], found that BCCs were the most common tumor undergoing MMS in both genders. In women, BCCs made up 72% of all tumors. In men, BCC made up 63% of all tumors. Women had more superficial BCCs and fewer basosquamous (metatypical) BCCs [7].

Squamous cell carcinoma (SCC) and SCC in situ (SCCIS) were the second and third most prevalent NMSC undergoing MMS. According to Lee et al. Women have fewer SCCs (16% of women vs 24% of men, $p < 0.01$) and SCCIS (8% of women vs 11% of men, $p < 0.01$). This data is in concordance with previous epidemiological studies [7].

In terms of tumor aggressiveness, female gender was associated with a moderately differentiated or well-differentiated SCC, whereas male gender was associated with a poorly differentiated or acantholytic SCC ($P = 0.002$). As expected, the poorly differentiated or acantholytic subtypes were also associated with larger tumor and defect sizes ($P < 0.001$), as well as significant subclinical extension ($P = 0.005$) [8].

In another paper [9], analysis of histologic subtypes by gender found that women referred for MMS were more likely to have morpheaform BCCs and basosquamous BCCs than were men, although the proportion of both histologic subtypes was relatively low overall. Men had significantly higher numbers of BCCs and SCCs.

Gender-specific behaviors that may explain this data is a higher engagement of tanning practices in women compared with men, which is likely to be intermittent and intense [10, 11] thus resulting in more BCCs than SCCs.

Male gender significantly increased the likelihood of extensive subclinical spread. Recurrent BCC in men had an OR of 5.3 compared with women requiring three or more MMS layers ($P = 0.001$). Tumors on the neck in men were also more than three times as likely (OR, 3.6) as those in women to demonstrate wide microscopic extension ($P = 0.02$) (See [9]).

22.5 Anatomical Location of Tumors

The nose is the most common anatomical location for tumors requiring MMS in both genders (22% of all tumors). Men are more likely to have tumors on areas exposed to sun by short or receding hair, such as the ears, temple, and scalp. This could be explained by gender specific alopecia patterns that subsequently affect the sun exposure patterns.

Female patients, in comparison with males, have a higher number of MMS procedures performed on other locations such as the forehead, nose, perioral region, and legs.

Women were found to undergo MMS in areas often treated by other modalities, such as the extremities, a fact that may be explained by greater concern for scar size [9].

22.6   Outcome of Surgery

Pain and anxiety associated with MMS was grater in females [12].

Using MMS defect size as a measure, it was found that patient factors including gender were overall not significantly associated with MMS defect size in both head/face and trunk/extremity tumors [13].

There is no difference in the presenting size of SCCIS, SCC, or keratoacanthomas. Initial areas of BCC are smaller in women when compared with their male counterparts as discussed later in this chapter.

There is no significant difference in the number of Mohs steps performed for any of the tumor types [6].

Most of the repairs in both genders are intermediate or complex linear closures.

22.7   Physician Bias

At the time of tumor removal, women are slightly younger when compared with men. In addition, initial areas of BCC are smaller in women when compared with their male counterparts. This may indicate that MMS is more liberally utilized in women in relation to men thus resulting in earlier referral to surgery. Nevertheless, Most MMS are performed on men because most skin cancers arise in men [14, 15].

Overall, females are more than twice as likely to be referred for reconstruction by a plastics subspecialty (See [6]). As discussed earlier, this cannot be explained by differences in tumor properties (size or location), and is most probably explained by differences in aesthetic considerations.

22.8   Mohs Practitioners

The exact distribution of gender among Mohs surgeons is not published.

Although surgical fields were traditionally predominantly male professions [16], The European society of Mohs surgeons (ESMS) reports that approximately 50% of its members are female.

Conclusion

Sun exposure patterns and aesthetic concerns lead to variations in the tumor biology and anatomy of skin cancer and thus many gender related differences are found in the treatment and outcome of patients with skin cancer undergoing MMS. Ultimately, the pattern of UV light exposure and aesthetic considerations may only partially explain the observed differences and other factors yet to be elucidated may be involved.

References

1. Shriner DL, McCoy DK, Goldberg DJ, Wagner RF. Mohs micrographic surgery. J Am Acad Dermatol. 1998;39(1):79–97.
2. Amber KT, Bloom R, Abyaneh MA, Falto-Aizpurua LA, Viera M, Zaiac MN, Nouri K, Hu S. Patient factors and their association with nonmelanoma skin cancer morbidity and the performance of self-skin exams: a cross-sectional study. J Clin Aesthet Dermatol. 2016;9(9):16.
3. Bowen GM, White GL, Gerwels JW. Mohs micrographic surgery. Am Fam Physician. 2005;72(5):845–8.
4. Reeder VJ, Gustafson CJ, Mireku K, Davis SA, Feldman SR, Pearce DJ. Trends in Mohs surgery from 1995 to 2010: an analysis of nationally representative data. Dermatol Surg. 2015;41(3):397–403.
5. Nosrati A, Berliner JG, Goel S, McGuire J, Morhenn V, de Souza JR, Yeniay Y, Singh R, Lee K, Nakamura M, Wu RR. Outcomes of melanoma in situ treated with Mohs micrographic surgery compared with wide local excision. JAMA Dermatol. 2017;153(5):436–41.
6. Lee KC, William Higgins H, Linden O, Cruz AP. Gender differences in tumor and patient characteristics in those undergoing Mohs surgery. Dermatol Surg. 2014;40(6):686–90.
7. Bastiaens MT, Hoefnagel JJ, Vermeer BJ, Bavinck JN, Bruijn JA, Westendorp RG. Differences in age, site distribution, and sex between nodular and superficial basal cell carcinomas indicate different types of tumors. J Invest Dermatol. 1998;110(6):880–4.

8. Leibovitch I, Huilgol SC, Selva D, Hill D, Richards S, Paver R. Cutaneous squamous cell carcinoma treated with Mohs micrographic surgery in Australia I. Experience over 10 years. J Am Acad Dermatol. 2005;53(2):253–60.

9. Batra RS, Kelley LC. Predictors of extensive subclinical spread in nonmelanoma skin cancer treated with Mohs micrographic surgery. Arch Dermatol. 2002;138(8):1043–5.

10. Wu S, Han J, Vleugels RA, Puett R, Laden F, Hunter DJ, Qureshi AA. Cumulative ultraviolet radiation flux in adulthood and risk of incident skin cancers in women. Br J Cancer. 2014;110(7):1855–61.

11. Kricker A, et al. Does intermittent sun exposure cause basal cell carcinoma? A case-control study in Western Australia. Int J Cancer. 1995;60(4):489–94.

12. Chen AF, Landy DC, Kumetz E, Smith G, Weiss E, Saleeby ER. Prediction of postoperative pain after Mohs micrographic surgery with 2 validated pain anxiety scales. Dermatol Surg. 2015;41(1):40–7.

13. Amber KT, Bloom R, Abyaneh MA, Falto-Aizpurua LA, Viera M, Zaiac MN, Nouri K, Hu S. Patient factors and their association with nonmelanoma skin cancer morbidity and the performance of self-skin exams: a cross-sectional study. J Clin Aesthet Dermatol. 2016;9(9):16.

14. Buster KJ, You Z, Fouad M, Elmets C. Skin cancer risk perceptions: a comparison across ethnicity, age, education, gender, and income. J Am Acad Dermatol. 2012;66(5):771–9.

15. Mora RG, Robins P. Basal-cell carcinomas in the center of the face: special diagnostic, prognostic, and therapeutic considerations. J Dermatol Surg Oncol. 1978;4(4):315–21.

16. Freischlag JA. Women surgeons—still in a male-dominated world. Yale J Biol Med. 2008;81(4):203–4.

Gender Differences in Facial Rejuvenation

Benjamin C. Garden and Jerome M. Garden

23.1 Introduction

The number of cosmetic procedures performed in recent years has greatly increased, as dermatologists and other physicians meet the demand of increasingly interested patients. Dermatologists performed over seven million cosmetic procedures in 2015, a 27% increase since 2012. Additionally, six in ten adults are considering a cosmetic procedure [1]. While the focus in this field has typically been centered on female patients, cosmetic procedures for men continues to grow as well, increasing 325% since 1997—totaling more than 1.2 million procedures in 2015 [2]. Men represent approximately 10% of those patients seeking cosmetic facial procedures. Successful cosmetic treatments of patients requires recognizing the gender differences in cosmetic desires, behavioral differences and facial anatomy.

B. C. Garden (✉)
Department of Dermatology, University of Illinois at Chicago, Chicago, IL, USA

J. M. Garden
Departments of Dermatology and Biomedical Engineering, Northwestern University, Chicago, IL, USA
e-mail: j-garden@northwestern.edu

23.2 Differences in Aging

Aging is due to both intrinsic and extrinsic factors resulting in the progressive changes to the skin and underlying tissue. Intrinsic factors, such as hormonal and genetic effects, and extrinsic factors, such as smoking and sun exposure, contributes to the clinical features of aging including rhytides, dyschromia, volume loss, and bony resorption. As these factors differ between genders, the process of aging varies amongst men and women.

As humans age, there is a reduction in sex hormone production, with differences in gender. Women after menopause experience a rapid decrease in serum levels of estrogen [3]. Most aging men, however, experience a more gradual decrease in testosterone, averaging a 1% decrease per year starting around age 30 [4]. Due to this subtle decrease, certain aging changes seen in male skin are more gradual than women. Mirroring the gradual decrease in testosterone, male skin thickness decrease linearly with age, whereas women experience a rapid decrease after menopause [5].

It is important to not discount behavioral differences between men and women that contribute to aging. Extrinsic aging factors include ultraviolet (UV) exposure, smoking, repetitive muscle movements and diet [6]. Smoking decreases capillary blood flow to this skin, depriving it of oxygen and nutrients. Additionally, smoking results in decreased collagen and elastin in the dermis, with a dose-response relationship between wrinkles and smoking [6]. Smoking is an independent risk factor for premature facial wrinkling after controlling for UV exposure [7]. Men smoke at a rate three times higher than women, increasing their risk for cutaneous aging and is strongly associated with their development of facial elastosis and telangiectasias [8].

UV light radiation contributes to skin aging through the degradation of dermal collagen and is estimated to account for 90% of visible skin aging. Men are more likely to have jobs requiring them to work outside, are less likely to use sunscreen and are more likely to develop sunburns [9–11]. Men's skin is also more prone to UV damage due to a reduced antioxidant capacity and increased UV-induced immunosuppression [12, 13].

These changes due to aging can cause patients to seek out facial rejuvenation. Additionally, as these treatments have gained greater social acceptance, men may feel a greater sense of permission to pursue these procedures. Men's desires for facial rejuvenation may be due to the belief that a more youthful appearance can allow them to gain a competitive edge in the workplace, although women in the workplace may have the same work pressures. Patient presentation for cosmetic treatments may vary between men and women. Men may suppress any emotional component in seeking care and just direct their questions exclusively to address a specific perceived flaw [14]. Both men and women may wish to enhance body image and self-esteem [15]. Understanding these factors may allow for enhanced patient experience and improved results.

23.3 Differences in Facial Anatomy

Sexual dimorphism refers to phenotypic differences between sexes of the same species. While differences in hair pattern, muscle mass and genitalia are more obvious, differences in facial anatomy is often less apparent (Table 23.1, Fig. 23.1). Men have a more angled jaw and equally balanced upper and lower facial proportions, which

Table 23.1 Gender differences in facial anatomy

	Female	Male
Forehead	Smaller, convex	Larger, flatter
Eyebrows	Arched, higher on orbital rim	Flatter, lower on orbital rim
Glabella	Narrow	Wider
Eyes	Smaller orbit, but larger in relation to skull	Larger orbit, but smaller in relation to skull
Cheek	Fuller, well-defined apex	Flatter, subtle apex
Nose	Narrow dorsum Supratip break Less nostril shown	Wide dorsum Absent supratip break More nostril shown
Lips	Lower lip larger than upper	Upper lip larger than lower
Jaw	Less prominent and narrow	Prominent and wide
Muscle movement	Less movement	Greater movement
Subcutaneous fat	More	Less
Blood vessels	Less	More

lead to a square face. Women have a smaller skull, approximately four fifths the size of the male skull, and with a gradual taper in the facial silhouette [16].

23.3.1 Forehead and Glabella

The male forehead is larger in size than in women. The male forehead has prominent supraorbital bossing inferiorly and a relatively flatter upper forehead. This contrasts with the nearly absent bossing and more continuous mild convexity found in females [17]. Men's eyebrows are flatter and tend to sit lower along the orbital rim [18]. The medial supraorbital ridge in men blends into the glabella, resulting in a larger glabellar prominence in men than women. In fact, glabellar projection were historically used for skeletal sex determination [19]. In women, the eyebrows have an arch that peaks in the lateral third and a medial downward slope which lies at or just below the orbital rim. As women age, their eyebrows begin to appear more masculine, as they become straighter and fall closer to the eye.

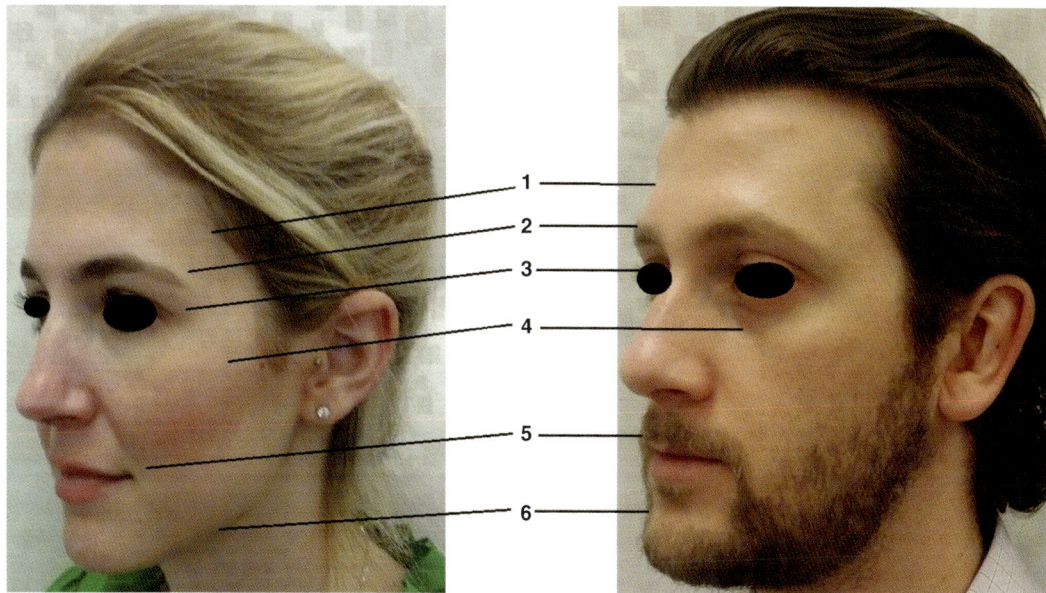

1) **Forehead:** Women have a smaller, more convex foreheads
2) **Eyebrows:** Women have more arched eyebrows that sit higher on the orbital rim
3) **Eyes:** Women have a smaller orbit yet is larger in relation to the skull
4) **Cheek:** Women have a fuller cheek with a more defined apex
5) **Lips:** Women's lower lip is larger than the upper, while in men the upper lip tends to be larger
6) **Jawline:** Women have a less prominent and narrower mandible and jaw

Fig. 23.1 Facial anatomical differences between genders

23.3.2 Eyes

The male orbit is larger and rounder in men, although it is proportionally smaller in relation to the size of the skull [20]. The male upper eyelid crease is positioned 8 mm above the lid margin, while in women it is measured on average at 12 mm. The male upper lid tends to be fuller and more redundant, and the lower eyelid tends to more severely shift downward with aging [21].

23.3.3 Cheek

The male cheek tends to be less prominent and flatter than the female cheek [22]. This is likely due to the frontal and zygomatic processes being wider in males [23]. The apex of the male cheek is more medial and subtle; while in females, the malar prominence has an apex located high on the mid-face, lateral to the lateral canthus.

23.3.4 Nose

The ideal male dorsal nose is wide and straight, compared to females in which it is narrow and laterally concave. The male nasal dorsum should approach a straight line from the radix to the nasal tip, while women tend to have more sloping line, often with a subtle 2 mm concavity [24]. The female nose has a supratip break, which is an inflection point before the tip starts to elevate, which is typically absent in men. There is also a slight upward rotation of the female nasal tip which results in more nostril shown than in men [24].

23.3.5 Lips

The upper lip is larger than the lower lip in women and older men, while young men have a larger lower lip. The ideal male upper lip projects 2 mm beyond the lower lip [24]. The upper lip is approximately 25% thicker in males compared to females, while the lower lip is 15% thicker [25].

With aging, the lips become smaller and thinner in both sexes [26].

23.3.6 Mandible

The male mandible, featuring a prominent jaw and chin, is one of the characteristic features of a masculine face [27]. The male chins tend to protrude with well-developed lateral tubercles that provide a square appearance [28]. Men also tend to have larger masseter muscles and a more prominent angulation of the mandibular rami, all of which provides more definition to a wide lower jaw [29].

23.3.7 Other Differences

There are differences noted regarding muscle movement, as well. Facial muscles are important in aging due to the lines formed in the skin during muscle contraction, leading eventually to rhytids at rest. Men produce larger facial expressions and have a great upward movement of facial muscles when smiling [30]. Additionally, men have less facial subcutaneous fat than women, while having higher rates of abdominal adipose [31]. Females exhibit 3 mm increased subcutaneous tissue in the medial malar cheek compared to males [32]. These differences in facial muscle movement and subcutaneous fat have clinical implications when comparing the severity and distribution of facial wrinkles. Men have more severe rhytides in all facial areas, compared to women, except the upper eyelid and nasolabial groove [33]. These differences contribute to men appearing, on average, 0.37 years older and women appearing 0.54 years younger than their true ages [34].

Other facial anatomical considerations between genders is that the male face contains a greater density of blood vessels than the female face. A perfusion study demonstrated greater facial blood flow in men compared to women [35]. This might be due to the presence on males faces of coarse hair which requires a dense vascular plexus and more capillaries in the dermal papillae to support. This might explain why men are more prone to

bruising after injections and post-operative bleeding following facial surgery [36].

23.4 Facial Rejuvenation with Neurotoxins

The cosmetic use of botulinum neurotoxin type A for facial rejuvenation has become popular as it is minimally-invasive, fast-acting and exhibits a great safety profile. The differences in male and female facial anatomy requires developing different injection techniques for male and female patients. As wrinkles tend to more severe in men compared to women, this requires adjusting the dosing of neurotoxin used. Studies have shown that men require higher doses than women to obtain equal efficacy [37, 38].

23.4.1 Neurotoxin for Glabellar and Forehead Wrinkles

The eyebrow depressor muscles are made up of the corrugator supercilli, procerus and the depressor supercilli. These muscles work together to move the brow downward and medially. This results in squinting and frowning and contributes to the dynamic wrinkles of the glabella. Injecting in this area requires staying at least one cm above the upper orbital rim and positioned medially to the mid-pupillary lines to avoid diffusion of toxin into the orbit which can result in eyelid ptosis [39].

The procerus muscle originates close to the nasal bone and extends vertically to the frontalis muscle above the brow. Treatment of the procerus requires a single injection placed carefully to avoid the medial portion of the frontalis; an injection too close will potentially cause elevation of the lateral brow when the frontalis contracts [39]. The corrugator muscles originate near the medial brow on either side of the procerus and extend laterally along the orbital ridge. The male corrugator muscles may extend more laterally than in women (Fig. 23.2). Failure to inject laterally enough in men, may allow contractibility at the distal portion of the muscle, producing an unnatural effect [39].

The frontals is the only muscle that elevates the eyebrows. It has no bony insertions and instead blends with the fibers of the procerus and corrugators. While the treatment of horizontal forehead lines due to the action of the frontalis muscle is off-label, it is commonly used for both males and females. Given the greater width, height and muscle mass of the male forehead, injection of neurotoxin requires a greater number of injection points and units. While in women, the injection pattern typically resembles a "V" shape, in men the pattern should be flatter and wider to accommodate for the wider forehead and flatter eyebrows (Fig. 23.3a, b). Treatment of the lateral portion of the frontalis is also recommended to prevent contraction of the lateral frontalis, which can cause arching of the outer eyebrow, producing a quizzical appearance. Additionally, if treating the glabella, then treatment of the lateral

frontalis is crucial in maintaining the flat male eyebrows. If the glabella is treated without treating the frontalis, the unopposed activity of the lateral frontalis can lift the outer brow, which in females can produce a desirable arch, while in men will produce a feminizing appearance [40].

An important consideration in males is the presence of a receding hairline. In these patients, the injection sites will need to extend higher and further into the scalp area to prevent an unnatural wrinkling in the alopecic scalp [40]. And although men require greater units to paralyze these muscles, the goals of the patient must be considered. A moderate amount of wrinkles on a male's forehead may produce a more distinguished look and therefore a natural look, with some movement, is generally being advocated for most patients.

23.4.2 Neurotoxin for Periocular Wrinkles

The periocular wrinkles, or "crow's feet", are caused by the contracture of the orbicularis oculi muscle. This broad circular muscle is divided into three portions—the lacrimal and palpebral portions involuntarily control eyelid blinking, while the orbital portion, which encircles the orbit, is under voluntary control. The contraction of the outer orbicularis muscle results in periocular rhytids with age. While many women desire these

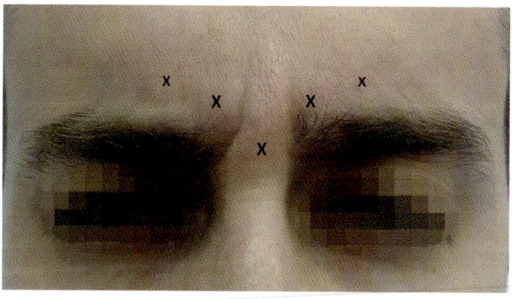

Fig. 23.2 Injection placement of neurotoxin in a male patient's glabella

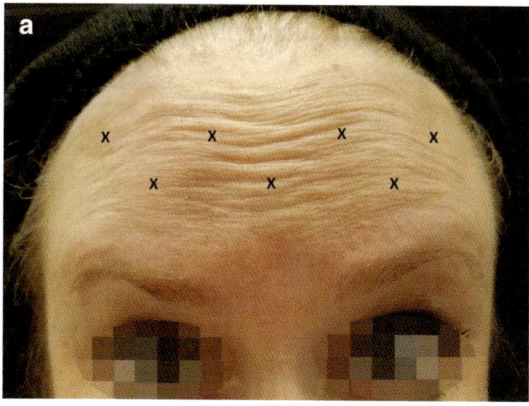

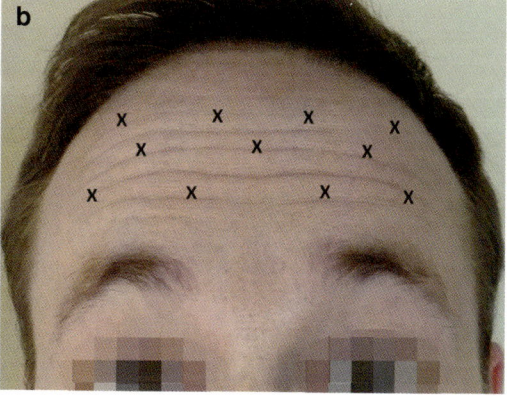

Fig. 23.3 Neurotoxin injection in female forehead (**a**) vs male forehead (**b**): In the female patient, note the "V" shape injection pattern to allow for arched eyebrows.

In men, the pattern is flatter due to eyebrow shape. Also note the injections higher on the forehead in this male patient with a receding hairline

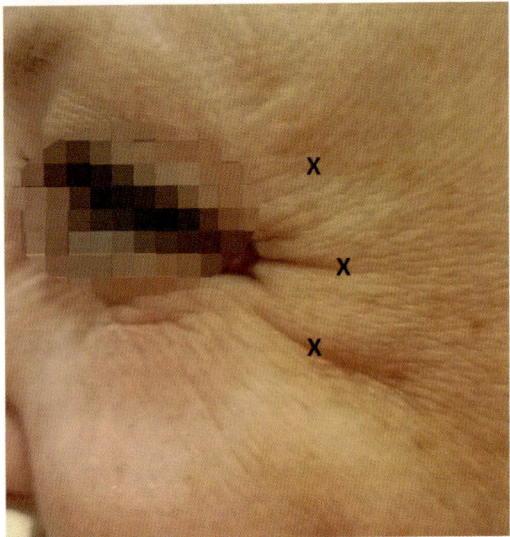

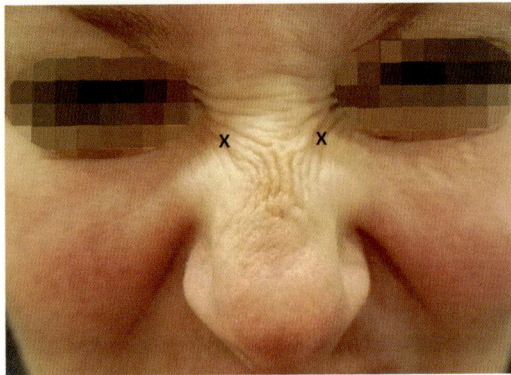

Fig. 23.5 Injection placement of neurotoxin in the nasalis muscles to treat a female patient's "bunny lines"

Fig. 23.4 Injection placement of neurotoxin in a female patient's "crow's feet"

lines to be completely gone, the presence of these wrinkles in men can indicate maturity. Thus, some men may desire just a softening of these rhytids.

In men, the outer orbicularis oculi muscle may be broader and more expansive than in women. Additionally, a greater activation of the zygomatic muscles in men, which elevate the cheek, results in a more lateral and inferior fanning of the periocular lines, compared to women having a more central or full pattern [41]. More injection points may be needed in men to accommodate the lateral reach of the orbicularis. Additionally, men's crow's feet may require a lower injection site and often near the insertion of the zygomatic muscles (Fig. 23.4). It is important to be aware of this and to avoid injecting into the zygomatic as this will result in a cheek droop or asymmetric smile. One method entails using more superficial injections for the inferior orbicularis, to avoid the zygomatic muscles with a deeper injection [42].

23.4.3 Neurotoxin for Nasal Rejuvenation

Depression of the nasal tip can cause an elongated look of the nose and unwanted ptosis. This depression tends to become accentuated with smiling. The depressor septi nasi muscle arises from the orbicularis oris muscle and inserts onto the nasal septum. When this muscle is hypertrophied or overactive, it can lead to nasal tip ptosis and upper lip shortening [43]. In one study, the most aesthetic nasolabial angle was 104.9° in females and 97° in men [44]. By injecting neurotoxin into the depressor septi nasi, one can elevate the nasal tip to an improved angle. Caution must be used to avoid paralysis of the orbicularis oris. Additionally, neurotoxin can be used in the nasal ala to reduce flair and in the nasalis muscle to treat "bunny lines" (Fig. 23.5).

23.4.4 Neurotoxin for Jaw and Chin

Men typically desire a wide mandible with a prominent flexure, contrasted with the narrow and rounded lower face of women. The masseter muscle at the outer corners of the jaw greatly contributes to the masculine appearance of a man's lower face. Off-label injection of neurotoxin into the masseter muscle is becoming increasingly popular in women to contour the lower face. In men, treatment of the masseter can potentially feminize the jaw. However, men can seek treatment for an asymmetric or aesthetically detracting prominence of the masseter. The use of neurotoxin in these men can lead to a smoother mandibular angle.

The placement of injections in the masseter depends on the number of bulges present when the jaw is clenched [45]. Have the patient clench their jaw and palpate the masseter to determine the number of bulges. Injection should be placed into the belly of the most prominent bulge, with one to three further injections depending on the degree of hypertrophy. The doses established for reduction of masseter mass have been determined primarily in female patients, but the dose needed depends on muscle thickness, regardless of gender. It may take 3–6 months to note significant recontouring. And while the complication rate is approximately 9%, such as an asymmetric smile, it appears to be higher with larger doses [45]. Therefore, a safe method would be starting with lower doses and re-evaluating at a 3-month follow-up.

Similar to the mandible, the chin in men is wider and projects more anteriorly than in women. With age, the loss of tissue and bone in the chin and cheek can decrease the projection of the chin and displace the mid face downward over the melomental folds, causing the oral commissures to turn downward. Injection of neurotoxin into the depressor angularis oris decreases the pull on the corner of the mouth, thereby elevating the oral commissures. Additionally, neurotoxin can be used in the mentalis to soften the chin clefts, which can give men an aggressive appearance [46].

23.5   Soft Tissue Augmentation

Volume loss in the aging patient, in either gender, can be quite apparent and is a frequent cause of patients seeking out cosmetic consultation. Men tend to have a greater loss of volume as they age. One study using magnetic resonance imaging to assess soft tissue amounts in the aging male quantified a 40% reduction in soft tissue thickness in the infraorbital area, compared to a 27% reduction in females [32, 47]. In males, the temples had a 23% reduction in soft tissue, the medial cheeks a 22% reduction and the lateral cheeks with a 15% reduction [47].

Dermal filler can be very useful in male patients who struggle with volume loss given their relative lack of subcutaneous fat. However, volume replacement carries the risk of feminization. It is important to assure the male patient that small amounts of filler can be used to volumize without overcorrecting or producing a feminine appearance. Further, filers can be used to augment masculine facial features or eliminate deep creases. Many of these methods are off-label uses and must be performed with a strong knowledge of the facial anatomy involved [48].

23.5.1 Filler for the Infraorbital Hollow

- The infraorbital hollow is composed of the tear trough, nasojugal fold and palpebromalar groove. The tear trough is defined as the depression of the medial lower eyelid, lateral to the anterior lacrimal crest and superior to the inferior orbital rim [49]. The loss of bone and soft tissue that occurs with aging contributes to the depression seen below the eyes. Before treatment, it is important to determine if there is excessive fat pad herniation or festooning above the orbitomalar ligament as this may appear worse after filler injection and is best corrected surgically. As previously noted, this area is the site of greatest soft tissue thickness loss seen in men [47]. One should use a more fluid hyaluronic acid (HA) fillers with a lower G' in this location and avoid poly-L-lactic acid (PLLA) or calcium hydroxyapatite (CaHa) as there is an increased risk of forming superficial papules [50].

23.5.2 Fillers for the Temples

The temples are a location of subcutaneous tissue loss in both the aging male and female [32, 47]. This loss causes a concavity to form at the temples. HA fillers with a higher G' can be placed in depots in a retrograde manner and massaged into place. PLLA and CaHa fillers has also been used in this area [51]. In the area of the temples, the superficial temporal artery and the temporal nerve can be found and injections must be performed above these structures, as there have been rare cases of blindness from presumed arterial injections [50].

23.5.3 Fillers for the Glabella

For glabellar lines that do not correct with neurotoxin, dermal fillers have been used to produce the desired effect. One must be aware of the vasculature in this area, including anastomosis of the internal and external carotid arteries, and the increased risks of tissue necrosis and blindness [48, 52]. It is essential to aspirate before injection in this area to decrease the risk of inadvertent injection into a vessel. Additionally, dermal fillers in the glabellar region can develop into papules and nodules. Correction of a glabellar line should be done with some amounts of a low viscosity HA filler using a microdroplet technique in the mid to upper dermis [50].

23.5.4 Fillers for the Cheeks

The cheek is a common area in which patients of both genders desire volume replacement. One must remember the anatomical differences in this area to properly fill these patients. While the female cheek is fuller medially, males have a more even distribution between the lateral and medial cheek. The male's cheek apex is more subtle and medial than the female [22]. Overcorrection of the male cheek may give a feminizing appearance. Fillers in men should be injected laterally along the zygomatic arch, avoiding too much volume in the anterior and medial cheeks [22]. Fillers injected in this area should have a higher G' to produce more lift. Having the patient animate after injection will allow identification of any bumps and gentle molding can be used immediately after injection to smooth any unevenness [50].

23.5.5 Filler for the Jawline and Lips

The jawline and lips are an important area to address while evaluating the male cosmetic patient. A strong chin with anterior projection contributes to the balance of the lower face and creates a masculine appearance. When assessing this area, one should use the Reidel plane, which uses a straight edge to determine chin projection in relation to the upper and lower lip [53]. Using this assessment, one can determine the need for filler for the chin or lips. In men, while the upper lip should be slightly more anterior than the lower, the volume of the upper lip should be about one-half the lower lip [54].

23.5.6 Fat Reduction

Another area that has become a target for facial rejuvenation is submental fat. This subcutaneous fat is found superior to the platysma and is caused by aging, diet and genetics. Deoxycholic acid is an injectable product that works by disrupting adipocyte cell membranes which leads to mild inflammation and phagocytosis [55]. Injection with this product has been shown to lead to improvement in the appearance of moderate to severe convexity or fullness associated with submental fat. The studies included both male and female patients with similar results [56]. Other non-injectable methods to target this fat include cryolipolysis, ultrasound, infrared and radiofrequency [57].

Conclusion

Facial rejuvenation continues to be a growing and expanding discipline in dermatology. While the products are the same, treating male and female patients can entail using different methods, dosing and aesthetic consideration. While approaching any patient for a cosmetic appointment, it is important to listen to their desires and reasons for seeking treatment. Understanding gender differences in aging and anatomy is essential to producing results that leave the patient satisfied.

References

1. American Society of Dermatologic Surgery. ASDS consumer survey on cosmetic dermatologic procedures. 2016. https://asds.net/consumer-survey/. Accessed 30 March 2017.
2. American Society of Aesthetic Plastic Surgery: statistics. 2016. http://www.surgery.org/media/statistics. Accessed 30 March 2017.

3. Friedman O. Changes associated with the aging face. Facial Plast Surg Clin North Am. 2005;13(3):371–80.
4. Bain J. Epidemiology, evaluation and diagnosis of andropause. Genetic Aging. 2003;6(Suppl 10):4–8.
5. Panyakhamlerd K, Chotnopparatpattara P, Taechakraichana N, Kukulprasong A, Chaikittisilpa S, Limpaphayom K. Skin thickness in different menopausal status. J Med Assoc Thail. 1999;82(4):352–6.
6. Kennedy C, Bastiaens MT, Bajdik CD, Willemze R, Westendorp RG, Bouwes Bavinck JN, Leiden Skin Cancer Study. Effect of smoking and sun on the aging skin. J Invest Dermatol. 2003;120(4):548–54.
7. Kadunce DP, Burr R, Gress R, Kanner R, Lyon JL, Zone JJ. Cigarette smoking: risk factor for premature facial wrinkling. Ann Intern Med. 1991;114(10):840–4.
8. Leow YH, Maibach HI. Cigarette smoking, cutaneous vasculature, and tissue oxygen. Clin Dermatol. 1998;16(5):579–84.
9. Buller DB, Cokkinides V, Hall HI, Hartman AM, Saraiya M, Miller E, Paddock L, Glanz K. Prevalence of sunburn, sun protection, and indoor tanning behaviors among Americans: review from national surveys and case studies of 3 states. J Am Acad Dermatol. 2011;65(5 Suppl 1):S114–23.
10. Falk M, Anderson CD. Influence of age, gender, educational level and self-estimation of skin type on sun exposure habits and readiness to increase sun protection. Cancer Epidemiol. 2013;37(2):127–32.
11. Thieden E, Philipsen PA, Sandby-Møller J, Wulf HC. Sunscreen use related to UV exposure, age, sex, and occupation based on personal dosimeter readings and sun-exposure behavior diaries. Arch Dermatol. 2005;141(8):967–73.
12. Damian DL, Patterson CR, Stapelberg M, Park J, Barnetson RS, Halliday GM. UV radiation-induced immunosuppression is greater in men and prevented by topical nicotinamide. J Invest Dermatol. 2008;128(2):447–54.
13. Ide T, Tsutsui H, Ohashi N, Hayashidani S, Suematsu N, Tsuchihashi M, Tamai H, Takeshita A. Greater oxidative stress in healthy young men compared with premenopausal women. Arterioscler Thromb Vasc Biol. 2002;22(3):438–42.
14. Ross A. Reflections on aesthetic facial surgery in men. Facial Plast Surg Clin North Am. 2009;17:613–24.
15. Rieder EA, Mu EW, Brauer JA. Men and cosmetics: social and psychological trends of an emerging demographic. J Drugs Dermatol. 2015;14(9):1023–6.
16. Garvin HM, Ruff CB. Sexual dimorphism in skeletal browridge and chin morphologies determined using a new quantitative method. Am J Phys Anthropol. 2012;147(4):661–70.
17. Whitaker LA, Morales L Jr, Farkas LG. Aesthetic surgery of the supraorbital ridge and forehead structures. Plast Reconstr Surg. 1986;78(1):23–32.
18. Gunter JP, Antrobus SD. Aesthetic analysis of the eyebrows. Plast Reconstr Surg. 1997;99(7):1808–16.
19. Keaney TC, Alster TS. Botulinum toxin in men: review of relevant anatomy and clinical trial data. Dermatol Surg. 2013;39(10):1434–43.
20. Pretorius E, Steyn M, Scholtz Y. Investigation into the usability of geometric morphometric analysis in assessment of sexual dimorphism. Am J Phys Anthropol. 2006;129(1):64–70.
21. Most SP, Mobley SR, Larrabee WF Jr. Anatomy of the eyelids. Facial Plast Surg Clin North Am. 2005;13(4):487–92.
22. Keaney T. Male aesthetics. Skin Therapy Lett. 2015;20(2):5–7.
23. Koudelová J, Brůžek J, Cagáňová V, Krajíček V, Velemínská J. Development of facial sexual dimorphism in children aged between 12 and 15 years: a three-dimensional longitudinal study. Orthod Craniofac Res. 2015;18(3):175–84.
24. Rohrich RJ, Janis JE, Kenkel JM. Male rhinoplasty. Plast Reconstr Surg. 2003;112(4):1071–85.
25. Gibelli D, Codari M, Rosati R, Dolci C, Tartaglia GM, Cattaneo C, Sforza C. A quantitative analysis of lip aesthetics: the influence of gender and aging. Aesthet Plast Surg. 2015;39(5):771–6.
26. De Menezes M, Rosati R, Baga I, Mapelli A, Sforza C. Three-dimensional analysis of labial morphology: effect of sex and age. Int J Oral Maxillofac Surg. 2011;40(8):856–61.
27. Brown E, Perrett DI. What gives a face its gender? Perception. 1993;22(7):829–40.
28. Thayer ZM, Dobson SD. Sexual dimorphism in chin shape: implications for adaptive hypotheses. Am J Phys Anthropol. 2010;143(3):417–25.
29. Loth SR, Henneberg M. Mandibular ramus flexure: a new morphologic indicator of sexual dimorphism in the human skeleton. Am J Phys Anthropol. 1996;99(3):473–85.
30. Houstis O, Kiliaridis S. Gender and age differences in facial expressions. Eur J Orthod. 2009;31(5):459–66.
31. Sjöström L, Smith U, Krotkiewski M, Björntorp P. Cellularity in different regions of adipose tissue in young men and women. Metabolism. 1972;21(12):1143–53.
32. Wysong A, Joseph T, Kim D, Tang JY, Gladstone HB. Quantifying soft tissue loss in facial aging: a study in women using magnetic resonance imaging. Dermatol Surg. 2013;39(12):1895–902.
33. Tsukahara K, Hotta M, Osanai O, Kawada H, Kitahara T, Takema Y. Gender-dependent differences in degree of facial wrinkles. Skin Res Technol. 2013;19(1):e65–71.
34. Bulpitt CJ, Markowe HL, Shipley MJ. Why do some people look older than they should? Postgrad Med J. 2001;77(911):578–81.
35. Mayrovitz HN, Regan MB. Gender differences in facial skin blood perfusion during basal and heated conditions determined by laser Doppler flowmetry. Microvasc Res. 1993;45(2):211–8.
36. Baker DC, Stefani WA, Chiu ES. Reducing the incidence of hematoma requiring surgical evacuation following male rhytidectomy: a 30-year review of 985 cases. Plast Reconstr Surg. 2005;116(7):1973–85.
37. Brandt F, Swanson N, Baumann L, Huber B. Randomized, placebo-controlled study of a

new botulinum toxin type a for treatment of glabellar lines: efficacy and safety. Dermatol Surg.
2009;35(12):1893–901.

38. Kane MA, Brandt F, Rohrich RJ, Narins RS, Monheit
GD, Huber MB, Reloxin Investigational Group.
Evaluation of variable-dose treatment with a new
U.S. Botulinum Toxin Type A (Dysport) for correction
of moderate to severe glabellar lines: results from a
phase III, randomized, double-blind, placebo-controlled
study. Plast Reconstr Surg. 2009;124(5):1619–29.

39. Ascher B, Talarico S, Cassuto D, Escobar S, Hexsel D,
Jaén P, Monheit GD, Rzany B, Viel M. International
consensus recommendations on the aesthetic usage
of botulinum toxin type A (Speywood Unit)--Part I:
Upper facial wrinkles. J Eur Acad Dermatol Venereol.
2010;24(11):1278–84.

40. Bloom JD, Green JB, Bowe W, von Grote E, Nogueira
A. Cosmetic use of abobotulinumtoxinA in men: considerations regarding anatomical differences and product
characteristics. J Drugs Dermatol. 2016;15(9):1056–62.

41. Kane MA, Cox SE, Jones D, Lei X, Gallagher
CJ. Heterogeneity of crow's feet line patterns in clinical trial subjects. Dermatol Surg. 2015;41(4):447–56.

42. Carruthers JD, Glogau RG, Blitzer A. Advances in
facial rejuvenation: botulinum toxin type a, hyaluronic acid dermal fillers, and combination therapies-
-consensus recommendations. Plast Reconstr Surg.
2008;121:5S–30S.

43. Rohrich RJ, Huynh B, Muzaffar AR, Adams WP Jr,
Robinson JB Jr. Importance of the depressor septi nasi
muscle in rhinoplasty: anatomic study and clinical
application. Plast Reconstr Surg. 2000;105(1):376–83.

44. Sinno HH, Markarian MK, Ibrahim AM, Lin SJ. The
ideal nasolabial angle in rhinoplasty: a preference
analysis of the general population. Plast Reconstr
Surg. 2014;134(2):201–10.

45. Xie Y, Zhou J, Li H, Cheng C, Herrler T, Li
Q. Classification of masseter hypertrophy for tailored
botulinum toxin type A treatment. Plast Reconstr
Surg. 2014;134(2):209e–18e.

46. Flynn TC. Botox in men. Dermatol Ther. 2007;20(6):
407–13.

47. Wysong A, Kim D, Joseph T, MacFarlane DF, Tang
JY, Gladstone HB. Quantifying soft tissue loss in the
aging male face using magnetic resonance imaging.
Dermatol Surg. 2014;40(7):786–93.

48. Sorensen EP, Urman C. Cosmetic complications: rare
and serious events following botulinum toxin and
soft tissue filler administration. J Drugs Dermatol.
2015;14(5):486–91.

49. Kane MA. Treatment of tear trough deformity and
lower lid bowing with injectable hyaluronic acid.
Aesthet Plast Surg. 2005;29(5):363–7.

50. Wieczorek IT, Hibler BP, Rossi AM. Injectable
cosmetic procedures for the male patient. J Drugs
Dermatol. 2015;14(9):1043–51.

51. Sykes JM. Applied anatomy of the temporal region
and forehead for injectable fillers. J Drugs Dermatol.
2009;8(10 Suppl):s24–7.

52. Khan TT, Colon-Acevedo B, Mettu P, DeLorenzi C,
Woodward JA. An anatomical analysis of the supra-
trochlear artery: considerations in facial filler injections and preventing vision loss. Aesthet Surg J.
2017;37(2):203–8.

53. Rosen HM. Aesthetic guidelines in genioplasty: the
role of facial disproportion. Plast Reconstr Surg.
1995;95(3):463–9.

54. Rossi AM. Men's aesthetic dermatology. Semin
Cutan Med Surg. 2014;33(4):188–97.

55. Dayan SH, Humphrey S, Jones DH, Lizzul PF, Gross
TM, Stauffer K, Beddingfield FC. Overview of
ATX-101 (deoxycholic acid injection): a nonsurgical
approach for reduction of submental fat. Dermatol
Surg. 2016;42(Suppl 1):S263–70.

56. Humphrey S, Sykes J, Kantor J, Bertucci V, Walker
P, Lee DR, Lizzul PF, Gross TM, Beddingfield
FC. ATX-101 for reduction of submental fat: a phase
III randomized controlled trial. J Am Acad Dermatol.
2016;75(4):788–97.

57. Dong J, Amir Y, Goldenberg G. Advances in minimally invasive and noninvasive treatments for submental fat. Cutis. 2017;99(1):20–3.

The Skin as a Metaphor: Psychoanalytic and Cultural Investigations

Shlomit Yadlin-Gadot and Uri Hadar

The skin is clearly, first and foremost, a material, biological entity. It is the enveloping surface of the body, the substance that both delineates and mediates what is internal to the body and what is external to it. The skin is the observed and perceived of the body, the encasement that implies the existence of one subject to another and, in many ways, the testimony the subject has of his own coherent, embodied existence. The psychic counterpart of this delineating function is the subject's experience of having an "inside" and an "outside" in relation to his psychic self. Thus, skin and self are inextricably intertwined.

Affected from within and without, skin is a metaphorical surface inscribed with social and cultural meanings, imbued and marked by psychic significance. Intimately known and experienced, the skin holds inscriptions of personal history, scars and pigmentations that record contingent happenings. Alongside the unique, the skin accommodates cultural constructions of sex, gender, age, race, religion, nationality and class. It exists as a political site constituted by cultural pressures, psychic tensions and the struggles of an outside grappling with a within.

This chapter will outline some of the significations that the skin has incarnated as the juncture of the somatic, the psychic and the cultural. Psychoanalytic and cultural theories have extensively explored the various meanings and functions of the skin, the former focusing on the individual development of the subject, the latter illuminating its socio-political nature. After presenting psychoanalytic theories that explore the skin through the prism of drive, emotion and relationality, we will present some cultural perspectives on the skin that emphasize political constructions of its various functions and characteristics. The Lacanian construal of the embodied subject will be suggested as providing a metaphorical space in which the intersection and struggle between the psychic and the political may be captured and discussed.

24.1 The Psychoanalytic Perspective

Freud's starting point in psychoanalysis was rooted in physiology, in the hypothesized workings of neural mechanisms. Construing the psychic as emerging from the body and its drives, Freud saw the skin as a crucial constituent of the early ego. He remarks: "The ego is first and foremost a bodily ego; it is not merely a surface

S. Yadlin-Gadot
Bar Ilan University, Ramat Gan, Israel

Tel Aviv University, Tel Aviv, Israel

U. Hadar (✉)
Tel Aviv University, Tel Aviv, Israel

The Ruppin Academic Center, Emek Hefer, Israel
e-mail: urih1@tauex.tau.ac.il

© Springer International Publishing AG, part of Springer Nature 2018
E. Tur, H. I. Maibach (eds.), *Gender and Dermatology*,
https://doi.org/10.1007/978-3-319-72156-9_24

entity, but is itself the projection of a surface" [1]. Clarifying this statement, an editorial footnote reads: "The ego is ultimately derived from bodily sensations, chiefly from those springing from the surface of the body. It may thus be regarded as a mental projection of the surface of the body" [1]. The human being does not come into the world with a ready-made ego. Instead, the ego must be brought into being through a variety of sensory experiences of the surface of the body.

Freud discussed both the sensorial and the protective functions of the skin but, unsurprisingly, he conceived of it primarily as an erotic organ: "... the skin, which in particular parts of the body has become differentiated into sense organs or modified into mucous membrane... , is thus the erotogenic zone par excellence" [2]. The emergence of the neonate into life is fueled by the instinct of survival, but no less—by pleasure. And pleasure's prime medium is the skin. In the very first stages of auto-eroticism, the infant's cause of bliss after a good feed is immediately transferred and attributed to his own skin, which he may continue to caress and to suck. The external world only gradually takes on a sense of 'being there' as an erotic object. Any part of the skin can become erotogenic, and the infant's own skin is the preferred site of his pleasure, always at his disposal.

The infant needs insulation to the same extent that he craves excitation, and his skin takes on the function of balancing and mediating. Here Freud merges ego and skin and places them on a par: both delineate, encase and create a space in which internal sensations are contained. After considering the workings of a 'contact barrier' in his model of the psyche [3], Freud introduces the idea of the ego's protective function against excitations from the external world. This "protective shield" [4] protects the mental apparatus from external stimuli that could overwhelm it. Freud describes the initial infantile situation as one of natural 'helplessness' (Hilflosigkeit) [5]. This helplessness demands protection and care that defend the fragile primal psyche-soma from traumatization. Thus, Freud addresses implicitly the role of the mother as a protective shield against stimuli, a function essential for maintain-

ing the internal balance in the child's psychic functioning, as well as in stimulating pleasure and desire.

Following Freud, Melanie Klein assumed that the early reality of the infant is wholly phantasmatic and internal. As she describes it, the infant's first objects are structured as part of his innate drives and create in his psychic world partial bodily images [6]. These phylogenetically determined preconceptions develop through such mechanisms as splitting, projection, introjections and identification. Moving from the paranoid-schizoid to the depressive position, the infant gradually differentiates internal and external worlds and integrates his experiences of love and hate.[1] The subject eventually coalesces and perceives both himself and his objects as whole. In her accounts, Klein did not consider the whole system of infant care and the surface of the body was absent from her theory. The skin function of 'holding' was re-introduced into mainstream psychoanalysis after Klein, by Winnicot [8], who assumed that the infant introjects patterns of containment provided by the mother.

Renewing Freud's engagement with the body's surfaces, this strain of thought integrated research findings from the field of developmental psychology into psychoanalytic theory. Most developmental psychologists came to regard the infant's first caregiver as the outer half of the infant, describing an integrated sensory progression from an experience of pleasurable symbiotic existence into emerging alterity. This process of separation-individuation is achieved gradually, as the mother defends the infant in the face of external stimulation. Spitz [9] spoke of the mother as

---

[1] Klein's positions refer to modes of mental functioning that last throughout life. Each of these positions has its own characteristic anxieties, defense mechanisms and configuration of object relations. Briefly, in the paranoid-schizoid position the infant's anxieties revolve around persecution and destruction; The caregiving object and self are split into 'good' and 'bad' parts, the former defending against the latter. In the depressive position, the infant's anxieties revolve around the guilt it feels over the rage and destructiveness it has directed towards its caregiving object; this object as gradually perceived as a whole person—both loved and hated—rather than as an assemblage of good or bad parts [7].

the 'auxiliary' ego, the symbiotic half of the mother–child unit, with the mother's body, the breast and milk experienced by the infant as his or her own body. Ethological research on attachment in young mammals and humans by Harlow [10] and Bowlby [11] has repeatedly shown that infants cling to their mother and maximize body contact with her, and fall into anaclitic depression when deprived of it. Harlow showed that a baby rhesus monkey preferred an artificial mother made of wire if it was cloth-covered and warm, even if it did not give milk. Bowlby's research on attachment and loss stressed the ways in which the infant needs and uses the early tactile relationship with the mother (or her substitute) to establish both security and gradual individuation.

Esther Bick [12, 13], focusing her work on this tactile dimension, considered the membrane that delineates inner from outer as a 'psychic skin'. Perusing what is logically demanded by the infant's initial helplessness, Bick showed the importance of the containing function of the mother for the earliest creation of the baby's sense of unity. The baby's 'psychic envelope' develops by the introjection of the mother's containing functions.

"The thesis is that in its most primitive form, the parts of the personality are felt to have no binding force amongst themselves and must therefore be held together in a way that is experienced by them passively, by the skin functioning as a boundary. But this internal function of containing the parts of the self is dependent initially on the introjection of an external object, experienced as capable of fulfilling this function. Later, identification with this function of the object supersedes the unintegrated state and gives rise to the fantasy of internal and external spaces … In its absence… all the confusions of identity attending it will be manifest" [12].

Following Freudian and Kleinian conceptualizations, Bick describes the first weeks of the newborn's life as fraught by primitive anxieties of death and disintegration. At this stage, the holding and soothing mother is experienced by the infant concretely as his own skin. A gradual introjection of her containing function allows the infant to experience himself as living comfortably within a skin envelope that contains and integrates his sense of self.

Various disturbances during this process of introjection may result in faulty development of the primal skin function. This can come about as a consequence of the actual object's inadequacy or from fantasy attacks on it. Flaws in the primal skin function may bring about the development of a 'perforated' mental skin—experienced as precarious and full of holes. This may lead to an image of self that is 'leaking', 'dripping' or 'dropping' in different forms, unprotected from external stimuli, be they tactile, auditory or emotive.

Against such faulty development in the primal skin function and the anxiety triggered by the experience of 'leaking' and 'dissolving' into space, defensive reactions begin. Here, the infant develops a 'second-skin', a defensive formation that–for the purpose of creating a substitute for the skin container function–replaces dependence on the object by a pseudo-independence, by the inappropriate use of mental functions or innate talents. Effectively, the ego defends itself against the fear of 'non-integration' by a 'pseudo independence' vis-à-vis the object, which generates catastrophic anxieties. This may manifest in hypertension and the creation of a chronic 'noise' envelope of babbling, head banging, repetitive motor rhythms etc. These create a secondary sensory experience of the boundary and bring stability by containment.

Wilfred Bion described the psychic envelope as a *container*. For Bion all primitive emotion is experienced in the form of unbearable bodily sensations, termed *beta elements*. These unbearable beta elements may be digested and transformed into bearable and thinkable elements (alpha), mediated by a 'mother-container' in an intersubjective event. This transformation is effected by means of the 'alpha function', a function carried out by the mother as the infant's container. The alpha function digests reality, transforms it into something that can be thought, and creates the links within this thought.

If the mother is able to contain the infant in this way, it will be able to create thoughts and eventually make use of alpha elements in order to think its own fears. The mental apparatus is predicated on this containment, and in optimal development will establish a double limit between the levels of the conscious and the unconscious, and between the internal and external worlds. Bion terms this limit a *membrane*, thus creating the ensuing analogy between sanity and the integrity of the skin [14]. The psychotic person is considered as having a *broken-skin*, resulting in a double confusion: one between the conscious and the unconscious experience and one between psychic and external worlds. By contrast, the neurotic is in possession of a "contact-barrier, owing its existence to the proliferation of alpha-elements by alpha-function and serving the function of a membrane which, by the nature of its composition and permeability, separates mental phenomena into … the functions of consciousness and … unconsciousness" [15]. For the psychotic "… no such dividing membrane exists" [15, 16].

The idea of faulty skin function has been employed also in the conceptualizations of autism. Tustin [17, 18] has posited sensations as the basis of both cognitive and emotional life. She describes the normal infant as developing a sensuous 'skin' that helps him to feel safe, and which is permeable for incoming and outgoing experiences. In contra-distinction and as a protection against trauma, the autistic child has developed an auto-sensuous insulation that blocks incoming and outgoing experiences in the form of a 'protective shell', an impenetrable, hardened skin [17, 18]. In her work with autistic children, Tustin [17, 18] described children "who [felt] skinless and disembodied. The skin has been replaced by the 'armor' of … autistic practices which help … to feel protected from the terrors of falling, of dissolving, of spilling …" [17, 18]. During therapy, "their body image begins to feel more substantial and intact [and] they begin to feel that they have an inner structure" (p. 235). In the same vein, Haag describes the therapies of autistic children and provides detailed descriptions of their experiences during the constitution or the restoration of the feeling of themselves within their skin [19].

Building upon the work of Klein, Tustin, Bick, Bion and others, Thomas Ogden explored the primary formations and organization of subjectivity in the psychic position he terms 'autistic-contiguous'. Adding this stage to Klein's paranoid-schizoid and depressive positions, Ogden suggested that the early existence of this subjective mode promotes the sustenance into maturity, alongside more developed modes. In the autistic-contiguous position, it is the experience of the body's surface that structures the form and content of the infant's inner world, which is his first incipient sense of self and meaning.

"In an autistic contiguous mode, it is experiences of sensation, particularly at the skin surface, that are the principal media for the creation of psychological meaning and the rudiments of the experience of self. Sensory-contiguity of skin surface and rhythmicity are basic to the most fundamental set of infantile object relations: the experience of the infant being held, nursed and spoken to by the mother … [Gradually], a rudimentary sense of 'I-ness' arises from relationships of sensory contiguity (i.e. touching) that over time generates the sense of a bounded sensory surface on which one's experience occurs" [20].

Ogden formulated an additional sense of 'groundedness', a sensory 'foundation' from which the infant can generate rudimentary forms of experience. Using Tustin's concepts of autistic objects, Ogden describes the creation of a sense of subjective 'boundedness' and 'edgedness', continuity and predictability, all generated by the experiences of feeding, when the infant's skin is in close contact with the mother's skin. In this position and within these rhythms, an infant may acquire a non-self-reflective sense of continuity and coherence "in which sensory need is in the process of acquiring features of subjective desire (the sensory-level beginnings of a subject wishing for something)" [20]. Once again, a stable sense of groundedness will enable healthy development, whereas in pathological development, autism will substitute petrification for this stability, and aim at the absolute elimination of the unknown and the unpredictable. This autism will provide the reliable comfort and protection that skin contact had failed to achieve.

The work of Didier Anzieu assimilates and elaborates ideas of his predecessors. Developing the notion of the skin as a protective shield, Anzieu develops the concept of the 'skin-ego', describing its functions and its evolution in the interface of mother and child. Anzieu's skin-ego is a representation of the boundary between the internal world and the environment, serving also as conduit, communicative envelope and the site of primitive, rudimentary thought. The skin ego serves also to screen exchanges with unconscious parts of the personality, in a way reminiscent of Bion's double limit.

The skin ego is a structure of the mind, 'pre-programmed' at birth in potential form, a precursor to the ego or the ego in its original state deriving, as Freud noted, from the body surface as a projection of that surface. It is "a mental image of which the Ego of the child makes use during early phases of its development in order to represent itself as an Ego containing psychical contents, on the basis of its experience of the surface of the body" [21].

But before it is the subject's own, Anzieu's skin-ego is a mental representation of maternal holding as it is experienced on the surface of the skin. In a sense, it contains both the mother's mind, which provides constant care to the infant's needs, and the sensations from body contact with her. The illusion of a shared skin is a maternal achievement in the sense that it is testimony to maternal attunement, to the mother's ability to create moments of mutuality in dimensions of touch, sound, eye contact and empathic emotionality. This illusion of a shared mind-skin is a chronologically intermediate structure between fusion with the mother and differentiation from her.

This 'shared interface' of a skin common to mother and child corresponds to a symbiotic fantasy which gradually gives way to a separation process through which the interface is internalized as a psychical envelope and a demarcated individual skin-ego. As the baby develops and as integration of self-progresses, the baby acquires a sense of the skin as the limiting membrane.

Introjecting the capacity for containment, a sense of individuality emerges from the dyad. The achievement of demarcation is simultaneously an achievement of tri-dimensionality, with the concomitant ability to contain and transform sensations and emotions into images, affects, and thoughts. Traumatic or untimely separations can give rise to pathogenic fantasies involving a rending of (common) skin, a secondary fantasy of invulnerable covering, or phantasies along masochistic and psychosomatic lines, in which the skin is imagined as bruised or beaten.

In developing his concept of skin ego, Anzieu cites a 'Freudian principle': that "every psychical function develops by supporting itself upon a bodily function whose workings it transposes onto the mental plane" [21]. He argues that contemporary psychoanalytic thought had neglected this principle, leaving the body as the great 'unacknowledged element' of contemporary thought, as the ignored "a general, irreducible, pre-sexual given, as the thing that all psychical functions lean on anaclitically" [21]. This emphasis leads Anzieu to posit direct links between the organic and the psychic, posing the psychic skin not only as a metaphor of the physical skin, but as its organic continuation. Anzieu describes nine functions of the skin-ego [21], discussing each function in its organic context and then transposing it to the psychic realm:

1. Maintenance: The body skin is a support for the skeleton and muscles. Correspondingly, the skin ego maintains and supports the entire psyche. Here Anzieu describes Winnicott's 'holding environment' and how the mother is the precursor of the child's being able to hold himself.

2. Containment: The skin has the function of covering the body. The skin ego, correspondingly, 'contains' the contents of the body. This sense of somatic containment is associated with the mother's correlative capacity for emotional containment and transformation, as described by Bion [14].

3. Protection: The surface layer of the skin protects the sensitive layers underneath. The skin ego, correspondingly, is the protective shield

against over-stimulation for both infant and adult. The mother's skin and body are offered for use as a shield against intrusive or excessive stimuli. The introjection of this protective capacity provides a source of security.

4. Individuation: The membrane of each cell protects the individuality of that cell. By analogy, one of the effects of the skin ego is to preserve the various self-functions and to provide a sense of connectivity and individuality. Skin boundaries are associated with psychic barriers that eventually differentiate the baby from the mother. Maternal dysfunction may compromise this development and lead to second-skin defenses [12], where individuality is not associated with real separation. Instead, it is achieved through secondary means of intentional mental effort that is analogous to muscular effort. This may reflect in such acts as excessive verbalization, alongside more direct emergency attempts to heal a perforated skin (paradoxically manifesting in piercing, cutting, tattooing, sado-masochistic sex, etc.).

5. Inter-sensoriality: The skin is a surface containing pockets and cavities. It is full of sense organs and integrates their diversity. In a like manner, the skin ego "connects up the body's sensations of various sorts and makes them stand out as figures against the original background" [21]. The skin-ego coordinates different sensations, associatively links auditory, olfactory, gustatory, and visual sensations with touch and creates a feeling of unity and coherence in what can otherwise be experienced as chaotic, multiple and fragmentary.

6. Sexualization: Parts of the skin-ego serve as support for the inborn drives and mediate their satisfaction. Reiterating Freudian insights, Anzieu describes skin contact as the source of pleasure and stimulation of the erogenous zones. The baby's skin contacts the mother's skin in a pleasurable way and the acquired skin ego holds this experience as the forerunner of the capacity for sexual excitation with another person.

7. Libidinal recharging: The skin surface receives ongoing stimulation from the out-

side, which regulates and stimulates the inside. The skin ego has the corresponding function of organizing and synthesizing the stimuli directed at the mind, controlling and regulating levels of stimulation.

The prohibition of touch enters here, as Anzieu describes the '*double taboo on touching*', which every child encounters and without which there is no possibility of moving from the skin-ego stage to that of thought. Anzieu emphasizes that, as the infant develops, touch remains fundamental only on condition that, at the right moment, it is forbidden. The taboo on touching is double in a number of ways. It controls both sexual and aggressive impulses; it concerns both internal and external contacts and forms a distinction or interface between them, separating family-space from that of the dangerous 'outside world'; it forbids the touch of the whole body (continued clinging to the mother) and, later, masturbatory touching with the hands; finally, it is bilateral, for its requirements apply to the adult who forbids as well as the child who is being disciplined. The taboo on touching is what sends us from an early echo-tactile form of communication towards a skin-ego that becomes the space of inter-sensorial inscription and gradually replaces the physical by the psychical [22, 23].

8. Inscription: Whereas the outer layer of the skin is a shield against external stimulation, the inner layer keeps a record of what has been experienced and contained. Registering tactile sensory traces, the skin-ego retains traces and inscriptions that are essential for the development of thinking capacity and symbolization. Elementary sensations and their associated phantasies present a register of early life experience: "The Skin-ego is the original parchment that acts as a palimpsest, preserving the crossed-out, scratched-through, overwritten drafts of an "original" pre-verbal writing made of traces on the skin." [21].

In Anzieu's formulations, '*formal signifiers*' encode sensory traces of early failures in maternal care that result in trauma for the child. In the early stages of the phantasized common skin, the mother digests and processes stimuli for the child. At this early pre-verbal stage, as there is no delineation between the conscious and the unconscious, the infant is not capable of repression or articulation. Therefore, intense impressions, sensations, and ordeals that hadn't undergone maternal processing and containment will 'petrify', constituting the elements out of which formal signifiers are built. Until able to verbally express early environmental failures of translating the sensual into emotional thought, these will remain signified through the 'sensate body'.

Formal signifiers don't take the form of a phantasy scene or an enactment, but rather the geometrical or physical transformation of a body that entails a deformation or destruction of form. The space in which they appear is two-dimensional and the patient senses them as external to himself. Anzieu gives examples: a vertical axis is reversed; a support collapses; a hole sucks in […] a solid body is crossed; a gaseous body explodes; […] an orifice opens and closes; […] a limit interposes; different perspectives are juxtaposed; […] my double leaves or controls me; […] a retreating object abandons me ([24]. see also [23]).

This conceptualization has clear therapeutic implications. When skin-ego deformations are understood as sets of formal signifiers, the analytic task is one of transforming body signals into a symbolic medium that allows thought and endows disturbance with meaning. Here the patient not only communicates his or her immediate sensations and body experiences, but also begins to talk and think about them. The analyst holds the patient with her attention, preoccupation and active intervention, and through these processes, provides for the patient the experience of being contained. Through counter-transference reactions, the analyst may intuitively infer early traumatic formations in the patient's history, and offer the patient understanding through integrative reconstructions.

In many ways, Anzieu seems to continue the work of his predecessors yet, as Lafrance [25] remarks, Anzieu's formulations are also revolutionary and significantly diverge from traditional

psychoanalytic thought. Firstly, the centrality of the skin in Anzieu's thought overturns the traditional privileging of 'depth' in relation to 'surface'. Secondly, the anaclitic relationship that Anzieu creates between the physical and the psychic skin emphasizes both the dimension of embodiment in subjectivity and the critical positioning of *relationality* in human development, namely, the manner in which early child development actively involves another person (usually the mother). This emphasis on relationality naturally leads us to examine the larger context of skin as a metaphor: the relation between the subject and his various social functions.

24.2 Cultural Accounts of Skin

Whereas psychoanalytic accounts of the skin focus on the creation of psychic space as an interiority (a self), cultural accounts of skin focus on the way that society, norms and history shape both skin and self. Foucault is probably the paradigmatic postmodern theorist who drew attention to the dominant discourses in society and the manner in which they prescribe norms in relation to which subjects regulate their bodies.

In his seminal '*Discipline and Punish*', Michel Foucault argued that the body must be explored as a subject of power relations. Foucault described 'methods' that operate meticulous controls over the body, which methods may clearly be recognized from the classical period onward, in rising intensities and ever growing levels of resolution. These methods "assured the constant subjection of [bodily] forces and imposed upon them a relation of docility-utility, might be called 'disciplines'" [26]. 'Disciplines' place the subject's body under minute control of social and economic forces. For Foucault "discipline is a political anatomy of detail", because it is everywhere. Its cunning aspect lies in the subject's complete obliviousness to his bodily subjection.

The subject's body is shaped by knowledge of which the subject is not consciously aware. The political technology of the body, the 'microphysics' of power, is encoded and may be deciphered only with effort and concentration, and only in the context of various systems of relations that are ultimately power relations. *The body politic* is a series of routes and weapons by which power operates. For Foucault, body is never superficial. Here, soul and consciousness are integral to the body, formed in its image and restricted by its constraints.

Foucault's micro-physics of power translate into disciplinary regimes such as makeup, dieting, dress, exercise and cosmetic surgery. Bodies are formed and regimented in ways that simultaneously comply with social norms and reinforce their dominance. Particular practices effectually create bodies that aspire to fit the social ideal, and thus major aspects of bodily identity are subject to social normalization. The social ideal defines the privileged position of certain bodies (in categories of gender and race) and the physical attributes that define what is male or female, black or white. These attributes cease to exist mainly as biological facts, but are rather realized by traditions, power relations and prescriptive practices—all appearing on the body's visible surface.

Butler [27–29], exploring the concepts of identity and subjectivity, takes the body as her point of departure and introduces the term of 'performativity'. For Butler, Preformativity redefines many of the things we have come to regard as natural. Focusing on issues of gender, Butler argues that the subjection of the body to normalizing practices expresses not only the way in which male and female bodies seek to approximate an ideal, *but the very process whereby sexed and gendered subjects come into existence at all.* Rejecting the view that gender differences have their origin in biological or natural differences, Butler describes femininity and masculinity as socially dictated bodily styles which our bodies incorporate to yield a gendered subjectivity. Like Foucault, she views discourses as producing the identities they appear to be describing.

In Butler's view, the proclamation of an infant's sex immediately accompanying birth is not a description of a fact, but rather a practice that constitutes gender. Many documentations [29–33] describe how this exclusionary binary and splitting action has often created trauma in

the name of normative order when employed in making decisions to alter the manifest gendered surface of a child's body. These decisions are directed by the overriding belief that a child's body must reflect one aspect of the binary, with gender construed as fixed and unidimensional. Underscoring these decisions as well is the belief that the child's physical conformity will aid in the child's adaptation toward a heterosexual system of complementary social relations [34].

From this perspective, materiality itself is always already artificially manufactured and holds no natural claims: "what I would propose in place of these conceptions of construction is a return to the notion of matter, not as site or surface, but as a process of materialization that stabilizes over time to produce the effect of boundary, fixity and surface, we call matter. The matter is always materialized as I think to be thought in relation to the productive and indeed materializing effects of regulatory power in the Foucoutian sense" [28]. Thus, Benthien [35], viewing skin as the site where identity is assigned, examines the ways in which skin forms define gender in different cultures, showing how male skin is perceived as thicker, resembling armor, whereas female skin is a diaphanous transmitter of emotion. Mythologically, the iron-skinned male often features a single area of vulnerability such as the heel of Achilles, which makes him human rather than divine, whereas the female equivalent is the *macula materna* or birthmark–a dark flaw in her semi-opaque softness and perfection.

The social imposition of norms upon the body reaches beyond gender, as described by Bordieu and expressed by the concept of *Habitus* [36]. Bourdieu's Habitus refers to the physical embodiment of cultural capital, namely, the deeply ingrained habits, skills, and dispositions acquired through our life experiences. The Habitus is a social property of individuals that orients behavior and provides a sense of practical expertise. And yet, it is not a conscious expertise; it is a state of the body and of being, a repository of ingrained dispositions that seem natural. Bourdieu calls this the 'bodily hexis', where the body is the site of incorporated history [36].

Predisposed practices tend to produce *doxa*, situations in which "the natural and social world appears as self-evident" [37] and the order of things remains unquestioned. All seemingly "natural" functions such as eating, caring, sexual relations etc. are actually forms of culturally inculcated norms of practice and belief. Regulation and determination of training and experience renders them so habitual and ingrained, that they are considered as natural instead of culturally developed. Thus, "every established order tends to produce (to very different degrees and with very different means) the naturalization of its own arbitrariness" [36].

In a complementary fashion, the established order defines its 'other' in terms of bodily appearance. Viewing the skin as the site for projection and exposure of deep seated cultural and political investments, Fanon, for example, describes racism as the "epidermalization of inferiority" [38]. Illuminating the inextricability of the body, the psychic and the social, Fanon describes the projection of inferiority onto the bodies of colored people in the colonial context through economic and cultural marginalization. These racist cultural values are then absorbed and introjected into the psychic life and embodied experience of the oppressed [38]. Fanon here is theorizing an "epidermal racial schema" (p. 92), with the skin serving as marker of social difference, human value and recognition. Benthien [35] catalogues experiments in the flushing-out of color pigments, the use of 'bleaching agents' today, and the existence of African-American 'bon ton societies' that admit only members whose skin is light enough to let their veins shine through. The ever increasing practice of body modification has been researched as highlighting gendered, racialized and sexualized dimensions of the subject, which are culturally-defined [39, 40].

As a sub-category of self-modification, the practice of tattooing is extensively discussed in cultural theory, documenting its various functions across eras and habits. In tribal societies, tattoos were formal components of initiation rituals, inscribing social transitions upon the flesh [41]. In modern Western society, particularly with adolescents, tattoos express stations or crises in the development of a consolidating identity. The tattoo signifies a certain degree of resoluteness [42]. It inscribes on the body an incontrovertible expression [43] and this permanent alteration of the body is experienced as more concrete, more forceful and more persuasive than any form of verbal expression. The experience of being tattooed with a self-made, visible decorative identifier can reinforce a sense of agency and control through the active manifestation of an otherwise passive experience [44]. Tattoos may also address the needs of affiliation, creating physical markers that indicate belonging to or separation from certain social or cultural groups. Furthering the function of skin as canvass from the personal to the public, Knopf describes the increasing acceptance and recognition of tattooing as a system of signification. At the extreme end, the tattoo is transformed from private symbol into artistic message, when artists use their own skin as canvass, blurring the boundary between the artist's body and his work, between what is personally and collectively owned [45].

24.3   Integrating Perspectives

As we have briefly and partially sketched above, skin has been inextricably tied to experiences of self and identity in both cultural and psychoanalytic theory. And yet, it seems that the interface of the cultural, the psychic and the organic remains the most difficult to describe and explore. Merleau-Ponty [46] asks: "Where are we to put the limit between the body and the world, since the world is a flesh?" (p. 248). Or, stating things the other way around: where, if anywhere, does the cultural end, and the biological or individual-psychic begin? And perhaps more importantly, how may we formulate their interrelations?

This question is not only of theoretical interest, but rather holds practical implications for diagnosis and treatment of physical and psychic malaise. While the cultural and psychoanalytic perspectives are clearly complementary, they may lead to divergent understandings of various phenomena. For example, whereas Anzieu may find piercing and tattooing to be symptomatic of failure in the function of the skin-ego and construe them as defensive and pathological configurations, cultural theorists may find these same practices as reflective of normative, sometimes prescriptive, behaviors. A third perspective, one that integrates the two, may find the same practice as constituting an autonomic stand in relation to cultural impositions. Zizek, for example, discusses the ways in which the potentially 'true' that resides in the unconscious, may be inscribed on the surface of the subject's body, thus becoming truth itself [47]. Merleau-Ponty had articulated this idea succinctly: "everything is both manufactured and natural in man, as it were, in the sense that there is not a word, not a form of behavior which does not owe something to purely biological being and which, at the same time, does not elude the simplicity of animal life" [46]. Accepting this point of departure, we do not aspire for an account that supplies us with unquestioned certainties that differentiate inner from outer and identify Zizek's 'truth'. Rather, we seek a conceptual framework in which we can contain several perspectives and describe their interrelations. We offer here the Lacanian perspective as one in which we can contemplate simultaneously the effects of culture and the constitution of psychic inner life as they interact on the organic surface of the skin.

The understanding of the Lacanian body is bound up with the understanding of the Lacanian developmental account and the three orders that constitute psychic life: The Symbolic, the Imaginary and the Real. We will therefore begin with their brief description.

24.4 The Lacanian Perspective

For Lacan, body image, identity and subjectivity are intimately inter-related, and formed only in relation to the pre-existing 'other'. Like Freud, Lacan emphasizes the fact that the human infant is born prematurely. This prematurity renders him totally helpless and determines his total and protracted reliance on others. Lacan describes the newborn's experience of himself as a dismembered limb, torn

and exiled from the mother's body. In this terrifying realm of disintegration and pending death, the infant is offered not the mother as auxiliary ego or common skin, but the irresistible lure of his own mirror image. This image presents the terrified infant with a unified whole, an integrated, coordinated totality. In a jubilant moment of 'Aha!', the infant identifies himself with this promising imago, thus creating the Imaginary nucleus of his ego [48].

Clearly, Lacan notes, this recognition in the mirror-image is nothing but an absurd 'misrecognition' that involves deep alienation. Alienation is, firstly, the consequence of the huge gulf that lies between the unified imago and the infant's fragmentary authentic experience. This imago is, secondly, steeped in the 'discourse of the Other', suffused with momentous implications and connotations that come from the desire and narrative of others as they encourage the child to recognize herself in the mirror ("What a strong boy!", "You're going to be beautiful, just like Mommy", etc.). Thus, from the start, the child's ego and body image are immersed in signifiers originating in the desires of speaking others. These signifiers are branded in the infant's flesh and form the contingent basis of his being. Lacan calls these first imprints 'unary traits', and I will later return to discuss their significance in the structure of the psyche.

Now, making matters worse, the infant quickly enters into an intense and ambivalent relation with his imago. This perfect, coherent image of himself arouses envy in the child, and he seeks to own it and put himself in its place. Simultaneously, the child feels that the image is there to usurp him, to further alienate and deplete his experience of self. This pattern of what Lacan terms 'narcissistic aggressivity' is the basic trademark of imaginary relations, the relations of the ego with others in the imaginary order. In the pattern of imaginary relations, the subject is never quite a definite self; he exists in relation to a specular other, a particular person, in relation to whom he · processes his own identity. In cycles of introjection and projection, a basic paranoid positioning is created, boiling down to the binary choice: "It's me or you".

These intense relations of love, hate and narcissistic rivalry remain a paradigmatic dimension in all future interpersonal relations. They are portrayed in the 'doubleness' we may find in endless stories, from Abel and Cain to Batman and the joker, always holding parameters of identification and negation, a rivalry that may be carried to the death, yet never quite gets there, because the annihilation of the other results in the annihilation of the undifferentiated self.

The entry into the Symbolic order, via the Oedipal complex and the transformation of the dyadic mother-child space into a triadic one, eases the aggressivity of Imaginary relations. Creating a third point of reference, it dissipates the immediacy of experience and allows mediation and thought. This transformative third is not necessarily a flesh-and-blood father. It is rather the Name-of-the-Father that forbids endless jouissance with the mother and constitutes the child as a desiring subject within the confines of language and the law. The Name-of-the-Father is, effectively, any symbolic object in the mother's discourse that causes the child to realize that he is not the one-and-only object of his mother's desire.

This realization may be construed as an emancipatory tragedy of sorts. On the one hand, the child is no longer the mother's 'all' and his primordial lack is brought back to him as a narcissistic injury that renews threats of disintegration. On the other hand, the child is freed from being the object of the mother's desire and is free to institute himself as a desiring subject in the Symbolic order. The other of the Symbolic order is marked by Lacan as the other with a capital O (dubbed 'the big other'): it is the order of language, culture and the paternal law.

The entry into the Symbolic order transforms the subject in several remarkable ways: firstly, the child renounces his incestuous desire to merge with the mother. This renunciation is effectually the primal repression that constitutes the unconscious and the child as its subject. Secondly, the child now transfers his desire to the father, and this new love will be expressed in the father's mode—as the love of ideas, culture and society. The initial bond with the mother will leave the child evermore haunted with an illusion of harmony and wholeness that he will always search for (and fail to achieve) in the realm of the Symbolic. This lack, constituted at birth, re-experienced when differentiating from the mother-child symbiotic dyad, is the source and the fueling of Lacanian desire. Thirdly, the initial alienation that allowed the subject to first recognize himself as individuated by means of his specular image is now further deepened in the realm of the symbolic and verbal representation.

Language does not arise from the individual, it is always there, in the world, outside; it awaits the newborn. When it reaches him, he is traumatized by it. Lacan believes that, while language initiates the subject into a human existence, it irrevocably tears him from his animal existence. It forevermore cuts his natural and direct connection with being, with the world, with his material body that had been immersed in the symbiotic jouissance (enjoyment) with the mother. This connection will always be mediated by language and fashioned by the culture that goes hand in hand with it. For this reason, something of the primal existence of a human being is truncated. All that man desires will be mediated in the (de) forms and the pre-given structures of the Symbolic order.

The Name-of-the-Father is the *master signifier* that inaugurates the subject into the world of language, law and desire. It terminates the formerly experienced jouissance of the maternal dyad and drives the repression of the desire of the mother, instating the father in her place and constituting the unconscious. This is the way that the barred subject of the unconscious is created as an effect of the signifier. The signifier castrates, divides and organizes both subject and his world within the confines and dictums of the law. The word kills the thing, as the father represses the mother, and the subject now is reconfigured around this vital void that lies at the center of his being, a transcendental absence that may never be filled. It is this void that drives man's desire.

By this developmental stage, the Lacanian subject is tripartite entity. He exists as subject in the triadic Symbolic order, defined by language and culture, social roles and norms that constitute his persona in the world. By distinction, in the imaginary order, he exists as 'ego', namely, as a conscious self, constituting his interpersonal relations with specific significant others. Within his experiential world, existing both 'within' and 'outside' of him, looms the third order—the Real, which is that part of experience that evades all representation, both Imaginary and Symbolic. The Real is all that lacks meaning and signification, appearing for the subject as uncanny, traumatic, uncontrollable and ineffable. Although the Real evades signification, it is indicated to the subject by such experiences as trauma, intense pleasure (jouissance), sexual difference and the collapse of the sense of self in the subject's innermost core.

The three orders function in complex synchronizations, coordinating in various ways the subject's identity in terms of cultural and social positioning, as well as intimate ties and conscious identity. The dynamics among the orders forms identity on the one hand, and the dimension of materiality or bodily being on the other hand. It is this materiality that holds the force and vitality of life and primal jouissance but, at the same time, remains unassimilated, traumatic and unsettling. Order is constructed in the Imaginary and the Symbolic registers and becomes undone by the Real.

The tripartite structure of mental life can be traced in the subject's experience of the body. The Symbolic body is tamed and dominated by the other (culture, language and the Law). Symbolic castration forces jouissance to be evacuated to the margins of the body, thus creating the classical Freudian erotogenic zones—oral, anal and genital. Whereas Freud understood these areas as epigenetically programmed, Lacan sees them as vestiges of jouissance, remainders of what had formerly been experienced by the body in its entirety. This Symbolic body is the body programmed and structured by cultural practices. It is carried and clothed in acceptable modes and answers particular ideals that are propagated by various social institutions such as schools, media and rules of conduct. These rules and ideals are not natural to the body and always remain alien in the manners described by Foucault's discipline and Bordieu's Habitus.

The Imaginary body may be equated with Anzieu's skin ego, i.e., with "a phantasy" [21], "a mental image" [21], of which the ego of the child makes use to satisfy its narcissistic need for an envelope and container. This is the body instated in the mirror image, a gestalt of the Imaginary order that had provided the infant with an illusion of mastery and control he will forever aspire to and never achieve. In the realm of the Imaginary and sexual relations, the subject will always search for what he lacks in the other, searching for a lost possibility of union and harmony that grants him narcissistic integrity, a possibility of self-recognition and love. The body here discussed is an imagined body, one that mediates all that the subject will ever know of closeness to his significant others.

This symbolic-imaginary body reflects the signifiers of the other and the existential need for boundary and grounding, but it leaves behind the terrors and the pleasures of the Real body. Alienation here is so complete, that it causes the subject not to recognize his own body when its Imaginary or Symbolic co-ordinates are thrown into question. When something of unknown origin appears on the skin or in a person's posture, we are immediately transported to the uncanny, and the anomaly perceived demands meaning and signification. Injury may bring about such a 'de-symbolization' of the body, resulting in a 'foreignizing' of the body, in making it foreign. Ironically, only in its foreignness the cultivated body may become organic to the subject. The organism lies on the underside of the Imaginary mirror image and on the beyond of the symbolic body. Here is the Real, fragmented body of old that had been sacrificed in Imaginary and Symbolic alienations in the service of allowing the subject to create himself as a recognizable entity in the social world. Fink sees the presymbolic Real as the "infant's body before it comes under the sway of the Symbolic order, before it is … instructed in the ways of the world" [49].

Lacan's formulations allow us to picture the struggle of the organic, psychic and cultural on the skin's surface. Here we may imagine a stratified life of the body. Our 'upper' symbolic body functions in accord with norms, rational behavior, courtesy, roles and aesthetics. Its functioning is often automatic, as we move, modify and position our physical being in automatic and programmed patterns. Managing daily our worldly dealings with others, we suspend our knowledge of the other's organismic body, the way it sweats, urinates and digests. Any intrusion of these contents can momentarily destabilize our sense of reality and bring forward the contingent, precarious and paradoxical constitution of ourselves and our world. Our 'intermediate', imaginary body holds our stability and certainty of self, the Imaginary fact of our individuality. It grants us a cohesiveness that allows us to deny our permeability, our lack of coordination and our limited mastery of bodily functions. It holds our knowledge and awareness of intimate dealings with the bodies of others. Our 'other' body, the unknown Real of our material selves is revealed in injury and trauma, through the effects of shock and dissociation, at times by means of comedy. It is invariably crude, abject, mesmerizing and uncanny. It holds vicissitudes that are encountered unplanned. It holds a 'beyond' that is inevitably tied to the root and essence of both life and death. It is the body at its birth, the body at the height of its forbidden incestuous jouissance, which knows no limits, not even the limits of self-preservation. The sublime enjoyment of jouissance distinguishes an experience of intensity, a loss of ego control and boundaries (which may be felt as horror or delight), from the temperate Symbolic-Imaginary pleasures of satisfaction.

As in the realm of psychic functioning, the coordination of the orders in the bodily domain is the hallmark of the embodied subject who has a chance at 'being', a chance to realize the possibilities of living. When coordinated across the orders, the subject's body may allow his stable and safe insertion in the social sphere, may grant him pleasures and intimacies with others, may instill in him the raw organismic energies that are at his disposal as a reservoir of life. Unravelled, the bodily life of the subject becomes depleted. It is made manageable by being subjected to Symbolic formalities and Imaginary pleasures, but it is vitalized by the indecipherable forces of the Real.

The above tripartite structure serves also to lend a unique meaning to the Lacanian symptom. For Lacan, the symptom holds, as a receptacle, the portions of desire and jouissance which did not find a culturally acceptable way of expression. A Lacanian analyst does not place himself in opposition to the symptom. Quite the opposite: he views the symptom as a reservoir of authentic, unedited potential life force, one that the patient seeks to express and yet is afraid to own. Allying himself with the symptom, the analyst tries to understand what symbolic prohibitions have denied the desire's expression, what prices the patient was loath to pay in lieu of their realization.

For Lacan, analytic interpretation seeks to free captured and stunted desires but it does not seek to completely eliminate the symptom. Every symptom has a kernel of pleasure and pain that does not answer to meaning and signification. This kernel may be understood as the subject's unary trait, a bodily inscription of the particular bodily experience that was generated by a particular mother's language onto the particular enjoying and pained body of her child. Acknowledging this 'pure' part of the symptom and acquiring the know-how of its assimilation into the subject's life heralds the final phase of analysis. Henceforth, its acceptance signals the subject's singularity, the parts of himself that will forever retain their alterity in relation to the Symbolic. The aim of the treatment is not to interpret the symptom *away*, neither is it the reconstruction of trauma. Instead, the subject is presented with a choice. Whereas formerly he had sought his identity and formulated it in the terms of the Symbolic conforming Other, he is now given the choice of identifying himself in terms of the *body* as Other, in terms of the bodily contingency that is wholly his own, in the terms of his particular economy of jouissance as given in the kernel of his symptom.

Lacan's final conclusion is that there is no subject without a symptom. Thus, the symptom receives a new meaning in relation to the goal of analysis. It is now taken to be that which defines mankind and it cannot be rectified or cured. It holds a singularity that doesn't conform; it demonstrates the particular jouissance of the real body of a particular subject. Identification with the kernel of jouissance given in the symptom is effectually the creation of what Lacan [50] calls 'sinthome'. The symptom (redubbed sinthome in relation to its binding function) will heretofore provide the binding of the three orders (Symbolic, Imaginary and Real) as their kernel or conjunction. Always involving the organism, it allows the subject to discover and formulate his secret, private name. In the next section we illustrate these insights through the analysis of Kafka's *Country Doctor'* and the manner in which a wound that appears on the skin becomes the kernel of the wounded subject.

24.5   The Skin in Kafka's *'Country Doctor'*

Kafka's universe is one that is torn. It is rendered fragmentary by magic, unknown forces that are always wild and uncanny. Yet, despite being unknown, these forces are also somehow familiar to those who are subjected to them. With a dry, clipped and seemingly rational narrative tone, Kafka creates his characteristic aura in this tale of a country doctor. The story portrays futile journeys, alienation and the disintegration of life. In our short analysis, we focus on the Doctor's body, as it dissembles into distinct, disjoint experiences that signal the doctor's death.

The story begins with a relatively mundane situation: a country doctor is summoned on an icy winter night to see a seriously ill patient. Already dressed up and equipped for his journey, the doctor finds himself helplessly stranded in his own snowy yard. His horse has died from overexertion and his servant Rosa had not been able to coax the doctor's neighbours into lending him a horse. Frustrated, the doctor kicks an old pigsty that had been unused for years, and from within it, miraculously, emerge two powerful, well-formed horses and a strange groom, crouched on all fours, naming the horses his 'sister' and 'brother'. Accepting this creature's gift of horses, the doctor orders the servant to assist him in harnessing his wagon to the horses. As she obedi-

ently does so, the groom wraps his arms around the girl, and when she flees alarmed to the doctor, he finds her cheeks marked red by two rows of teeth. The doctor threatens the groom with the whip, but immediately checks his wrath, recalling that the creature is a stranger and, moreover, the only one who offered him help. As the groom claps his hands and the horses fly off at an incredible pace, the doctor realizes that he has left Rosa at the mercy of the groom. Rosa flees into the house, locking doors to defend herself against the groom's onslaught, but as the horses fly the doctor hears how the door of his house is breaking down, leaving Rosa to her inevitable fate.

The intense unfolding of the story introduces the reader to the Symbolic, Imaginary and Real orders of the doctor and his world. The protagonist does not have a name and is referred to as 'doctor'. Defined by his position in the Symbolic order, he is required to answer requests for help. If he cannot attend to his patient, if he cannot venture from his yard, he cannot be a country doctor and remains stripped of his raison d'etre. He must attend to the patient who has called upon him in order to maintain his identity. Yet, an unknown force hinders his progression toward that which is not only his livelihood, but his Symbolic life itself.

What is this force that threatens to deprive the doctor of his Symbolic definition? As in many of Kafka's stories, the protagonist has a number of 'doubles' who define him in different ways. The first double in our story is the servant, Rosa, who serves to define the Imaginary person of the doctor. Then there is the groom, a semi-human creature that appears crouched on all four and is blood-related to the horses. The groom here embodies the real, animal-like aspect of the doctor's existence. His uncivilized nature is brought out as he bites the servant and proceeds in his intention to rape her. The doctor, stripped of his natural energies, alienated from them in his Symbolic roles, finds himself depleted, 'horseless' and immobile. Alienated from his organic existence, the doctor's body is passively transported by the force of norms and habits that devoid it of vitality. As he arrives to the patient's home, the doctor is rushed in by the patient's family.

Rosa co-produces the Symbolic by virtue of her social role as servant, but being the only character in the story bearing a name, she instates the Imaginary, her name triggering color and visual images. The doctor is clearly fond of her and yearns for her. She offers the doctor personal recognition and relational intimacy. The groom violates her specular position by marking her skin with his teeth. The doctor's decision to maintain his Symbolic positioning and desert the object of his affections deprives both him and Rosa of their Imaginary skin. Rosa becomes a pure physical being, a sacrificial lost 'thing', violently subjugated to the Real. As the Imaginary home the doctor and Rosa shared crashes under the groom's onslaught, Rosa's wound, soon re-found in the doctor's patient, remains uncannily inscribed in the reader's consciousness, like the smile of the vanishing Cheshire cat in Alice's wonderland, a metonymic echo of a cheek, a damsel, a relation of love.

The doctor's Symbolic husk is brought to its destination in the sickroom. He looks at the young man in his bed: "Thin, without fever, not cold, not warm, with empty eyes, without a shirt, the young man under the stuffed quilt heaves himself up, hangs around my throat, and whispers in my ear, "Doctor, let me die"". Indeed, it seems that in a limbo of neutrality and sterility, lacking any distinctive and singular identifying trait, the patient is already dead. There is nothing alive about him. At this moment the patient is revealed as an additional double for the doctor. Both lack vitality; both are but husks in their Symbolic roles of doctor and patient. Their bodily functions are 'dead' to the extent that the doctor's perceptual apparatus does not function. He sees nothing. Not even his patient's illness.

In the abyss of this lack of vitality the doctor recalls his Rosa. His wish to save her makes him bitter with his Symbolic calling: "I am employed by the district and do my duty to the full, right to the point where it's almost too much. Badly paid, but I'm generous and ready to help the poor. I still have to look after Rosa, and then the young man may have his way, and I want to die too". It seems that the young man's lack of life and lack of desire to live reflects to the doctor his own loss

of life. He envisions for a moment the physical life he might have shared with Rosa, had he not devoted himself so exclusively to work. He understands the way the Symbolic had drained his desire for pleasure, his ability to have an embodied relation with another. The doctor tells us that such a life was a possibility just as he acknowledges that this possibility no longer exists: "With the help of my night bell the entire region torments me, but that this time I had to sacrifice Rosa as well, this beautiful girl, who lives in my house all year long and whom I scarcely notice–this sacrifice is too great…".

The memory of Rosa and his imaginary existence enliven the doctor's body enough to restore something of its lost functions. The doctor now finds what he had formerly missed—his patient's wound: "On his right side, in the region of the hip, a wound the size of the palm of one's hand has opened up. Rose colored, in many different shadings, dark in the depths, brighter on the edges, delicately grained, with uneven patches of blood, open to the light like a mine". This wound, intricately described, with a detail found nowhere else in the story, bleeds color into the formerly grey and white scenery of the story. Juxtaposing the vision of life represented by Rosa and the perception of the formerly missed wound, its significance is made clear: it holds the energy of life in its texture, in its color, in its depths and in its hypnotic quality. Indeed, the wound is inhabited by forms of life: "Close up a complication is apparent. Who can look at that without whistling softly? Worms, as thick and long as my little finger, themselves rose-colored and also spattered with blood, are wriggling their white bodies with many limbs from their stronghold in the inner of the wound towards the light". The wound is the only living thing in the pale nondescript boy. The worms are described as birthed beings from within this wound, searching for light. As the doctor discovers this Real of life, the desire to live takes hold of the boy: ""Will you save me?" whispers the young man, sobbing, quite blinded by the life inside his wound".

This wound is the break in the skin that holds the body, that claims individuation and that holds ordinary significations. The break in the skin allows the doctor to see and to experience both his patient and himself. It allows the obscene and terrifying beauty of life to manifest itself, as it cuts through the regular fabric of life and habit. The habituality of life is shown in its deadening potential, as the equation between the skin's integrity and way life is undone. The living dead are both blinded by the life that is exposed in the wound which, like an organism, opens up and turns to the light.

The doctor acts again in the logic of doubles when he realizes that the boy's malaise is his own. Like the doctor, the boy lacks a backbone, as the neighbor's children taunt him with their song: "Take his clothes off, and then he'll heal, and if he doesn't cure, then kill him. It's only a doctor; it's only a doctor". Stripped of both his Symbolic and Imaginary skins (respectively, his ability to heal and to love) only the chaotic Real remains. This Real juncture means both life and death. Despite its despicable, traumatic nature, it also holds the beauty of life. We see this double nature of the Real in something else, namely, the position of the wound in its Symbolic reverberations.

There is a moment in the book of Genesis when Jacob prepares himself to re-meet his estranged double/brother—Esav. He spends the night alone on a riverside. There, a mysterious being, considered to be an angel or God, wrestles with Jacob, striking him painfully in the hollow of his thigh. This locus in Jacobs body gets sanctified as the mark of god by the prohibition of eating the thigh tendon (which appears later in Genesis). Thus, the wound encapsulates not only the Real (in its uncanny and paradoxical nature), but also the Symbolic (as emblem of a godly touch) and the Imaginary (as the echo of Rosa's bitten cheek). The wound, then, encapsulates both the fragmentation of human existence and the possibility of its rebinding. It holds the potential for reaching a new integration between body and subjectivity, matter and meaning.

The doctor is stripped of his clothes, put to bed with the boy, laid down on the side of his wound. It seems here that this wound serves to surpass the imaginary delineation of bodies, creating a potential of shared life, an additional

potential that is not realized in the story. The boy is angry and derisive, furious with the doctor's impotence to heal him. And yet, he grasps the beauty of his wound: "I came into the world with a beautiful wound; that was all I was furnished with". This seems to echo the deep knowledge the doctor has of symptoms, knowledge reflected in both his fascination with this particular wound and with the general aim of his calling. *The doctor in search of a symptom is a subject searching for the real.*

The doctor replies enigmatically, yet in a way that apparently comforts the boy and allows him to die peacefully. He says to him: "Young friend," I say, "your mistake is that you have no perspective. I've already been in all the sick rooms, far and wide, and I tell you, your wound is not so bad. Made in a tight corner with two blows from an axe. Many people offer their side and hardly hear the axe in the forest, to say nothing of the fact that it's coming closer to them." Only one thing carries a clear meaning in the doctor's opaque narrative: the doctor tells the boy that people seek this, this blow, this wound, this something that they offer themselves to receive and oftentimes miss, losing the possibility of the meaning it may grant.

The doctor exits the scene when the boy dies. But he will not make it home: "Naked, abandoned to the frost of this unhappy age, with an earthly carriage and unearthly horses, I drive around by myself, an old man. My fur coat hangs behind the wagon, but I cannot reach it, and no one from the nimble rabble of patients lifts a finger". The doctor here is bereft of all skin. He has come apart, he has shed his Symbolic and Imaginary skin, and he has left behind the seething life of the symptom. Not owning his symptom is the signal of his impending death.

Conclusion

It seems we have traversed much territory in order to reach a point where we may approach any itch, bruise, allergy or lesion with curiosity. We have presented skin's ambiguous potential, its functions as a border and a cloak, as a mirroring of self and as its mask. Interfacing the self and the world, the skin acts as locus and site of inscriptions—cultural, psychic and contingent. The skin can be marked to include or ostracize, to register personal history, collective histories and traumas. It is always a part of both the Real and the Symbolic, as organ and as art. Its history as a memory space and a sensual organ is implicated in personality formation and our relations with others. We have investigated the skin in its opacity as well as in its permeability; as a medium of communication as well as a mediator between the internal and the external. We have explored its function as a representative of self, alongside its nature as a site of sensuality and eroticism.

Encountering a symptom upon the skin, we enter a realm of multiple significations and meanings. We may be forced to examine what we conceive as natural, what narratives we adhere to, how we comprehend the unravelling of the Symbolic, Imaginary and the Real and what may be our role in their method of re-harmonizing. A patient with a symptom always ails. Yet, we do not know *what* ails. We encounter, as have healers of soma and psyche for years, the mixture of bewilderment and anxiety, pain and pleasure, which arise when a person encounters upon his flesh the uncanny and the incomprehensible. Irregularity of the skin always carries a message that is formed in the disharmonized juncture of organism, psyche and society.

We do not advocate an idealization of symptoms. But we believe that the symptom acts as a transitional phenomenon: it reshuffles our familiar ways of being in the world. The symptom calls for a change that is sometimes interior and sometimes manifest. Sometimes the symptom requires deciphering in order to understand its message. But at all times, it expresses energy that is vital, restless, seeking. The symptom signals both our resilience and our malleability. It testifies to questions, to possibilities of change and modes of rebellion. Symptoms may need healing, but they may also demand a closer appreciation of their function. A symptom is a message from the Real, dissatisfaction with the prescribed and the normative, even

when these are pleasurable. It urges us to reconsider the metaphors we live by. It calls upon us as doctors–as subjects of the Symbolic–to pay attention to the Real.

References

1. Freud S. The ego and the id, vol. 19. Hogarth Press: London; 1923. p. 3–63.
2. Freud S. Three essays on the theory of sexuality, vol. 7. London: Hogarth Press; 1905. p. 125–71.
3. Freud S. Project for a scientific psychology, vol. 1. London: Hogarth Press; 1895. p. 283–344.
4. Freud S. Beyond the pleasure principle, vol. 18. London: Hogarth Press; 1920. p. 1–65.
5. Freud S. Inhibitions, symptoms and anxiety, vol. 20. London: Hogarth Press; 1926. p. 77–175.
6. Klein M. The psychoanalysis of children. In: Klein M, editor. Contributions to psychoanalysis. New York: Mcgraw-Hill; 1932. p. 1921–45.
7. Klein M. A contribution to the psychogenesis of manic-depressive states. Int J Psychoanal. 1935;16: 145–74.
8. Winnicot DW. The theory of the parent-infant relationship. Int J Psychoanal. 1960;41:585–95.
9. Spitz RA. The psychogenic diseases in infancy—an attempt at their etiologic classification. Psychoanal Stud Child. 1951;6:255–75.
10. Harlow HF. Love in infant monkeys. Sci Am. 1959;200(6):68–74.
11. Bowlby J. The nature of the child's tie to his mother. Int J Psychoanal. 1958;39:350–73.
12. Bick E. The experience of the skin in early object-relations. Int J Psychoanal. 1968;49:484–6.
13. Bick E. Further considerations on the function of the skin in early object relations. Br J Psychother. 1986;2(4):292–9.
14. Bion WR. Attention and interpretation: a scientific approach to insight in psycho-analysis and groups. London: Tavistock; 1970.
15. Bion WR. Learning from experience. London: Tavistock; 1962.
16. Bion WR. Transformations: change from learning to growth. London: Tavistock; 1965.
17. Tustin F. The perpetuation of an error 1. J Child Psychother. 1994a;20(1):3–23.
18. Tustin F. Autistic barriers in neurotic patients. London: Karnac; 1994b.
19. Haag G. Fear of fusion and projective identification in autistic children. Psychoanal Inq. 1993;13(1):63–84.
20. Ogden TH. On the concept of an autistic-contiguous position. Int J Psychoanal. 1989;70:127–40.
21. Anzieu D. The skin-ego. London: Karnac; 2016.
22. Segal N. The other French Freud: Didier Anzieu—the story of a skin. Paper presented at Freud, archives and legacies, centre for German-Jewish studies, University of Sussex; 2006.

23. Segal N. Consensuality: Didier Anzieu, gender and the sense of touch. Amsterdam: Rodopi; 2009.

24. Anzieu D. Psychic envelopes. London: Karnac; 1990.

25. Lafrance M. From the skin ego to the psychic envelope: an introduction to the work of Didier Anzieu. In: Cavanagh S, Failler A, Hurst R, editors. Skin, culture and psychoanalysis. London: Palgrave MacMillan; 2013. p. 16–45.

26. Foucault M. Discipline and punish. New York: Vintage; 1977.

27. Butler J. Gender trouble, feminism and the subversion of identity. London: Routledge; 1990.

28. Butler J. Bodies that matter: on the discursive limits of sex. London: Routledge; 1993.

29. Butler J. Undoing gender. New York: Routledge; 2004.

30. Colapinto J. As nature made him: the boy who was raised as a girl. New York: Harper Collins; 2000.

31. Diamond M, Sigmundsen K. Sex reassignment at birth: along-term review and clinical implications. Arch Pediatr Adolesc Med. 1997;151:298–304.

32. Kessler S. Lessons from the intersexed. New Brunswick: Rutgers University Press; 1998.

33. Money J, Green R. Transsexualism and sex reassignment. Baltimore: Johns Hopkins University Press; 1969.

34. Corbett K. Gender now. Psychoanal Dial. 2008;18(6):838–56.

35. Benthien C. Skin: on the cultural border between self and the world. New York: Columbia University Press; 2002.

36. Bourdieu P. Outline of a theory of practice. Cambridge: Cambridge University Press; 1977.

37. Bourdieu P. Structures, habitus, power: basis for a theory for symbolic power. In: Dirks NB, Eley G, Ortner SB, editors. Culture/power/history: a reader in contemporary social theory. Princeton: Princeton University Press; 1994. p. 155–99.

38. Fanon F.. Black skins, white masks. Translated by C.L. Markmann. New York: Grove Press; 1963.

39. Johnston RA. The skin-textile in cosmetic surgery. In: Cavanagh S, Failler A, Hurst R, editors. Skin, culture and psychoanalysis. London: Palgrave Macmillan; 2013.

40. Lemma A. Under the skin: a psychoanalytic study of body modification. New York: Routledge; 2010.

41. Van Dinter MH. The world of tattoo: an illustrated history. Amsterdam: KIT Publishers; 2005.

42. Rosenblum DS. Adolescents and popular culture. Psychoanal Stud Child. 1999;54:319–38.

43. Hewitt K. Mutilating the body: identify in blood and ink. Bowling Green: Bowling Green State University Popular Press; 1997.

44. Grumet G. Psychodynamic implications of tattoos. Am J Orthopsychiatry. 1983;53:482–92.

45. Knopf K. An interminable cretan labyrinth. In: Rosenthal C, Vanderbeke D, editors. Probing the skin: cultural representations of our contact zone. Newcastle upon Tyne: Cambridge Scholars Publishing; 2015.

46. Merleau-Ponty M.. Phenomenology of perception. Translated by C. Smith. New York: Routledge; 1962.

47. Žižek S. Enjoy your symptom! Jacques Lacan in Hollywood and out. New York: Routledge; 1992.

48. Lacan, J. The mirror stage as formative of the function of the I as revealed in psychoanalytic experience. In: Ecrits: a selection. Translated by A. Sheridan. London: Tavistock; 1949. p. 1–7.

49. Fink B. The lacanian subject: between language and jouissance. Princeton: Princeton University Press; 1995.

50. Lacan, J. Seminar XXIII: Le Sinthome. In: Miller JA, editors. Translated by L. Thurston; 1975–6. Source: http://www.lacanonline.com/index/wp-content/uploads/2014/11/Seminar-XXIII-The-Sinthome-Jacques-Lacan-Thurston-translation.pdf.

Index

© Springer International Publishing AG, part of Springer Nature 2018
E. Tur, H. I. Maibach (eds.), *Gender and Dermatology*,
https://doi.org/10.1007/978-3-319-72156-9

Printed by Printforce, the Netherlands